STRETCHING
& FLEXIBILITY

KIT LAUGHLIN

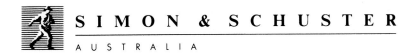

SIMON & SCHUSTER

AUSTRALIA

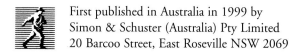

First published in Australia in 1999 by
Simon & Schuster (Australia) Pty Limited
20 Barcoo Street, East Roseville NSW 2069

A Viacom Company
Sydney New York London Toronto Tokyo Singapore

National Library of Australia
Cataloguing-in-Publication data:

Laughlin, Kit, 1953- .
Stretching and flexibility.

Bibliography.
Includes index.
ISBN 0 7318 0602 6.

1. Stretching exercises. I. Title.

613.71

Cover, internal design and illustrations by Jeremy Mears
http://announce.com/~jeremy
Photographs by Kit Laughlin

Set in Garamond 11/14

10 9 8 7 6 5 4 3

The exercises and advice given in this book are in no way intended as a
substitute for medical advice and guidance. Because of the differences
from individual to individual, your doctor should be consulted to check
that the information given is safe for you. Consult your doctor before
beginning this or any other exercise program. The author takes no
responsibility for any injury that may be caused as a result of applying
the information in this book

To the students and teachers of *Posture & Flexibility,* wherever you may be

Contents

Illustrations viii

Foreword

A new direction ix

Preface

Why should we stretch? 1

How this book is set out 2

How to use this book 3

Cautions 4

Introduction

Background to the approach 7

The Posture & Flexibility approach to increasing flexibility 10

(i) The Contract–Relax (C–R) approach 11

(ii) Partial poses 13

(iii) Partner-assisted 14

How Posture & Flexibility evolves 15

How to breathe in the exercises 16

What happens when we stretch? 17

The 10 principles of using the P&F approach effectively 20

Contact details 21

Muscles of the body 22

Chapter One

Lessons 1–7 25

Lesson one: the daily five (plus two) 25

1. Floor clasped feet middle and upper back 25

Middle and upper back from chair 27

2. Backward bend from floor 28

3. Lying rotation 30

4. Standing side bend 32

5. Seated hip 34

6. Chin to chest 37

7. Neck side bend 40

Lesson two: shoulders 42

8. Partner lying rotation 42

9. Arm across body 44

10. Partner front arm 46

11. Partner arms up behind back 48

12. Partner arm up behind shoulder blade 50

13. Arm behind head 52

14. Wall middle and upper back backward bend 54

15. Floor neck rotation 56

Lesson three: calf and hamstrings 57

16. Floor face down arm and leg lifts, and abdominal curls 58

17. Partner floor single leg forward bend 60

18. Floor folded leg calf (soleus) 62

19. *Wall standing calf (gastrocnemius)* 63

20. *Floor single leg calf* 64

21. *Buttock and hip flexor* 66

22. *Lying hip (piriformis)* 68

Exercise 8, Partner lying rotation, revisited 70

Standing alternate leg forward bend warm-up 71

Exercise 17, Partner floor single leg forward bend, revisited 72

LESSON FOUR: HIP FLEXORS, QUADRICEPS, TRUNK BACKWARDS AND HAMSTRINGS 75

Free squats warm up, partner or solo 75

23. *Floor instep* 77

24. *Standing quadriceps* 78

25. *Standing suspended hip flexor* 79

Exercise 2, Backward bend from floor, suspended variation 81

Exercise 1, Floor clasped feet middle and upper back, revisited 82

26. *Seated/lying single leg quadriceps* 83

27. *Partner backward bend over support* 85

Exercise 4, Standing side bend, hanging version 88

28. *Partner lying hamstring, knee flexed* 89

LESSON FIVE: LEGS APART AND ROTATION 92

Standing legs apart warm-up, bent and straight legs 93

29. *Floor side bend over straight leg; other folded* 95

30. *Wall seated knees apart* 97

31. *Partner/solo kneeling knees apart* 98

32. *Partner/solo wall lying bent legs apart* 100

33. *Wall lying straight legs apart* 101

34. *Wall seated straight legs apart* 102

35. *Partner floor middle and upper back bend* 103

36. *Partner/solo floor lying bottom leg folded rotation* 105

LESSON SIX: HIP FLEXORS, BACK BEND AND ROTATION 108

37. *Abdominal curls over support* 108

38. *Lying rotations* 110

39. *Partner hip flexor* 113

40. *Partner seated/lying single leg quadriceps* 115

41. *Partner standing suspended hip flexor, with support* 116

Exercise 2, Backward bend from floor, revisited 117

42. *Floor feet held back bend* 118

43. *Folded legs clasped knees upper back* 119

44. *Partner shoulder depress* 121

45. *Upper back on all fours* 123

LESSON SEVEN: HAMSTRINGS, HIP FLEXORS AND PARTIAL FRONT SPLITS 124

Free squats warm up, with held positions 125

Exercise 21, Buttock and hip flexor, revisited 128

46. *Partner floor hip and hamstring* 129

Exercise 17, Floor single leg forward bend, revisited; folded leg variation 132

47. *Partner partial front splits, off support* 133

48. *Floor forward bend over bent legs* 135

49. *Partner all fours rotation* 136

50. *Partner shoulder depress with flexion and lateral flexion* 137

THE UNNUMBERED LESSON: CHECKING YOUR PROGRESS 139

CHAPTER TWO

LESSONS 8–15 150

LESSON EIGHT: HAMSTRINGS, LEGS APART, AND BACK BEND 151

51. *Standing clasped single bent leg hamstring* 154

52. *Partner/solo standing single leg forward bend* 155

53. *Partner wall standing hamstring* 156

54. *Partner wall squat knees apart* 156

55. *Partner seated legs apart* 157

LESSON NINE: UPPER BACK, NECK AND SHOULDERS 162

Standing rag-doll warm up 162

56. *Sideways bend across support* 165

57. *Lying legs behind* 166

58. *Partner bar shoulder flexion with hip traction* 168

59. *Partner/solo shoulder internal rotation* 170

60. *Partner/solo shoulder external rotation* 171

LESSON TEN: LEGS APART AND TRUNK 174

61. *Partner wall seated knees apart* 175

Wall standing legs apart warm-up 176

62. *Partner wall seated legs apart, facing wall* 177

63. *Legs apart, off support* 179

64. *Seated or standing bent leg rotation* 182

65. *Partner kneeling arms up and behind* 182

LESSON ELEVEN: BALANCING AND STRENGTH 184

Free squats warm up, knees apart, revisited 184

Standing suspended hip flexor (ex. 25) and buttock and hip flexor (ex. 21) warm-up .185

66. *Partner lying 'Y'* 187

67. *Floor feet sequence warm up* 188

68. *Standing horizontal one leg support* 190

69. *Standing 'Y' one leg support* 192

LESSON TWELVE: CALF, WRISTS, TRUNK, AND HIP (PIRIFORMIS) 195

70. *Partner floor single leg, both legs calf* 197

71. *Floor wrist and hand sequence* 198

72. *Kneeling elbow on floor rotation* 200

73. *Partner floor wall seated side bend* 201

Free squat ankles clasped bottom position 202

74. *Seated legs folded knees apart forward bend* 203

75. *Seated clasped bent leg upper back* 204

76. *Partner floor external hip rotator* 205

LESSON THIRTEEN: HAMSTRINGS, QUADRICEPS, HIP FLEXORS, FRONT SPLITS 208

77. *Partner bar standing calf* 209

78. *Floor forward bend over straight leg, hurdler's variation* 210

79. *Standing forward bend over bent and straight leg* 211

80. *Wall and floor kneeling/straight leg outer hamstring* 213

LESSON FOURTEEN: NECK, WRISTS, ANKLES, WHOLE BODY 216

Exercise 55, Seated legs apart, solo version 222

Free squat bottom position, ankles clasped, straighten legs sequence 224

LESSON FIFTEEN: A FINAL CLASS OF MAJOR POSES 225

81. *Partner wall reverse legs apart forward bend* 226

82. *Wall lunge rotation* 228

83. *Partner floor back bend, off support* 230

84. *Wall squatting rotation* 232

85. *Partner floor backward bend* 233

CHAPTER THREE

END POSES 236

86. *The ultimate quadriceps stretch* 236

87. *Partner floor hamstring and lower back* 238

88. *The ultimate back bend* 239

89. *The ultimate bent-leg hip adductor* 240

90. *Balancing straight legs apart* 241

91. *The ultimate legs-apart stretch* 242

92. *Sitting and standing peacocks* 246

93. *The ultimate front splits* 247

94. *The ultimate abdominal workout* 248

95. *Ultimate quadriceps and hip flexor* 249

96. *Forward bend over straight legs* 250

CHAPTER FOUR

RECOMMENDED EXERCISES FOR SPORTS 252

Racquet sports 252

Football codes 253

Court sports 253

Martial arts and gymnastics 254

Cricket 254

Golf 255

Swimming 255

ACKNOWLEDGMENTS 256

TECHNICAL NOTES 258

RECOMMENDED READING LIST 260

GENERAL INDEX 262

INDEX OF NAMED EXERCISES 268

ILLUSTRATIONS

Muscles of the body, front view..22

Muscles of the body, back view...23

Muscles of the neck, side view, flexed...37

Muscles of the neck, side view, extended....................................38

Muscles of the neck, in side-bend position..................................39

Muscles of arm and chest, arm lifted behind...............................42

Muscles of arm and back, arm lifted to side................................43

Muscles of the neck, head rotated...56

Muscles of the leg, side view..60

Muscles of the leg, inside view..60

Muscles of the legs, from behind...61

Muscles of the lower leg...62

Muscles of the thigh..66

Sciatic nerve passes under piriformis..68

Part of sciatic nerve pierces piriformis..69

Psoas, iliacus and quadratus lumborum......................................75

How 'turnout' helps hip abduction..92

How tight ilio-psoas alters shape of spine.................................108

As leg extends, hip joint ligaments tighten around neck of femur......113

Levator scapulae details and Class II lever................................122

A NEW DIRECTION

Flexibility and strength are critical in life—for all of us, at all ages—and not just for the professional or amateur athlete. Of the two, flexibility is the more important, in my experience. I'd go further, and say that a lack of flexibility is the main reason for the muscular injuries that affect top-flight athletes in all sports, and this is as true today as it was when I was playing. And everyone knows that injury is the most common reason an athlete's career stops. More generally, we might say that flexibility and strength are the physical attributes underlying the essential qualities of suppleness and resilience necessary for a good life. But how do you go about developing these?

Many people go to the gym these days and make a conscious effort to improve their physical well-being. Quite a lot is known about how to get stronger and fitter and, to a greater or lesser extent, you can see this information being put into practice. The interesting thing is that people, and sports people in particular, treat stretching in an entirely different way from other aspects of fitness—the sort of thing that can be ignored entirely or treated as a sort of add-on to 'real' training—a sundry activity as it were. Whenever you go to a gym, you see people sitting around doing their warm-up or cool-down stretches with nothing like the focus they display when lifting weights or doing an aerobics class. They stretch while looking out the window, or chatting to a friend, or they simply tune out as they go through the motions. One of the reasons is they don't find it enjoyable. Perhaps another reason is that people make slow progress, if they make any at all. Many assume that they were 'born stiff' and give up quickly.

Kit's new book *Stretching & Flexibility* will change your way of thinking about flexibility and will certainly improve the way you go about achieving it. Everyone will find exercises to suit his or her body type and level of flexibility. What I like most about the book is that the people demonstrating the exercises look just like you or me—to paraphrase H. G. Nelson, they are ordinary people doing extraordinary things. Kit would say, though, that being flexible is nothing special; it just feels good to be that way. I could not agree more. I think that becoming flexible physically is one of the best ways to acquire emotional strength, too, and when we feel good about ourselves, we are more likely to be understanding of others. Together with a good diet and a moderate lifestyle, this book will provide you with the tools to become healthier, in all senses of the term.

When we first met, I said to Kit over the phone that I could spare only 15 minutes. Three hours later, we were still sitting on the grass in a park, ideas flying backwards and forwards as we discussed how we would like to influence change in the world. I still laugh when I remember his response to my saying that the key to a healthy life was 'all things in moderation'. 'Especially moderation,' he replied. I am certain that this book will revolutionise the way we go about becoming more supple. Enjoy yourself, and learn something profound about how your mind and body works.

Greg Chappell

WHY SHOULD WE STRETCH?

These days everyone knows that they *should* stretch: you cannot open a magazine without coming across articles promoting stretching as the best way to decrease injuries, help you lose weight, decrease recovery time from workouts at the gym, reduce stress, and improve posture—stretching is even being promoted as the latest way for bodybuilders to increase muscle size! And stretching long has been the choice of self-help therapy for many practitioners who deal with neck, back and other musculoskeletal problems. But a number of questions remain: which positions are best for what part, what kind of stretching, done what way, and how often? This book will answer these questions and more besides. Before we start to look at answers to these questions, though, I want to emphasise what I have found to be the most important reason to stretch—it simply feels wonderful to do. This reason is almost never mentioned yet, if you are to continue any activity, it must feel good, regardless of any other benefits it may have. Part of what this book is about is exactly how this subtle dimension can be maximised.

I realised there was a need for a book that takes a beginner through a number of classes, similar to the way we teach *Posture & Flexibility* at the Australian National University Sports Union, where these classes have been running for more than 11 years. I have found earlier books that dealt with stretching unsatisfactory, and here I have tried to write the book that I would have found helpful when I started. How many books have you seen that feature some lithe, apparently boneless, individual performing spectacular feats of flexibility (and balance and strength, too), yet nowhere could you find a stretch for an arm muscle, or that particularly tight muscle at the side and back of your neck? The answer must be many, if my experience is any guide.

And most books on the subject simply present separate exercises; the how-to-put-it-all-together section is buried at the back somewhere. What I do here is start at the beginning: I assume that you are a normally flexible adult. In other words, touching your toes could be a challenge some days. It is a little-noted physiological fact, I believe, that the toes *are* further away some days! So we will begin with simple, yet effective, exercises, and will feature the warm-ups we use, movements that you can really do properly, that feel good to do, and that will prepare you for more difficult poses later on. In each lesson, exercises are linked in some logical or functional way and many of the later classes revolve around particular themes. You will be able to move through the material at your own pace and, by the time you get to the end, you will have done one semester (15 weeks) of our course. I guarantee that your flexibility will be markedly improved, you will know your body better than ever before, and your movements in daily life will have become more graceful. You will simply feel better.

If you are already flexible, at this point you may be feeling that you have picked up the wrong book, but do not despair. Many of the exercises presented here are new or substantial modifications of exercises you know. There will be a few staples, of course; there are only so many ways that the body can be moved, after all. But even our advanced students can get an excellent stretch when they drop into one of the *Beginners'* classes, and we have found that returning to a simpler version of an exercise you know well can reveal new insights if it is done a slightly different way.

I have presented the material as I would in class. Essential anatomical information is contained in the relevant section of a lesson; all photographs refer to the text of a section, and so on. You will find simple cues to the essential aspects of what we have found to be good form in larger type, so you can read them when the book is alongside you as you practise. I decided to use photographs instead of drawings because a drawing can depict any position and this does not inspire confidence or trust. With photographs much information is provided in addition to the basic positions and you know that the person writing the book can do the recommended exercises too.

The question of precisely how to present the wealth of material that comprises *Posture & Flexibility* occupied all of the teachers for several months, requiring a large number of occasionally rowdy meetings, and resulting in the generation of charts, spreadsheets, diagrams and lists. The problem we set ourselves was this: what is the most user-friendly and *efficient* way to present the huge number of warm-up movements, partial poses, end poses, and movements that defy simple characterisation? Many of the teachers are professionally employed in research institutions and feel that they understand something about the problems of categorisation; in the end, though, we felt that we needed a new way of presenting the material that would achieve both goals simultaneously.

The breakthrough came when one of the senior teachers, Dr Carol Wenzel, told us of the reaction of one of her students to the proposition of presenting the material as a series of end poses, with the required steps documented within that section. She likened this approach to the generation of lists of different ingredients (and perhaps not very different from other books on stretching exercises); what was needed, Carol realised, was the particular organisation and presentation of the ingredients that result in the recipe that is *Posture & Flexibility*. This suggestion was unanimously approved by the teachers. I asked them all to make known their preferred ways of organising and presenting the materials; this resulted in the generation of as many variations on exactly how new students should be taken through a 15-week semester of *Posture & Flexibility* as there are teachers. I have taken the best of these variations—in other words, the material is presented here so as to emulate as closely as possible the experience you would have if you enrolled in one of our courses.

How this book is set out

The *Introduction* begins with a description of how the *Posture & Flexibility* classes came to be, the criteria by which we selected the movements that comprise the set of exercises we use, and how the classes are run at the Australian National University. We hope that this can become a model for classes in your area.

Chapter one comprises the first seven classes that a newcomer would experience, were they to join a *Beginners* class. Each class builds on the one before and, by the time the seventh class is complete, the main elements that distinguish *Posture & Flexibility* from other approaches to stretching have been taught. Each class teaches the warm-up movements that are related to the theme of that class. In later lessons, exercises from earlier classes are presented again as repeats. These smaller photographs are marked with an '*R*' and the relevant page number for easy revision.

Chapter two comprises the final eight weeks of a typical 15-week course. In this second term, some reasonably difficult exercises are presented, more difficult versions of earlier poses are taught, and our particular approach to enhancing flexibility is added to the basic positions. As far as possible, each class is slightly more difficult than the one preceding. Every class has an organising theme (for example, one might be mainly concerned with forward-bending movements), and so a particular class may be more difficult for you than another if that class focuses on your tight areas. Generally, however, each class may be thought of as self-contained, as there will be additional movements that counterbalance the emphasis of that class's theme, and hence balance the effects on the body.

Chapter three departs in style from Chapters one and two. Each section of this chapter shows how to get into and out of a standard stretch, or end pose. Appropriate warm-ups for each stretch will be indicated; these may include an easier version of the stretch that has been taught in an earlier class. These exercises comprise the elements of a typical *Intermediate* class and a few from the *Advanced* series of classes, but are not organised in the order they might be taught. By this stage, the reader will be able to pick and choose from among this array to achieve a particular effect or to prepare him or herself for a particular activity.

Chapter four lists collections of small photographs of warm-up positions and end poses related to sporting or martial activity. All are numbered so you can refresh your memory of how to do them—if necessary by turning back to the relevant pages. If you are a runner or a basketball player, for example, once you have worked your way through the elements of the list (either by going through all the classes in the order of presentation, or by turning back to the relevant earlier class or section) you can use it to review at a glance the exercises we have found to be most effective for your sport.

The next sections of the book are *Acknowledgments, Technical notes* and a *Recommended reading list.* The Reading list is annotated and will guide you to the books that I have found inspiring or effective. This list will allow you to gain a deeper understanding of the anatomy and physiology, or even the neurobiology, that underlies the basic task. All the recommended books have been useful in the development of the approach of *Posture & Flexibility.* The Acknowledgment section lists many of the current *Posture & Flexibility* teachers who have helped me construct the system presented here, and lists our web-site address which provides the most up-to-date list of teachers (many of whom are working around the world) and their locations, if you wish to attend their classes. The web site also gives details of our educational aids, such as video and audio tapes.

Either the *Table of Contents* or the final part of the book, the *Index,* may be used to locate a stretch for a particular muscle or group. For example, if you want to find a *biceps* stretch, it will be listed in the *Table of Contents* as such (10. Partner front arm), or you may use the *Index* to locate stretches grouped by particular functions (for example, all exercises that may be considered as bending the body backwards) or by muscle name (for example, if you know that you need to stretch *tensor fasciae latae*). The *Index* duplicates much of the *Table of Contents*, but is organised differently.

How to use this book

Although you may use the book (via the *Index* or *Table of Contents*) to locate a stretch for a particular part of the body, by far the best effects will be gained if you work your way through the book in the order that the material is presented, because some of the effects we are trying to achieve occur through the *conjunction* of poses or series of poses. Progress in the first few classes will be slower than subsequent ones, but this will be to your advantage in the longer term. The early classes contain more instruction than later ones—the early ones concentrate on teaching the method, which requires some explanation for comprehensiveness and safety. As those aspects are learned, the pace of subsequent classes picks up, and more exercises will be featured. Additionally, you will be able to apply the *Posture & Flexibility* method to any exercises not described here, and which may be essential to your activity.

I suggest you begin with lesson 1 and do a new lesson every week. As we recommend stretching only twice per week to begin with (the exceptions being the five trunk and spine exercises that can be done every day, and which are taught in lesson 1), do a complete lesson, and choose the most **difficult** exercises out of the lesson to try again at a subsequent, shorter session. In the beginning, I suggest that the old adage 'less is more' be your guide. I will expand on the reasons behind this advice in Chapter one.

Cautions

I strongly suggest you discuss your intention to begin a stretching exercise program with your coach or your health care professional, if you are seeing one. It may be that embarking on a stretching exercise program may work against whatever program or treatment you are receiving and you will need to know whether that is the case. If you have neck or back problems, you may wish to consult the book *Overcome Neck & Back Pain,* now in its third edition; this book deals directly with these problems and contains many specialised exercises that will not be found here. Your health care professional may have reasons for recommending for or against particular exercises, and it is a matter of safety, as well as courtesy, that you discuss your intentions.

On using the book itself, do not rely on the photographs alone. Each exercise consists of photographs that indicate the suggested form of an exercise, plus descriptions of how the exercise is to be done or the work to be done when in the final position. Sometimes the precise way of getting into or out of a pose is particularly important. These details will be found in the text. Read the **entire** description of each individual exercise while referring to the accompanying photographs, examine any illustrations that may accompany the photographs for relevant anatomical detail, then lie the book on the floor and get to work! Your enjoyment of any pose will be enhanced greatly if you know precisely where you are to feel any particular effect and what part of your body needs to be held which way *before* you try to do it.

Once you have read the text, the **Cues** point out the major style or effort aspects of an exercise. These are displayed in a typeface large enough to be read when the book is on the floor next to you, but do not rely on these alone. Before doing an exercise, make sure you know how long the final position is to be held, and how many breaths in and out are suggested for best effect.

It may be that when you look at an exercise you know that you can do a more extreme version. I recommend strongly, however, that you begin with the easier-looking version. In our *Advanced* classes, we have found that returning to an easier version of a pose than the one we would normally use always gives the student new insight and new sensations. This is just because the student can actually *do* the pose (achieve it technically); accordingly, the student can attend to the more subtle aspects such as breathing in particular ways or concentrating on the sensations coming from the body—and it is in these subtleties that many of the large-scale effects of a pose reside.

And finally, let me make a few practical suggestions. When practising at home, make sure that you can concentrate on what you are doing: turn off the television, and pull the telephone jack out of the wall. The former ensures that your concentration is on *you*; the latter that you will not be disturbed in the middle of doing something difficult. Similarly with children and pets: you will not be able to concentrate with your two-year-old climbing all over you or with your dog licking your ear (lying on the floor is an open invitation!). So, it may be that a short practice after putting the children to bed, or at some other convenient time during the day, will be best. I will expand on the best time of the day to stretch, and how best to incorporate stretching into your other activities, below.

Make sure that you go to the toilet before beginning your practice. We suggest that you do not eat for an hour-and-a-half or so before practising, but a small snack half-an-hour before beginning will not usually do any harm. These prescriptions are really a matter of comfort—some of the rotation and forward-bending movements are simply unpleasant to do if your stomach is full. Wear clothes that permit easy movement: track suit pants and a loose top, or tights and a leotard are suitable. Have a strap, belt, dish towel or similar to hand, as you will need something to use to hold onto your feet if you are not particularly flexible. Many of the poses use equipment that we have made, but I will suggest substitutes that you will find around the house or in any gym that will do the job.

The most important caution is to urge you to concentrate on the sensations coming from your body while practising. I will develop this theme in detail as we go through the classes, but the latest research strongly suggests that it is the re-mapping of the brain's image of its own physical capacities that is the main result of the correct stretching technique, and which directly produces the increases in the range of movements of the body that we recognise as 'becoming more flexible'. This is not the whole story, but it is a major part, and to facilitate this process we need to *feel* what is happening; that is, be strongly aware of the suite of sensations coming from the body. Accordingly, you must get into every stretch position *slowly*—not primarily for safety reasons (although important), but to maximise the sensory information coming to you from your body. I will expand on this theme later, too.

And last, when you look at the photos and try to emulate the shapes being depicted, attend to the *form* of the exercise being demonstrated, not the teacher's *performance* of it. You may well be able to achieve a more extreme position than the one demonstrated, or you may be less flexible, but the purpose of the photographs is to show the crucial elements of an exercise—*how* to do it. For example, the essential form of a seated forward bend may be that the movement needs to be achieved by bending *only* at the hip, and the trunk and the legs are held straight. If you bend forward (and let us say that you can place your forehead on your knees) but your back is rounded, you will have missed the point of the photograph completely. This is the main reason I have insisted you read the entire text for an exercise. In the one described, for example, if the body is not held in the suggested shape, it is very likely that you will have felt the stretch in your back as well as the back of your legs—which is totally undesirable. Each exercise will describe precisely where the effects *should* be felt, and what work you will need to do—in the example, you need to hold the trunk straight, and bend forward only at the hips until you feel the stretch at the back of the legs; conversely, the back will need to bend if that is what we want to stretch. We have a perhaps hackneyed saying in the exercise classes: 'Rome wasn't built in a day'. So take your time and *enjoy* the journey of self-discovery you have embarked upon.

The *Introduction* describes how we have arrived at the positions we advocate, and also describes how the classes at the Australian National University are organised and run. You may turn straight to Chapter one and begin the first lesson if you like, and return to the material in the *Introduction* at a later time.

BACKGROUND TO THE APPROACH

I began stretching at the Australian Academy of Ballet in Sydney—but certainly I was no dancer. In fact I had the distinction (at the age of 26) of being the least flexible student in the early morning *limber* classes, held every day before the real classes started. Picture the scene: a very fit, very stiff adult male in a class of young dance students, all of whom had perfect flexibility in the usual sense (side splits and front splits used to warm-up for the warm-up class!), and the students going through a relaxed stretching program to a piano, or sometimes recorded music. The instructor would call out in a beautifully projected voice, 'Now, fold your body onto your legs for a count of eight. One, two ...', and everyone except me would do just that. The term 'frustrating' would not begin to cover what I felt: a moderately competitive middle distance runner, capable of putting up good times on the right day, *and not able to touch my toes*. What was I doing here?

Like many people, I had realised at an earlier point that a lack of flexibility probably had something to do with the discomfort I experienced living in my fit and strong body. So, I tried all sorts of classes to try to make myself more flexible. I kept going to the *limber* classes for two years before work, but I made only slow progress. In fact, for the first six months, I could not see any measurable progress and I wonder now why I stuck with it for so long. It could only have been that the sheer grace displayed by the young dance students fascinated me and it was clear that these slender bodies were strong, too. Overall, though, it was the quality of movement that they all displayed that most interested me: ease, beautifully coordinated—in all, the best word is *graceful*. And I wanted that for myself. In terms of teaching an adult how to become flexible, however, the classes left much to be desired, and it was not until I realised that all of these students had become flexible at much earlier ages (often having started dance classes when they were five or six years old) that I understood that these students were correctly using the classes I was attending. They used the *limber* classes as an extended warm-up and to practise moving in certain ways in preparation for the day's work, whereas I was trying to make my body imitate the patterns of flexibility that they already had. It became clear to me that I needed methods that would alter my patterns, and this realisation is where my search for efficient stretching methods really began.

My thoughts turned to the problem that I was facing: how do you make an *adult's* body flexible? For many reasons, this is an entirely different task from making a child's body flexible. It is not just a matter of a child's body having looser ligaments and more supple muscles (although these are the sorts of conventional reasons that are offered whenever discussions like this occur), for to say this is merely to restate the problem a different way. Why is it that adults' bodies are so much tighter, why do adults display such individual postural signatures, and why aren't adults' bodies soft, supple and graceful, the way young children's are? And the most important question: can the adult be brought back into this state of gracefulness and, if so, how? The answer to the question of whether the adult body can be returned to its earlier suppleness is an unqualified yes, and the answers to the question of 'how' are what we are concerned with in the remainder of this book.

When I watched one of the young dancers folding a perfectly straight body over straight legs, again and again, without effort, I realised that the experience for her of doing that movement was completely different from the experience I had when I attempted the same movement; my body simply refused to move that way and, once the end of my range of movement had been reached, it was my *body* that stopped me from going further. How then could my body (using the conventional separation between mind and body for a moment) be made to do what my mind wanted? It became obvious that force would not work (if it had, my body would have been perfectly flexible a long time ago), and simply holding the end position of a stretching movement produced some results, but the discomfort in the muscles involved was off-putting. Moreover, the effects of this kind of stretching are felt for days afterward: the muscles can be very sore. This suggested that this approach was altering the muscles, but were the results worth the pain? Many people have tried conventional approaches to becoming more flexible and have decided that the answer to that question is no. These are the people who decide that they were born stiff, and they are the ones who drop out of classes everywhere.

A minor breakthrough in understanding occurred during a four-year stay in Japan. I had been working with an extremely flexible woman who was the translator at the *shiatsu* school where I was studying. She was the last remaining *shihan* (senior teacher) of an exercise form named *Jikyo Jutsu* (which loosely translates as 'self-help method'). The form is characterised by various dynamic and repetitive movements (including percussive techniques) to stimulate various glands around the head and neck and to direct pressure on particular internal organs, as well as dynamic stretches for the arms and legs. The woman explained that *Jikyo Jutsu* makes the practitioner flexible *not* by stretching the body (as it might appear) but by regulating the flow of internal energy, called *ki* in Japanese. Because I was studying *shiatsu* and immersing myself in the theory of Oriental medicine (one theory underpins all modern Chinese and Japanese traditional medicine, with some variations) I found the explanation convincing in that context. In time I became a *shodan* (first dan or black belt, but in Japan that signifies the most junior of teachers), but my flexibility had not improved significantly. And the attitude of the teacher was essentially one of disbelief: how could someone who had practised martial arts as long as I had not already *be* flexible? Here was the same old problem, expressed in a different way.

Watching her work, I realised that in some way my body was organised differently from hers; and the differences reminded me of that time I spent working out with the young dance students. Once again I became aware that movements which for me provoked the strongest sensations in my body had no such effect on her. Sliding her legs into the full side-splits position gave her the same sensations in her legs and hips as when I touch the back of my head with my hand: mere awareness of the movement involved. Suddenly I knew that my *experience* of trying to imitate a movement like side splits was completely different from hers, even though the movements might look the same to an observer. She explained that all she felt was the movement of her legs; the same movement for me produced feelings of alarm, fear that I would injure myself, and pain. I wanted to have the same expanded range of movement that I admired in the dancers and in this teacher. Like most people, I could touch my knee to my chest if my leg was bent at the knee, but had no capacity to do the same hip movement if the leg was straight. Clearly, there was no joint limitation; the limitation was somewhere in the muscles, nerves, or perhaps the *fascia* that permeates the entire structure. The task remained: how could I change the way my body mapped its available movements, so the desired movements would be as easy to do as all of my other movements?

One day, working out in the small local gym near my traditional Japanese house, a glimmer of deeper understanding occurred. I was attempting a forward-bending movement with the legs apart, and I happened to be sitting opposite a piece of equipment that presented a bar to me at hand height. I reached out to hold it to help me hold my back straight. I grasped it, lifted my chest to help straighten my back, and, as I did, I became aware of the increased sensations in the inner and back thigh muscles, the ones limiting the movement. I decided to apply a reverse tension to my hands, using these muscles that were sending such strong sensations to me. I pulled gently back on the bar using the muscles at the back and inside of my legs for a while. I noticed that as soon as I began to pull back, the uncomfortable pain-like sensation in the back of the legs diminished slightly; in fact, holding the end position of the movement became more bearable immediately. But, as soon as I stopped the pulling movement, I became aware of something quite different: the sensations that initially had prevented me from going deeper into the stretch position were no longer present. Cautiously I took in a breath (all the while feeling a little anxious), tried to calm myself and let the body go limp while still holding myself in position and, very slowly, pulled myself a little closer to the bar. On moving further forwards, I could feel the old sensations come back, but it was clear that I had moved further into the stretch. I continued to go forward until the sensations returned. I waited a while, and began the process again. A greater range of movement was achieved. After trying this a couple more times I could feel that no further movement forwards was going to occur.

I was tremendously excited by this event, because once I came out of the new end position and tried going back into it again I could feel that my body's reactions and sensations in this position had changed. The initial point in the range of movement that ordinarily would stop me from going further had definitely receded; I could feel that something had happened to the way my body felt about that point, but it would be many years later before I realised what was behind this change. In the meantime I experimented with this approach, and devised ways of applying it to all the stretches I knew. Within weeks my flexibility began to improve noticeably.

Years later, in a book shop in Canberra specialising in remaindered texts, I came across a book entitled *Proprioceptive Neuromuscular Facilitation*, in which a partial explanation for the effect I had observed was found. The original textbook was written by two physical therapists, Knott and Voss (1968), and it describes a large number of complex movement patterns. Originally developed at the Kabat-Kaiser Institute in the United States in the late 1940s, the technique was designed to re-educate the movement patterns of people with cerebral or spinal injuries. Typically, the handbook describes 'spiral-diagonal' patterns, such as the complex chain of movements the body makes when you roll on to one side before getting up out of bed. A short paragraph describes the Hold–Relax approach to increasing the range of movement of an affected limb, where the patient applies an *isometric* contraction against an increasing force applied by the practitioner: a static contraction against resistance (Knott & Voss, 1968, p. 98). Most who use the term PNF stretching are referring to this fragment of the whole technique. The same paragraph describes two other approaches, both of which we have tested, and neither of which affects the body of healthy individuals to anything like the same degree.

I decided to call my approach to increasing flexibility **Contract–Relax (C–R)**, even though, in the original book, this term referred to the use of *isotonic* contractions (a moving contraction against resistance), and despite the fact that my approach to using this technique is different from the original in a number of significant ways. My reasons are that the name Contract–Relax describes the crucial elements succinctly, and that the PNF approach was once a core idea in physical therapy and hence will seem familiar to many. I also dislike the coining of new terms when perfectly acceptable ones exist. The authors do not expand on the mechanisms behind what they describe (that is, they describe what happens when the techniques are used, not why), and it would be many years before I came across what I found to be a convincing explanation, which I shall address below.

The Posture & Flexibility approach to increasing flexibility

When I returned from Japan in 1985, I opened my clinic, the *Shoshin Centre,* and enrolled at the Australian National University (ANU). I wanted to make sure that I did enough stretching for myself, and in 1986 I decided to start a class at the Sports Union. I had intended to teach my own approach to yoga, but there were a number of yoga teachers already operating there, and the manager (a large ex-Olympic water polo player, René Bol) asked me what was distinctive about my approach. I explained the use of the Contract–Relax approach in a context of standard hatha yoga postures, and that practice would make the student more flexible, and improve his or her posture. He suggested that we call it *Posture & Flexibility,* and I began with one class that semester. By the end of the first year, I was teaching five classes a semester and had taken on a number of student teachers. Now, 13 years later, we have about 27 classes a week: 19 or 20 *Posture & Flexibility* classes, (depending on how many of the teachers are available) and 6 to 8 *Strength & Flexibility* classes where the emphasis is more on efficient strength improvement. Outside the ANU we run in-house classes for various government departments, classes at Sydney, Adelaide and Newcastle Universities, specialist courses for elite athletes in various sports, and courses at other locations, including in countries other than Australia.

After years of experimentation and development, the *Posture & Flexibility* approach is offered as a stand-alone method to increase awareness and flexibility. In its simplest conception, any potential *Posture & Flexibility* exercise must satisfy **two constraints**, and most exercises comprise **three elements**.

The two constraints are safety and effectiveness. The first of these, **safety**, is paramount. We have trialled a great many exercises, and estimate that, of the 100 or so routinely used forms, we have probably rejected as many, mainly on the basis of not satisfying this constraint. We constantly monitor the feedback from the classes to this end. For this reason we do not use many extended poses in our *Beginners'* classes (by extended, I mean poses where the body's weight is supported on straight arms or legs, where the elbows or knees are themselves not supported). Similarly, any exercise shape that imposes rotational torque on the knees is not used in *Beginners'* classes, and generally our backward bends are done over supports.

Effectiveness is assessed with respect to the over-arching goal of increasing flexibility, and is measured by *results gained for time spent.* For example, I will recommend later that major exercises (ones that stretch large muscle groups, such as the hamstring or the *quadriceps* group) be done only twice per week. Although it is often said that one needs to stretch every day in order to become flexible, I tested this claim while teaching in Japan. I found that the groups of students who stretched these muscles once or twice per week made consistently faster progress than those who stretched the same muscles every day, or every second day. These were groups of adults, however, and as I mentioned above, adults' bodies are different in many respects from those of children.

The three comprising elements of *Posture & Flexibility* are (i) the use of the *Contract–Relax* (C–R) approach, within a structure of (ii) *partial poses,* many of which are (iii) *partner-assisted.* I will deal with each of these elements in turn.

(i) The Contract–Relax (C–R) approach

As mentioned above, the Contract–Relax (C–R) technique is one of three described in the original PNF handbook. Explicitly, it is a set of techniques to be used by a practitioner on a patient. We have found that the approach as described in the handbook can be improved, and this is what I will describe here. There are three steps to successful implementation of the C–R approach. First, the limb is taken into a stretch position, either by the student, or, in the case of a partner-assisted exercise, by the partner. This initial stretch position needs to be relatively comfortable; we have found no advantage to the final stretch end point by beginning with a more extreme stretch position. If anything the contrary is true: if you begin the process in a strong stretch position, all surrounding musculature will contract to a greater degree than otherwise, and this increased whole-body tension works against the final step. I recommend holding the initial position for 10 to 30 seconds. We have found that the larger the muscle being stretched, the longer all steps should be held. Again, this determination is based on much experimentation, and these recommendations are based on what seems to provide the greatest improvement in end position.

The second step requires the student to *contract*. This means that the student pushes or pulls the limb being stretched in precisely the opposite direction to that used to get into the initial position; alternatively, the student pushes or pulls the muscle(s) in which the stretch is felt. The length of this contraction can be varied to suit the size of the muscle being stretched; the larger the muscle, the longer the contraction. Generally, a contraction will range from a few seconds (in the case of neck muscles, for example) to half a minute (in the case of hamstrings or *quadriceps*). The strength of contraction has been tested over a long period. For beginners, I recommend a gentle contraction; sometimes just enough to actually feel the muscle concerned. It is often the case that a beginner cannot feel a stretch sensation in a particular muscle (the hip flexors, *psoas* and *iliacus* are common examples) and we have found that a very gentle contraction can make the student aware of the location of a muscle immediately, whereas a stronger contraction produces an almost overwhelming sensory feedback from a much larger part of the body as surrounding muscles become involved as well, to stabilise the body. As the student progresses, and is further able to distinguish between the stretch sensation and pain, stronger contractions may be used for the larger muscles of the body.

The final step has two parts. Once the contraction phase is over, the student will need to *relax*. This is a much more difficult instruction than merely reading or hearing will suggest. The original PNF handbook is silent on this element, but I can say that without effective techniques to make the body relax at this point, the C–R technique will produce indifferent results. We have found that attending to one's breathing is the key to this essential aspect. We make no recommendations for breathing in the contraction phase, for experience has shown that most people will automatically brace themselves using the *Valsalva manoeuvre* (holding the breath against increased tension in the abdominal and other trunk muscles). However, the same reflexive behaviour militates directly against effective stretching so, after the contraction, the teacher will direct the class to take a full breath in and, except for any muscles being used to support the position, to let the whole body go soft and *relax*. Then, *as the student breathes out,* the final phase, the restretch, is performed. In this second part of the relax phase, the student or the student's partner assists in achieving a new stretch position, which will always be further into the range of movement than before. The new position is held for a duration that depends generally on the size of the muscle being stretched, but usually from 15 to 45 seconds.

The three-part C–R approach may be repeated. We have found that the most commonly reported experience is that no further increase in the range of movement can be achieved beyond three repetitions. In fact, if the student has a breakthrough in a tight muscle and is able to move well into a new range of movement (for example, a 10 or 15 degree improvement in the session) they will notice themselves tightening up within minutes of achieving the new movement, even if only one cycle of the C–R approach has been used to that point. Such improvements are cumulative however and, once a breakthrough has been achieved, stretching the same muscle at a subsequent session (assuming sufficient recovery) will produce sensations that are qualitatively altered. Most students report that a significant fraction of the increase remains and is noticeable at the next session.

The C–R approach has a number of advantages over conventional stretching, both *ballistic* (using momentum to increase the range of movement) and *static* (holding the end position of a stretch without movement). Ballistic stretching (for example, performing high kicks to the front or side) is inherently dangerous for the untrained person, because the end point of the movement is both hard to predict and difficult to control. Momentary over-stretching is a common cause of shoulder, *biceps* and hamstring muscle group injuries, as reported in the sporting press daily. Research has demonstrated that the body's capacity to produce muscular contractions that could prevent over-stretching at the end of the range of movement in fast, power-based activities is significantly reduced, compared with strength that can be applied in the normal range of movement. However, many sports require powerful ballistic movements, and these will need to be practised. There are two kinds of sensing mechanisms in muscles and tendons; one kind sensitive to position, and the other sensitive to time *and* position. Acquiring flexibility using the C–R approach will improve your ballistic flexibility to a significant extent, but the student who needs ballistic flexibility in their particular activity will need to do these specific fast movements in addition to the slow, careful exercises recommended in this book. For further information on how to improve ballistic flexibility, consult the book *Stretching Scientifically*, by Thomas Kurz (1994).

Static stretching, the approach most commonly used to increase flexibility, is typified by holding a position where a stretch sensation is felt for 10 to 30 seconds. A number of these stretches are performed in the one session. Reasons to support the use of this technique are that it is safe and that it tends not to aggravate any existing injuries. The disadvantage of this conservative approach is that, for the inexperienced individual, the end point in the range of movement is difficult to determine (that is, exactly when in the range of movement is a stretch being experienced?) and there may be difficulty distinguishing that further point in the range of movement where pain, or even injury, may be felt. People unused to stretching will feel pain and the stretch sensation at the same time if the static method is used, and will be unable to distinguish between these sensations. This is especially so if the student has been suffering muscular or other types of pain for long periods. The C–R approach distinguishes these sensations quickly, often the first time it is used, and awareness (*proprioception*) is enhanced immediately. The difficulty of determining the optimal end point of the range of movement experienced in static stretching has two consequences: either the student does not stretch far enough and does not improve, or the student does not acquire the enhanced sensitivity to the range of movement between stretch sensation and injury. We call this range the 'stretch window'. How it may be opened is dealt with in detail in subsequent chapters.

A further advantage of the C–R approach is that its use develops strength at the very end of the range of movement, which is left unaltered by conventional stretching and resistance training. This is due to the contraction phase of the approach, which is an *isometric* strengthening effort. Research shows that isometric contractions produce increases in strength at the points in the range of movement at which they are used. Isometric means that the muscles are exerting effort on the limb concerned, but no movement is produced. It is usually contrasted with *isotonic,* where the effort results in movement. Accordingly, when you use the C–R approach, not only do you become more flexible, but you also develop increased strength, especially at the end of the range of movement.

(ii) Partial poses

The second element in the *Posture & Flexibility* approach to stretching is the use of partial poses, or parts of standard exercises. We have broken down many complex exercises into an elemental vocabulary of what I call 'functional units of flexibility'. This term denotes the reduction of a multi-joint movement into smaller parts, the classification of which is pragmatically determined—we stop reducing when the effect of a partial pose still can be assessed as being effective in terms of the desired outcome. Functional units are logical elements based around single joints initially and which then include multiple joints and more complex movements. For example, a standard stretching exercise for the hamstring muscles (the large muscles at the back of the leg between the hip and the knee) is to sit on the floor with outstretched legs and to fold the upper body over the legs by bending forwards from the hips. One can see this exercise being done poorly at any gym, any day. Because the untrained individual lacks flexibility in the hamstring muscles, the final position is achieved by bending the spine strongly forwards.

We begin by using a couple of stretches for the two calf muscles. Loosening the calf muscles, especially *gastrocnemius*, can result in a startling improvement to bending at the hips, *even though these muscles are not directly involved in the movement.* Just why this is so will be explored in the forwards-bending class below. Next, we stretch the hip muscles (*gluteus maximus* and *piriformis*, in particular). We stretch the hip joint and *gluteus maximus* to signal to the body that a certain range of movement is possible at the joint; the reason for stretching *piriformis* will be covered below. The student then proceeds to do one or two *single-leg* hamstring stretches. We do one leg at a time because, although most people are not strong enough in the trunk to hold the trunk straight against the combined forces of *both* hamstring muscle groups, everyone can do so if only stretching one leg. Another reason is that stretching one leg at a time reduces the total sensory input; it is easier to hold any final position as a result. Following this, we would do a lower-back, and possibly a middle-back and upper-back, stretch, and then try the complex whole-body movement (the forward bend over both legs) again.

In all people to date, their performance in the whole pose is noticeably improved over their first attempts, even allowing for warm-up effects. In addition, the student will have become aware of which are their tight muscles in the chain of muscles required to do the exercise—and they will have learned the most efficient partial pose to alter these tight muscles and a simplified description of the essential anatomy. In the inexperienced person, there is often a great deal of difficulty in working out exactly which muscles are limiting movement; the movement simply feels stiff and uncomfortable. The 'functional unit' approach identifies these areas precisely. We have also run simple experiments which suggest that identifying one's tightest areas in a chain of muscles, and using the partial pose approach to altering these, improves the student's performance of the whole pose significantly faster than the same amount of time spent practising the whole pose. We always practise the whole pose at the end of the partial-pose session to realise any holistic benefits the pose may have, and to mimic most closely the functional demands of the complex movement. The final benefit of the partial pose approach is that all students, regardless of their overall level of flexibility, will be able to practise the elements in some suitable form, and this helps their confidence and shows them that they are improving.

(iii) Partner-assisted

The final element of the *Posture & Flexibility* approach is partner-assisted stretching. This has many advantages over solo stretching. In the contraction phase, the student can concentrate on just the sensations of using the desired muscle to do the work against the partner's support. Another advantage is that the student does not need to make the effort to hold him or herself in a final, or difficult, position, and can concentrate on the subtle details of good form and the essential element of breathing. The partner, who is another member of the class, can check the student's form and provide essential feedback. We have found that alerting the partner to form considerations is an extremely effective way to make them aware of the same details when the pairs change over. In time, our classes become self-correcting, all of the students becoming as aware of good form as the teachers.

Objections have been raised that partner-assisted stretching is dangerous, and a number of contemporary books on stretching recommend against partner work on this basis. We have overcome this objection by designing the majority of partner exercises so that the person being stretched (the *stretchee*, in our terminology—the one neologism of this book) is in control of the end position, and not the partner (or *stretcher*). This satisfies the safety constraint and we stress this point in one of the early classes. We note that the students are adults, and that the best teacher in the world cannot know what the student is experiencing. Accordingly, we inform out students that, as we will teach them only exercises in which they control the end point, we expect them to be responsible for themselves. This may seem somewhat peremptory, but we want our students to take control of themselves; indeed the essence of the approach we advocate is self-awareness—and self-awareness cannot be achieved without embracing this responsibility.

There are also substantial psychological advantages of partner-assisted stretching over solo stretching. The students find that they tend to hold the end position of a stretch for longer than they would if on their own and this is often volunteered in the course of a class. It simply feels good to be supported by another when concentrating on difficult positions, and enduring the sometimes powerful sensory stimulations one's own body is producing in the big hamstring and *quadriceps* stretches is eased enormously if one has a partner to help; this will have to be experienced to be appreciated.

There are, of course, many occasions when the student must work alone. I will show an individual version of most stretches, and provide the essential cues for good form. Often though, the subtlety of a stretch will be felt more strongly when you practise with another and, when you have felt these sensations doing partner work, they are much more easily recaptured when doing the stretch on your own. If only for this reason, it is worth attending a class from time to time if you can. When choosing a partner in class, try to find someone approximately your own size and weight. We have had little trouble teaching people to assist well, but we often spend as much time teaching the stretcher as the stretchee; they have a basic relationship and both play a fundamental role.

How Posture & Flexibility evolves

We have no tradition, which I believe is to our advantage. Tradition in an exercise form can lead to stagnation—in my experience, the originators of most of the major approaches to body work around us today were insightful, and uncovered novel and interesting ways of working with the body. What can happen is that the subsequent generation of teachers becomes rigid in its approach, and some contemporary exercise forms explicitly discourage innovation, claiming that the originator's method is complete. The irony is that the originators of most of these forms created new systems precisely by breaking away from their own teachers, or by striking out in a direction that was new at the time. Further, there is a serious temptation to become overly enamoured of one's own creation and blind to its shortcomings. In my own system, I hope that I have avoided these shortcomings, mainly by the strictest adherence to an *impersonal* objective: the principle of using whatever techniques appear to work in achieving our goal of increased flexibility, within the dual constraints of safety and effectiveness. Orientating oneself to this objective, rather than protecting the boundaries of one's own creation, seems to be the best way to proceed.

Early in my attempts to refine the *Posture & Flexibility* approach, one of my then teachers expressed reservations about teaching the method to all who wished to learn. He was concerned that teachers of other systems would take the ideas and incorporate them into their own systems. I believed then, as I do now, that any attempt to protect the 'purity' of a system will fail, and that having explicitly permeable boundaries around one's work is the only sensible alternative. We invite the teachers of other approaches (yoga, aerobics, pilates, physiotherapy, martial arts, athletics and others)—anyone with an interest in stretching—to participate. My feeling is that we have learnt at least as much as we have taught and, because of our stated goal, feel no misgivings about taking and using anyone else's techniques that appear to help us achieve that goal.

Our classes are graded *Beginners*, *Intermediate* and *Advanced*. There are other classes too: a 'Neck, Shoulders & Relaxation' class, which comprises 15 to 20 minutes of relaxation practice added to a gentle mix of neck, upper-back, and arm and shoulder exercises (office workers and academics love these); an 'Over 40s' class, which features a slightly slower pace, and which includes many students under 40; and a 'Dynamic Forms' class which teaches basic tumbling and balancing movements in addition to stretching. Most classes are an hour-and-a-quarter long, some an hour, and the *Advanced* is an hour-and-a-half long. The students spend the first 15 minutes of each class practising their own work (we encourage them to practise their *worst* poses—and the diligent ones do) and this provides teachers with a unique opportunity to judge the effectiveness of their own teaching styles—are the students practising in good form? If not, the teacher corrects the student and (I hope) rethinks the approach of their previous classes. The only rule in the class once the formal teaching period is underway is that students may not talk while the teacher is instructing.

All teachers in the local area are required to attend the *Advanced* class once a week. The teaching of this class is rotated among the teachers equally and new techniques are encouraged. In addition to the teachers being creative individuals, they attend workshops in different areas and disciplines and bring back new ideas. Many suggestions for the improvement of existing exercises come from students, too. The only rule in the evolution of new techniques in *Posture & Flexibility* is that a teacher *must* 'road test' a new exercise or part of an exercise in the *Advanced* class. In this way, all the teachers can assess the idea and usually improve it on the spot. If an idea passes this scrutiny, it is approved tentatively as an acceptable exercise. Subsequent experience will, perhaps, reinforce this impression and it may become part of the core technique. Like evolution proper, many do not. As I mentioned in the *Preface*, we have rejected at least as many exercises as we have taken on. We hold no exercise or technique immune from this scrutiny and, because we do not owe our ideas to any particular discipline, the current body of work is robust. We are not particularly attached to any form and nor do we mourn its passing: we are interested only in what works. I cannot overemphasise the extent to which these simple rules have contributed to a dynamically evolving form. For example, I came across a particularly effective *piriformis* exercise by accident while I was warming up to teach the *Advanced* class one evening and this excited me so much that I decided to make it the focus of that class. By the time we had finished, we had three variations (some looking quite different in form) on the basic movement and had discovered that over a third of the teachers were very tight in this area.

A great many teachers of other approaches have come to work with us over the years. When someone trained in another form works with us, we ask them to teach a guest class in their style from time to time, so we might learn something new or have our ideas challenged by another perspective. Egos are remarkably absent in this process, exactly because our focus is on what I call 'the impersonal objective': the goal of becoming flexible.

One more aspect of our approach deserves note. All techniques are based on my understanding of anatomy, the one area of Western medical enquiry unquestioned by any other form of medicine, or any of the complementary forms within our own culture. I chose to attain this level of understanding because of its commensurability with the largest number of approaches to body work and because it gives us a basis for talking to practitioners of all sorts of other modalities, who traditionally may not have communicated with each other. This grounding also avoids the infuriating response I so often encountered in my own study of various forms: when asking why something was done a particular way, the answer often was 'that's the way we do it', or 'that's how my teacher did it'. This is not good enough for me. If the form of an exercise cannot be justified by, or anchored in, anatomical understanding, there still, of course, needs to be a reason for doing it a certain way—it may be as simple as, 'If you try it like this, compared with that way, it feels better.' Some explanations and many experiences do not yield to the scientific method, after all.

How to breathe in the exercises

Breathing cannot be separated from effective stretching. I have previously covered the specifics of how to breathe, but I wish to return to this important component of the stretching experience from a slightly different perspective. The way we breathe is so much a part of all of life's activities that we tend to ignore it, except in extreme circumstances. However, because the way we breathe is fundamental to the experience of being alive, techniques that can help us to become more aware of this vital process, and perhaps improve its efficiency, are crucial. Attending to this aspect can have dramatic effects on the quality of one's life.

Think back to the last time you felt angry. Let us say you were driving to work and someone thoughtlessly and dangerously cut in front of you. What were your first responses? You took in a breath, all the trunk and neck muscles tightened, and you may have felt a flood of adrenaline through the body. Your pulse and respiration rate went up, and you became strongly aware of how you felt. Does this sound familiar? It is such patterns of increased tension and altered breathing that form our emotional responses, a theme I will return to below. And, in this typical example, how would you go about calming yourself? You would take a few deep breaths in and out; as you did so your body would settle down to its more comfortable rhythms.

When you are stretching, you need to realise that holding the breath in, or breathing in an unusually shallow way (usually referred to as *tidal* breathing), is one of the body's primary protective mechanisms. That is, when threatened or in pain, you will tend to hold your breath, and your muscles, of your trunk in particular, will display elevated tension. In any case, electromyographic studies have shown that tension in the muscles is slightly elevated with every breath in, and that this decreases as you breathe out. These facts about how the body works suggest strongly that any stretching effort will be best made as you breathe out. If you take a deliberate breath in before you stretch, the effect is heightened; in addition, you will be teaching the body to associate the sensation of being stretched with the action of a deliberate breath out and, once learned, this association will help you stay more relaxed in all other parts of your lives.

It must be obvious, but worth repeating, that it is not possible to feel relaxed while the muscles of the body are tense. By 'tense', I mean having elevated muscle tension, for some tension (called *tonus*) is necessary for all of the normal body functions (from holding oneself up during the day to digesting food) and the absolute degree of normal muscle tension and its range vary from person to person. When I refer to tension, I mean changes to one's usual patterns, wherever they may be found on some universal scale. Western medicine recognises two ways of reducing muscle tension to desirable levels: the use of one of the *benzodiazepine* prescription medications, and the development of techniques that lead to the relaxed state. The benzodiazepines achieve their anti-anxiety effects mainly by reducing muscle tension—one's state of mind alters as one's physical state changes. I have dealt with the state of relaxation in some detail elsewhere (see Laughlin, 1995); here it is enough to say that there are a great many approaches to acquiring this state, among them yoga *nidra*, the many approaches to meditation, biofeedback and self-hypnosis. For an excellent non-technical introduction to these concepts, see Benson (1976).

There is a third way of acquiring an enhanced state of relaxation at will: the use and practice of the right stretching exercise. By 'right', I mean efficient, but any stretching exercise will have this effect, to a greater or lesser extent.

I mention the two recognised ways of altering one's state of mind to feel more relaxed to make the point that attending to your emotional state and the accompanying breathing patterns while you practise will lead to significantly heightened awareness. There is no doubt that acquiring this sense will improve your flexibility (in the sense of what might be observed by someone else), but of far greater importance is what you will learn about yourself in the process—knowledge that simply cannot be gained any other way. I will expand on this idea below.

What happens when we stretch?

Conventional explanations of the cellular changes accompanying the phenomenon of becoming more flexible would draw on terms such *sarcomeres*, *A-bands* and *I-bands*, *Z-lines* and *H-zones*. These kinds of explanations have been covered in detail by other authors and references will be found in an annotated section at the end of this book. Although flexibility is a property of muscles, ligaments, tendons and bones, it is not principally controlled within these parts of the body. The brain is a major part of what we 'stretch' when we do stretching exercises. Further, to the extent that muscles *do* stretch, the main changes occur through the remodelling of connective tissue, or *fascia*, the most abundant of the materials comprising muscles.

In this section, I shall only sketch the physiology involved; for sources of more detail, see the *Recommended reading list* at the end of the book. All textbooks on stretching claim that muscles can contract to about 70 per cent of their resting length and can be extended to about 130 per cent of this same length. A muscle's capacity to contract decreases as it is extended beyond its resting length and, at around 120 per cent of its resting length, the two components of muscle tension—connective tissue resistance to elongation and active contraction by the muscle—are about equal. Accordingly, while you can still generate tension in the muscles, the brain and nervous system impose the significant limitations on how far you can stretch. This is one reason we advocate the **C–R** approach.

Of interest here is the neurological phenomenon called *postcontractive reflex depression (*Kurz, 1994, p. 19) or *autogenic inhibition* (Alter, 1988, p. 49)—immediately after a sufficiently strong contraction, the muscle's resistance to elongation is momentarily reduced, and we can stretch further than would otherwise be the case. We have found that once someone becomes accustomed to using contractions to help their stretching, strong contractions are not necessary. As mentioned above, we have found that gentle contractions can elicit an improved end position, and we suggest that this may be due to a *reduced* overall level of excitation in the neural system. As a student advances, however, stronger contractions may be included from time to time, partly to experience the different sensations that result and partly to increase strength in particular muscle groups. Strong contractions seem to be required to achieve both the side-splits and front-splits extreme positions, and this may be related to the strength needed to support the intermediate positions that one must use along the way. Another reason may be that the brain is aware of the propensity for injury in these movements and will not facilitate relaxation until it is aware that there is sufficient strength to support the extended positions.

Once we can no longer voluntarily generate appreciable force in the muscles we are stretching, it is likely that we are working more on the connective tissue. About 60 per cent of the weight of muscles is composed of this interesting substance. Each bundle of *myofibrils*, the smallest unit of each muscle's system, is encased in a thin wrapping of it, and numbers of bundles are grouped and further encased in it, at all scales up to the complete muscle. The outermost casing of *fascia* forms the tendons that join the muscle to its bony attachments. Connective tissue also forms large sheets of *fascia*, on which muscles pull, and which also act to separate muscles and provide movement between them. Our skin is largely composed of connective tissue. Connective tissue is formed of *collagen*, the longest molecules in the body and the substance which provides its tensile strength, and *elastin*, which gives it its elasticity. Both kinds of fibre are located in a ground substance, a *mucopolysaccharide* which allows the fibres to move over each other with little friction and, at the same time, acts as a glue to hold them together. Connective tissue exhibits a property called *thixotropy*: the capacity to become harder or softer, depending on what force or energy is acting upon it. Heat softens it, and this may be one of the reasons that having a hot bath makes a perceptible difference to how far you can move when you stretch. As you age, your connective tissues become generally tougher, drier, harder, and shorter. The process has been described as being very like tanning of leather: the collagen fibres become increasingly *cross-linked*, a term describing additional hydrogen bonds. Cross-linking reduces the movement between the collagen molecules—the connective tissue becoming tougher, but increasingly prone to damage. Underuse *and* overuse will alter connective tissue; the former facilitates the hardening of the ground substance and the latter damages the fibres comprising the connective tissue itself.

Connective tissue is injured when we pull a muscle. Although rich in nerves, connective tissue has a poor blood supply, particularly at the junctions with bones and muscles. During the healing process, collagen fibres are laid down randomly (electron microscope scans reveal that the fibres form no pattern) but, as tension is experienced at the site, the collagen fibres move to align with the forces acting on them. If healing is complete, the new material is incorporated into the old seamlessly. Scar tissue is unorganised, low-strength connective tissue. Tension needs to be applied gently, increasing from very light forces to the sort of forces that the part will experience during normal activities. Stretching provides the right kind of forces, providing you are sensitive to the feedback—the *sensations* of stretching.

The final aspect of stretching I wish to discuss now is the most problematic and the one about which the least is known, but which may yet prove to be its most important dimension. In 1942, Reich claimed that character armouring was 'functionally identical with muscular hypertonia', and that altering this tension altered the patient's emotional trauma (1989, p. 270), and a great many schools of body work have elaborated the ways in which this might be brought about. Emotional states have their physical correlations—as everyone knows—but the idea that physical states (muscular and visceral) may be fundamentally *constitutive* of emotion, and an essential part of what we call rationality, is a recent development. Further, it may well be the case that the memory of emotions is located not in the brain but in patterns of proprioceptive activity in the muscles, tendons and skin of the body (Damasio, 1996). I am certain that one's postural signature and the varieties of the individual's responses to stress emerge from this relationship; that is, one's experiences are literally embodied, as Reich suggested, and the mechanisms described by Damasio may be the key to further understanding this aspect of our existence. More generally, it seems the body is being moved from the periphery of academic interest towards the centre, if somewhat uneasily. For example, the operators of classical logic (*and, not* and *or*) have been derived directly from the body's experience of learning about the constraints to its movement in the physical environment and, further, the body's awareness of itself appears to be essential to thought (Johnson, 1987).

Stretching is one of the most efficient ways of exploring ourselves and our inner states. If the approach as outlined here is followed, you will be able to experience yourself completely in the present, as each instant of time goes by. When you stretch—if you pay attention—the flood of sensory feedback is so strong that you will not be able to think of anything else. By making subtle alterations to your position, you can make extremely fine changes to these sensations, and will be able to move them in the direction of more pleasurable sensations or greater comfort. You will feel the point at which stretching is no longer necessary for that place and will move onto the next. Finally, you will feel 'done' and the session will be over. You will have a strong impression of completeness, or closure, and a sense of oneness with yourself that is unique in my experience. At this point, your prevailing emotion will be a sense of calm—a feeling far from the absence of emotion. It is a feeling of balance achieved, a kind of deep satisfaction. In the terminology of physiology, your resting *tonus* is reduced, and you are relaxed. But it is far more than this, because the state was achieved *actively*. As you practise, you are remaking the proprioceptive maps of yourself, and you are finding ways to resolve those places in your body that suffer the reactions to the stresses of daily life. In a real sense, you are remaking your emotional responses and how these affect you, bringing them closer to what you feel comfortable with. When those same stresses are re-encountered, they most likely will trigger the same responses but, because your awareness of your internal states is heightened, you will find that you are able to let any unwelcome responses go more easily. Too many students have reported similar experiences over the years for this to be coincidental. It is time to get started; below you will find a summary of the key principles of the approach.

The 10 principles of using the P&F approach effectively

i) **Maintaining the form of the exercise is the fundamental principle and takes precedence over all others.** The text and the photographs are intended to illustrate the *form* of each exercise. Your performance will depend on your flexibility and, in some movements, your strength—you may well be more flexible than the model in some cases. Make sure you understand where the stretch is to be felt, how the position is to be stabilised, and which muscles have to do what work.

ii) **Always hold the final position for the recommended time; if you cannot, you are overdoing the stretch.** All of us have seen someone at some time (often at a party, and frequently after a drink or two) drop down into the splits to show off how flexible they are (or used to be). This can cause injuries. Unless you can hold a position, you do not own that flexibility. The usual recommendation for the length of time to stay in an end position will be expressed in breaths; one breath being a normally paced breath in and out. Ten breaths is around 30 seconds if you are working hard, and is the minimum time the end position should be held. You may benefit from a longer time, especially if large muscles are involved.

iii) **When using the C–R approach, do not let the limb against which the contraction is being performed move at all.** We have found that any movement in the limb reduces the final stretch position, often significantly.

iv) **When using the C–R approach, do not push too hard.** The original PNF textbook recommendation is based upon maximal resistance of an isometric contraction (Knott & Voss, 1968), but we may assume that, as this method was intended to be applied in the clinical or hospital setting, no great force in absolute terms was expected. We have found that gentle contractions (from the stretchee's perspective) are all that are required, and that stronger contractions actually work against the desired outcome. This is probably due to the necessity that many other muscles be involved in stabilising the body if the forces generated are high. One's own mass is often sufficient if the contraction is soft. We recommend that, generally, between 20 and 30 per cent of the possible contraction force be used; less if the person has muscular problems.

v) **Only the muscle(s) used to contract will experience the stretch effect.** In many contraction movements, it is possible to use different muscles to move the limb. For example, in exercise 3 (a lying rotation) it is possible to use the hip muscles to press the leg towards the ceiling, or the waist and lower back muscles to rotate the hips in relation to the shoulders. Whichever muscles generate the force experience the release.

vi) **If you have a clear left–right pattern of flexibility, always begin by stretching the tighter side first, stretch the looser side, then restretch the tighter side.** This principle applies to any exercise that permits a comparison of left and right in any plane of movement. Stretching this way means the tighter side will experience twice the work, and will adapt faster. Once both sides are approximately the same (this may take some time), do equal work for each side.

vii) **If an exercise requires one of a matched pair of muscles to contract to produce the stretch, repeat the first side's stretch for a few seconds to relax the last-used muscles.** This principle mainly relates to solo rotation and side-bending movements. For example, rotating the trunk to one side uses half of the trunk's muscles to produce the movement, which stretches the other half. Turning to the other side contracts the just-stretched side, so to ensure the whole trunk is relaxed, turn back to the first side for a few seconds.

viii) **Always bend forwards after bending backwards.** Once in class, after giving this instruction, a young wag asked, Do we have to bend backwards again now, to compensate for the forward bend? I replied that he could if he wanted to, and he was welcome to keep going if he could not decide where to end the process. The point here is that the muscles of the spine tend to tighten when bending backwards, so bending forwards for a moment relieves this situation; this is simply the way the body is organised. The front (anterior) muscles do not usually tighten when bending forwards (although in the very first exercise we do, a forward-bending movement, I do say to lift the hands above the head if the stomach muscles have cramped while doing the movement). The main goal is that the body feel comfortable after particular stretches, which means a compensating movement is sometimes necessary.

ix) **When returning from an extended (stretched) position, use muscles other than the ones you have been stretching.** A moment's thought will tell you that if you are stretching a muscle, then, *by definition*, it is out of its normal range of movement. A muscle asked to do work out of its normal range is much more prone to injury; accordingly it is sensible (and feels much better) to use other muscles to return the body to the start position.

x) **Using a contraction will locate a muscle, and help you focus the stretch effect.** It is often the case that you will not feel a stretch in a desired muscle. This is most likely (paradoxically, perhaps) if this is one of your very tight muscles, or an area that you have injured in the past. The reasons are probably related to the way the body protects itself and its dissociation from sensory feedback from areas that long have been a problem. Performing a gentle contraction really brings this area back into your conscious focus, and will enhance the stretching effect considerably.

Contact details

I would like to hear feedback, of any kind. If one does have an interest in the worth of what one teaches, criticism is at least as useful as praise. Additionally, if there is sufficient interest in learning more about what we do, we will come to you to present workshops.

Kit Laughlin
LPO Box 159,
Australian National University,
Canberra, ACT 2601
AUSTRALIA
E-mail: kit.laughlin@anu.edu.au
Web page (URL): http://www.posture-and-flexibility.com.au

MUSCLES OF THE BODY

The following pages present a front and back view of the surface muscles of the human body. Most of the important muscles we will be stretching in the lessons below will be found here. Relevant additional details of parts of the body will be presented in the lessons.

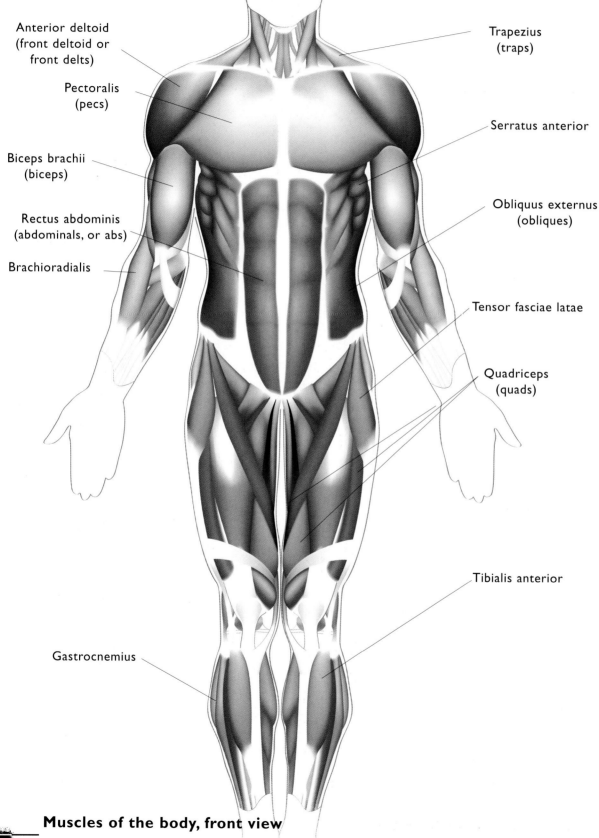

Anterior deltoid (front deltoid or front delts)

Pectoralis (pecs)

Biceps brachii (biceps)

Rectus abdominis (abdominals, or abs)

Brachioradialis

Trapezius (traps)

Serratus anterior

Obliquus externus (obliques)

Tensor fasciae latae

Quadriceps (quads)

Tibialis anterior

Gastrocnemius

Muscles of the body, front view

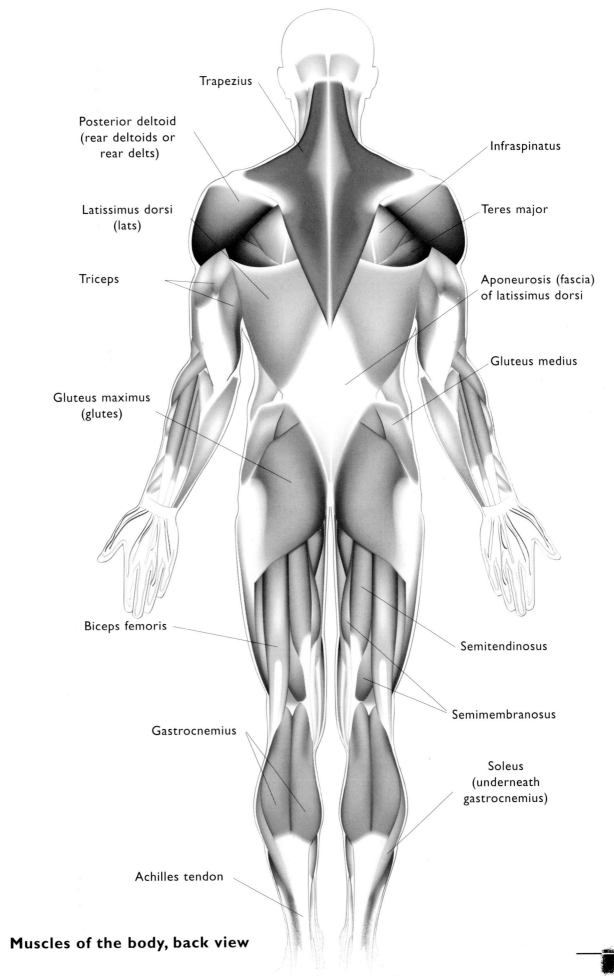

Trapezius

Posterior deltoid
(rear deltoids or
rear delts)

Infraspinatus

Latissimus dorsi
(lats)

Teres major

Triceps

Aponeurosis (fascia)
of latissimus dorsi

Gluteus medius

Gluteus maximus
(glutes)

Biceps femoris

Semitendinosus

Semimembranosus

Gastrocnemius

Soleus
(underneath
gastrocnemius)

Achilles tendon

Muscles of the body, back view

CHAPTER ONE

LESSONS 1–7

In the *Preface* we have covered how the method developed, a few practical cautions about clothing, the timing of meals and so on. Let us now turn to the first exercises we teach, and the reasons we teach them.

LESSON ONE: THE DAILY FIVE (PLUS TWO)

As I mentioned in the *Preface*, we do not recommend that stretching exercises for the major muscle groups of the body be done every day, but there are five that may be done daily—mainly to keep the spine mobile and to rid the body of the effects of the stress of daily life. A great deal is known about the biochemistry of stress—the classic fight or flight syndrome (for the original, and still completely relevant, text that began the field of research, see Selye, 1976)—and hundreds of books have been written about occupational stress (see, for example, Albrecht, 1979, for one of the seminal books in this field), but there is remarkably little written on the muscular effects of stress. Put simply, the major effect of stress is increased tension. Everyone—as you know—holds elevated tension in various muscles around the body. (These are the places you love to have massaged!) In time we will teach specific stretches for these areas, but today we will learn some compound movements that will stretch most of the muscles that attach to the spine (and therefore move it), and we will move the spine in all of its major directions. In addition, we will show you one of the best stretches for the hip region; just why this can be important we will leave until a later lesson. The lesson finishes with two effective neck stretches.

1. Floor clasped feet middle and upper back

This exercise stretches the middle to upper back, depending on your proportions. In addition to the paravertebrals (the muscles running alongside the spine), this exercise stretches *trapezius* and *rhomboideus*, and the movement is also one of the few solo stretches available for a muscle that lifts the shoulder, *levator scapulae*. As one end of levator scapulae attaches to the shoulder blade and the other to the side of the cervical spine, this muscle either elevates the shoulder or flexes the neck to one side. Consequently, this exercise can also be used as an indirect neck stretching exercise. The movement stretches the spine and all its posterior ligaments. Exercise 1 is also great to do after backward bending, to make the body feel completely comfortable.

Head placement is critical, both to avoid possible neck injury and to ensure that the stretch is felt in the correct muscles. Those who are relatively inflexible may find it difficult to get into the starting position; if so, try placing your forehead, instead of the top of your head (the standard direction) on the floor. Bulky people will find it difficult to get into the starting position unaided, but using a strap around the feet will help (shown in the last photograph in the series).

In the easiest version, kneel down as shown. While supporting yourself with one arm, reach through the knees (notice that the knees are further apart than the ankles) and hold the foot of the same side, by reaching around the arch to hold the side of the foot. Lean forwards and place the top of the head on the floor, resting some of the body's weight on the head. This locates the shoulders with respect to the hips. Now reach through the knees with the other hand, and hold the other foot. If you cannot hold your feet, use a strap. Ensure that the top of the head is resting on the floor. Breathe normally. Gripping the feet (or the strap) firmly, slowly and gently push the hips forwards. Because the hands are holding the feet, the middle and upper back are drawn into a forward curve, as in drawing a bow. Generally, this will not irritate the lower back if back pain is your problem—for most people, all of the stretch is felt higher in the back. If this position is not possible for you, a version that can be done on a chair or bench is described immediately below.

In the final position, breathe in and out for about five breaths. Let the stretch go by letting the hips return to the start position. Take one hand off one foot, and place it in the support position. Now breathe in and hold your breath while you use the support arm to lift yourself back to the beginning position. Holding your breath in as you get up will stop your face going red and, if you have low blood pressure, will stop you feeling faint as you get up, which is always a possibility when exercising with the head below the heart. Resume normal breathing. Do not lift yourself up into the start position using the muscles of the back. As a general rule, when returning from any extended (stretched) position, use muscles other than the ones you have been stretching. You may move the main locus of the stretch further down to the middle of the back by holding the feet from outside the legs; this variation is detailed in lesson 4, page 82.

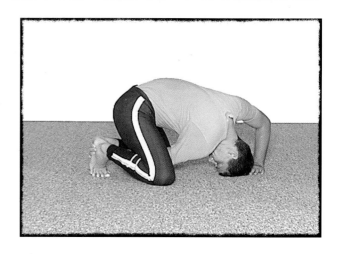

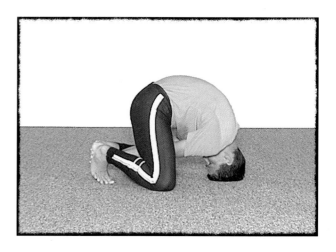

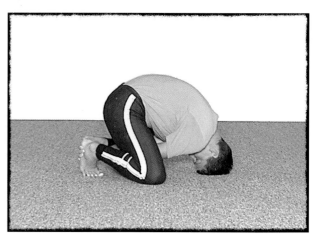

Cues

kneel and hold one foot
lower head or forehead to floor
hold other foot
gently push hips forward
breathe normally
hold breath in as you return to the start position

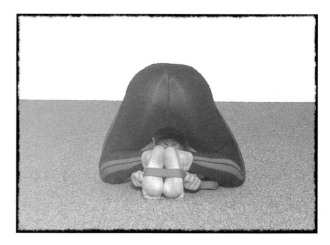

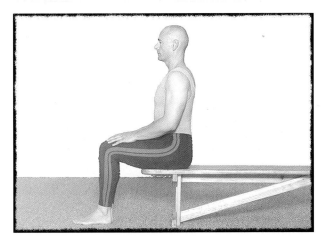

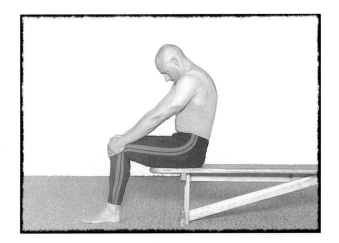

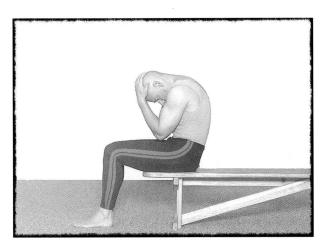

Middle and upper back from chair

If you cannot get into the starting position for exercise 1, you may achieve a similar stretch for the middle and upper back using a bench or chair. Look at the first photograph in the sequence. Sit on a stable chair, and let your neck bend so that your chin comes towards your chest. You may feel a stretch down the middle of the back by doing only this. If so, hold the position breathing normally for five breaths or so. If you want to increase the stretch, move your hips closer to the front of the chair and reach your hands up and clasp them behind your head. Slowly let the weight of your arms come onto the back of the neck; this will increase the stretch. If you want to increase the effect even more, let your hips roll *backwards* as you let the upper body slump forwards, as shown in the second photograph. Because your neck is already stretched forward, slumping in this manner gives a pleasing stretch in the middle and upper back. Hold the final position for five normal breaths in and out. In time, the neck and back will loosen sufficiently to let you do exercise 1.

An alternative movement may be better, depending on your pattern of flexibility and your proportion. Look at the photographs. Sit on the front of a stable chair, and hold your knees. Let your chin go towards your chest slowly. Two movements will give the desired stretch. The first is to use the arms to gently *pull the shoulders towards the knees*—note that the trunk does not move at the hips. The second movement requires you to roll the hips backwards to increase the stretch. Varying the strength of the two bending forces will change the main focus of the stretch, so play with these elements.

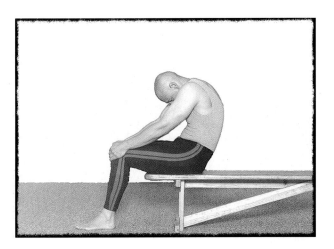

Cues

chin to chest

let hips roll backwards

to increase stretch, hold knees

gently pull on knees with hands

2. Backward bend from floor

The next exercise is described in two forms, because your proportion (lengths of body segments) substantially influences the final effects of the pose. As you become more flexible, the stretch will be felt in the abdominal muscles. The critical aspect of this pose is in keeping the lower-back muscles completely relaxed while using only the arms to lift the shoulders and incline the upper body backwards.

This exercise, in various forms, has been a popular recommendation for lower-back problems. A disadvantage is that backward-bending movements commonly irritate the back pain sufferer, probably through compression of the facet joints. Such compression sensations will be exacerbated by any tension in the muscles running along the spine, so my advice is try to keep all the back muscles relaxed while using the strength of your arms to get into the position. The conventional way to approach this stretch (the cobra pose from yoga) is to tense the buttock muscles before starting and to hold these muscles tight during the pose. The problem with this approach is that the untrained person cannot avoid tensing the lower back muscles as well—the very thing we are trying to avoid.

In the easiest version of this exercise, the starting position is lying face-down, legs together, with your forearms flat on the floor in front of the shoulders. Deliberately relax the whole body. Rocking the body from side to side will help to relax the trunk muscles. Take a deep breath in and, as you begin to breathe out, elevate the upper body slowly onto one elbow at a time, leaving the front of the hips on the floor. Rest on the elbows with the head in a neutral position with respect to the trunk, and let the front of the body sink as close as it can to the floor. Breathe 10 slow breaths.

In the intermediate version, start the same way, but extend the arms. If you think you may not be flexible enough to extend the arms fully if you have them under the shoulders, place your hands further out to the sides, so that the shoulders will not be lifted quite as high when the arms are straightened. If you can keep the lower-back muscles relaxed, this is an effective and comfortable stretch for the front of the body. As soon as you have reached maximum arm extension, pause and breathe in and out a few times, trying to keep the body as relaxed as possible. Breathe in and draw the shoulders as far back as you can, using the

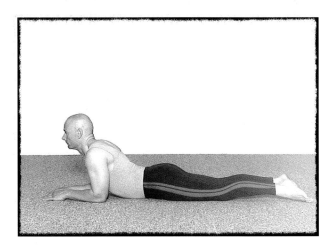

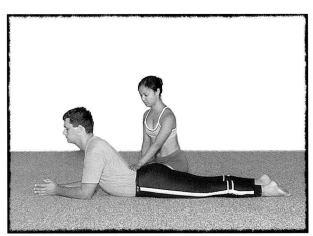

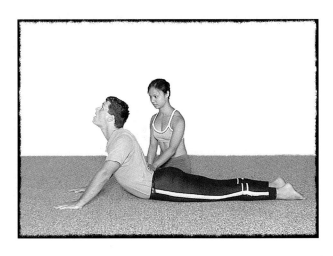

Cues

keep back muscles soft

use only arms to lift shoulders

breathe in a relaxed way

take head back with mouth open

roll up to recover

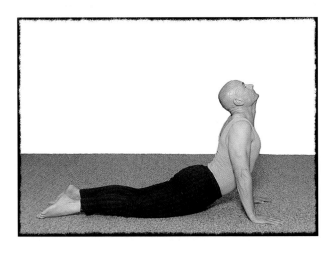

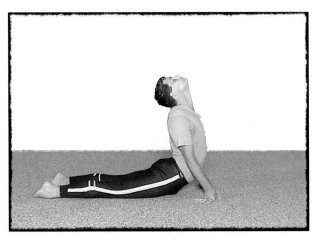

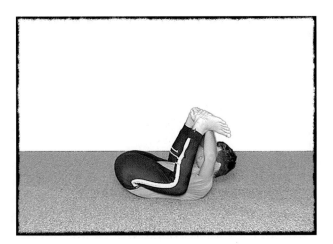

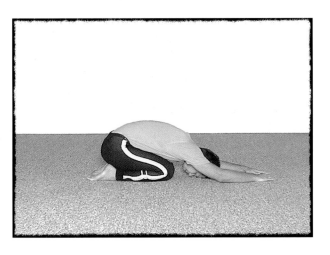

muscles of the shoulder blades and upper back. Be careful that this action does not tense the muscles of the lower back. If it does, lower yourself to the floor and begin again, concentrating on the first part of the exercise only. Hold the final position for 10 breaths.

If you have someone to help, the tension in your lower back muscles can be monitored. In the photographs, Julie is kneeling alongside Mark, with her hand placed on his lower back, just above the hips. As he lifts himself higher, she can feel whether the muscles tense; if they do, she tells him to lower himself out of the stretch a little, and to roll his body from side to side gently. Once the muscles have relaxed (this may take a few attempts) she tells him to try again. The final position of the stretch can be understood as the point just below where the muscles tighten.

Once comfortable in the final position, the stretch may be enhanced by opening the mouth and tilting the head back. Once the head is back, slowly close the mouth. Hold this position for a few breaths. I am showing an intermediate-level backward bend and Mark is showing a more advanced one.

The recovery position is shown in the third photograph. Always finish backward bending by coming out of it slowly and immediately rolling over onto your back, clasping the bent knees to the chest. This action will gently stretch the lower back muscles, which usually (despite one's best efforts) will have tightened up a little during the pose. Hold the knees to the chest until the lower back feels relaxed.

Alternatively, you can let the body relax over folded legs, as shown in the last photograph.

Don't forget that exercise 1, middle and upper back, can always be used for the same purpose.

3. Lying rotation

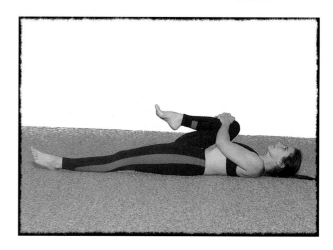

Lie face up, as Jennifer is demonstrating. Gently pull one knee towards the chest, and see what that feels like. Some people trap the tendons and muscles of the hip flexors if they pull the knee straight back to the chest. If you feel an uncomfortable pinching sensation in the groin of the bent leg, or the front of your pelvis makes contact with the top of that thigh (common among women), check to see whether overly tight clothing around the top of the leg might be a contributing factor. If loosening the clothing does not remove the irritation, let the leg go away from the chest until at arm's length, and let it move more to the *side* of the body. Then bring the knee back to the body again, but this time in the direction of the armpit. Bringing the knee towards the body, but more from the side, usually avoids the sensation of compression in the hip joint.

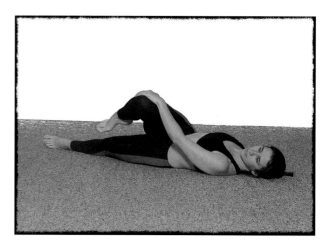

Now, gently pull the knee into the chest (or armpit) using both hands, as shown. You may feel the stretch variously from behind the leg (top part of the hamstring muscle) to inside the leg (the adductors), and you may also feel the stretch in the bottom muscles on the bent-leg side. Pulling the knee to the armpit is part one of the movement.

After holding the stretch for about 10 breaths, let the leg go to arm's length. Hold the outside of the thigh with the hand of the opposite arm, as shown. Roll the leg across the body. As soon as it passes over the vertical centre-line of the body, take some weight on the bottom leg, and shift the bottom hip across in the opposite direction. This ensures that the spine, as seen from above, remains straight. Most floor rotations do not include this refinement and, as a result, the spine is both rotated and hyperextended (arched backwards) in the final position; the two movements together are often sufficient to cause pain in someone with back problems.

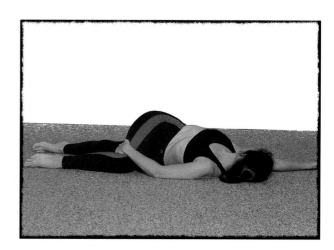

Slowly take the top leg across as far as it will go. The limit is when the opposite shoulder begins to lift off the floor. You may grasp a sturdy table leg to hold the shoulder down, but do not force the stretch. Concentrate on breathing and relaxing. Notice that, as you breathe in, the leg tends to rise and, as you breathe out, it tends to go closer to the floor. You may rest the knee of the bent leg on a cushion if the end position is quite a way from the floor, as shown in the last

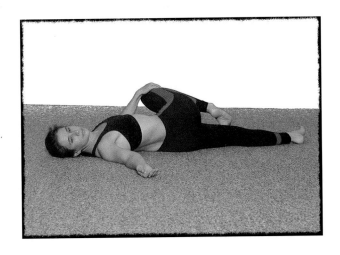

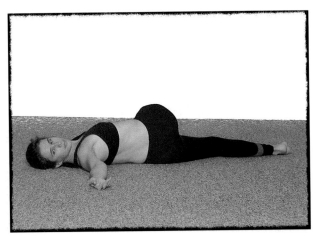

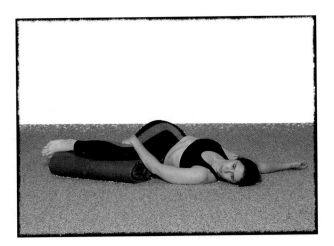

Cues

knee to armpit to stretch hip

hold outside of knee

roll bottom hip underneath

breathe and relax

photograph. This will enable you to hold the position comfortably. This is part two of the movement.

As you become more flexible, reduce the thickness of the cushion until it is no longer necessary. In all but the last photograph, Jennifer is demonstrating the intermediate version of the exercise; her knee is on the ground, and her shoulders are on the floor. Give yourself time and you will reach this position too. In the exercise, look at your outstretched hand. Hold the final position for about 10 breaths, then return the leg to the starting position.

If one side of the body is tighter in this movement in either part one or part two, we can use the Contract–Relax (**C–R**) approach to even them up. In the final stretch position of part one, hold the bent leg with both hands and very gently try to press it away from you against the resistance of your arms for five seconds or so. *Do not let the leg move at all.* We have found that the extent of the improvement in the final position depends crucially on this point being observed. Be sure to push back *gently*; if you push back too hard, many other muscles will tighten to stabilise your position and, again, the extent of the final position will be compromised. After the contraction phase, stop pushing, take in a deep breath and, *as you breathe out*, gently pull the knee closer to the chest. Hold this new position for five breaths in and out.

To improve part two, hold the outside of the bent leg as before. In this contraction, push the leg towards your hand. Rather than the hip muscles, use the *back and waist muscles* to press, in order to maximise the stretch in these muscles. Remember, the muscles used to generate the contraction force will be the muscles that experience the stretch effect. Relax, breathe in, and on a breath out, slowly press the leg closer to the floor.

The next spinal movement we will do bends the body to the side. In addition to the muscles of the waist, it stretches many hip and back muscles.

4. Standing side bend

Using a wall in this movement ensures correct alignment and provides support. The aim is to stretch all of the side waist muscles, the obliques, in the first instance. As these become more flexible, the exercise will also stretch *quadratus lumborum* and the deep spinal muscles. The abductors of the leg will also be stretched, including *tensor fasciae latae*. As one extends the arm above and across the head, *latissimus dorsi* and other back muscles are added to the stretch. Jennifer is demonstrating this exercise, too.

Standing with the weight evenly on both feet, lean the body against a wall. Maintain the whole body in contact with the wall during the exercise. Lean to one side as far as you can, and place the hand on the hip. Alternatively, you may grasp the leg firmly. Choose the position that gives you the best support. The best feeling in the end position in this movement will be experienced *only* if the upper body's weight is supported completely on the arm. If this does not occur, the very muscles we want to stretch will have to hold you up.

Once comfortably leaning on the support arm, reach the other arm out and over the head as far as you can—the locus of the stretch will extend from above the hip you are stretching to the whole of that side. Try to reach the hand out past where it stops, as though you are trying to grasp something just out of reach. This will increase the effect noticeably. Hold the final position for five breaths only.

To come out of the stretch, very slowly roll the top shoulder away from the wall, trying to increase the sidewards stretch all the while. As you rotate the shoulder forward, your apparent flexibility at the waist will increase noticeably and you will need to increase the lean to the side just to maintain the stretch sensation. The locus of the stretch will move too, from just above the hip to further towards the spine itself as the shoulder rotates forward. If you find a position that feels particularly good in this transition move, pause there for a breath or two. Repeat for the other side. To relax all the muscles just worked, stand away from the wall and, with your weight over both feet, swing your arms around behind you to both sides. This turning action gently uses all the muscles stretched and compressed by exercise 4.

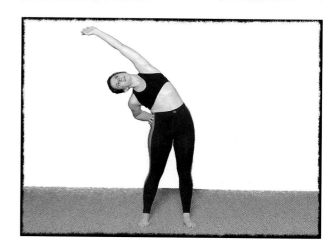

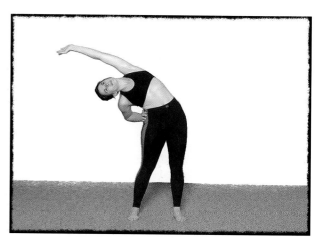

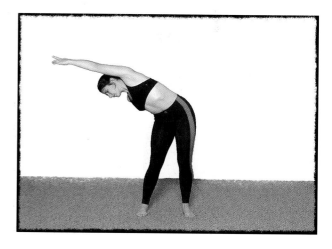

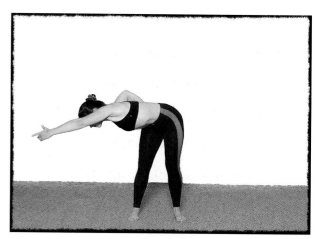

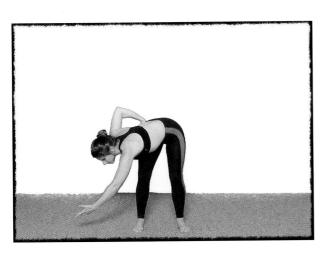

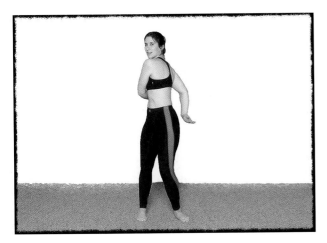

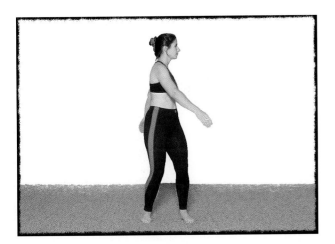

Cues

lean sideways onto support arm

reach out top arm

slowly roll top shoulder forwards

stretch other side, then

bend knees and swing arms

5. Seated hip

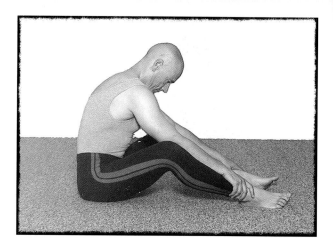

Inflexible hip muscles (in particular *gluteus maximus*, the main muscle of the bottom, and *piriformis*, one of the external hip rotators) can contribute significantly to back pain in some people, and to dysfunction in many more. This stretch is one of the best to loosen this area. Anatomical details are shown in the illustration accompanying exercise 22, on page 68.

Before we attempt the movement, I wish to introduce a technique that helps isolate many hip and hamstring movements. We call the movement a 'negative thrust', to distinguish the movement from a standard, or 'positive', thrust, in which the hips are moved forwards. Look at the photograph. I am sitting on the floor with the legs about shoulder width apart and the knees bent. Sit this way and try to feel the bottom bones pressing on the floor. Now arch the lower back backwards, and you will feel the pelvis rock forward and the bottom bones contact the floor more directly. If you have a partner they can assist you by placing their hands on your lower back to assist in the movement. Rolling the pelvis forwards in this fashion is the core idea behind the negative thrust. The main sensation will be experienced in the hamstring muscles (between bottom and knee, at the back of the legs) if they are tight. If this is the main sensation, bend the legs further at the knees and repeat the movement.

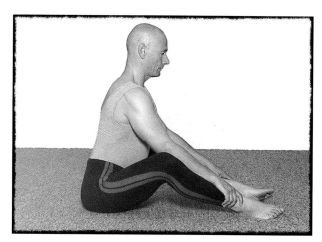

This rolling of the pelvis is the key to isolating various muscles, usually on the back (posterior) side of the body. Later I will describe the positive thrust that can be used to isolate particular muscles on the front (anterior) side of the body. In some poses the direction 'lift the chest' will be made, and this often achieves the same effect as arching the middle and upper back backwards. Rolling the pelvis like this moves the bottom bones (the *ischial tuberosities*) further away from the knees and lengthens the hamstring muscles in the process. The movement also exposes some of the external hip rotators to greater stretch, and this effect will be felt in the next exercise.

Cues

hold ankles; let body slump

arch back backwards, and

feel the pelvis roll forwards

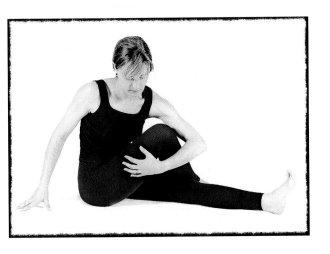

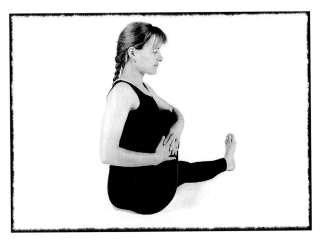

Cues

hold knee with opposite elbow

negative thrust; lift chest

C–R: press knee into forearm

restretch: draw knee to armpit

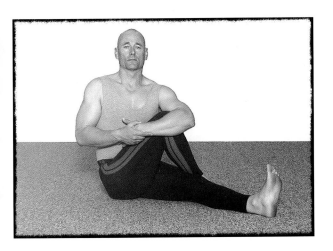

With this technique in mind, we are ready to do the seated hip stretch. In the easiest version, sit on the floor as Petra is demonstrating, with one leg outstretched. Bend the other leg at the knee and place the foot on the outside of the straight leg. Check that your back is held straight (lift the chest to make sure) and grasp the knee with the opposite shoulder's arm. As you breathe out, gently bring the knee back to the chest. Ensure that you can feel the floor through *both* bottom bones—the most common error in this pose is that you inadvertently lift the bottom bone of the leg you are holding off the floor as you bring the knee to the body. If your form is good, you will feel the stretch in the hip of the held leg.

A **C–R stretch** can be used here. You may care to review the C–R principles on pages 11 and 12. To restate briefly, a C–R has three main elements: first stretch the limb gently, and hold for a short while. Hold the limb, and *without letting it move*, press it away from you for six to ten seconds. Stop, breathe in, and on a breath out, relax the muscles involved, stretching a little further as you breathe out. If the hip is tight, you may prefer to use the stronger grip position I am demonstrating in the third photograph. Hold the new position for five breaths (20–30 seconds) or so.

This exercise is a good one to practise the **C–R stretch** technique because it is easy to hold the leg yourself. Hold the knee in your best position for a few breaths in and out, getting used to the feeling in the hip. Now gently press the knee away from you, holding it all the while. The leg you are pressing away from you *must not move* at all. Press for a count of six (count one, two, ... and so on to yourself slowly), then stop pressing—again do not let the leg move from this position. Take in a deep breath, and on a breath out, relax the hip muscles completely, slowly drawing the knee closer to your chest in the direction of your armpit. *Make sure that the hip of this leg stays firmly on the floor.* Hold the new final position for 20–30 seconds, breathing normally. Rest for a moment and stretch the other side. Note which side is tighter in this movement, and next time you stretch, begin with this side. Do the looser one next and finish by stretching the tighter side once more. In time, the differences between left and right will be reduced. If both sides feel the same, do each side once.

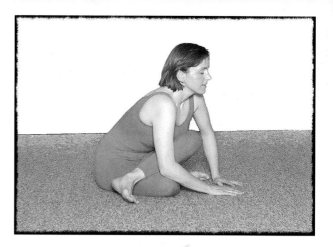

If the version just described does not give you a strong enough stretch in the hip, you may try the folded leg version, demonstrated by Carol. In all respects other than the starting position, this intermediate version is the same. Look at the photograph. Do not sit on the folded lower leg, but keep it sufficiently outside the line of the body to permit both bottom bones to contact the floor firmly. If you are not loose enough in the hips to sit like this (insufficient *external rotation* of the hip of the leg closest the floor is the most common reason) stay with the version above. Lean your upper body forwards on the bottom bones until it is inclined towards the leg in front of you, and feel how this presses the bottom bones into the floor. Carol has her eyes closed to better feel the sensations. Because this is an important point, you may wish to try this version sitting on a hard floor without any mat or cushion the first few times you try the exercise. Move subtly from side to side in the starting position until you are sure that both bones are pressing on the floor equally. Clasp the knee as close as possible to under the armpit of the opposite shoulder while keeping your back straight. Now slowly sit up straight, as long as you can hold the form. The stretch will be felt in the hip, but more strongly than in the straight-leg version, because folding the second leg forces stricter form on you—it is easier to hold the lower back straight.

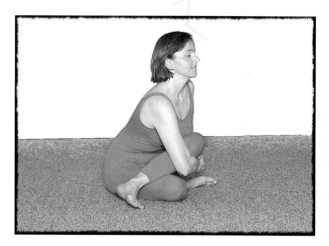

A **C–R stretch** can be achieved by pressing the leg away from you as for the previous version above. Stretch both sides, and make a mental note of which one is tighter. When you practise next time, begin with the tighter side, do the looser one, and repeat for the first side. In this way the tighter side will loosen more quickly and both sides will become similar.

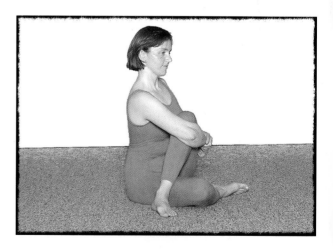

The next two exercises, 6 and 7, are not part of the daily five. Many people hold tension in the neck area, however, and any of the neck exercises may be included in your daily routine if you wish.

Cues

ensure both hips on floor

negative thrust and lift chest

C–R: press knee to forearm

restretch: draw knee to armpit

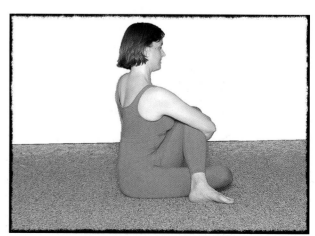

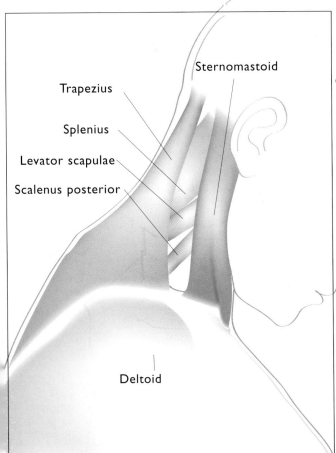

Trapezius
Sternomastoid
Splenius
Levator scapulae
Scalenus posterior
Deltoid

Muscles of the neck, side view, flexed

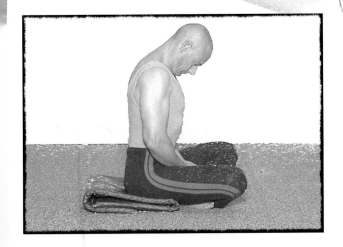

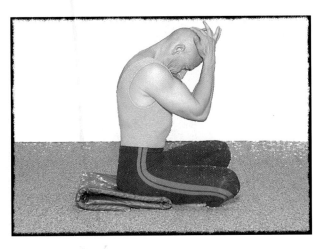

6. Chin to chest

There are a number of ways to sit for this exercise. If you can sit on your folded legs, it is easier to hold the back straight, but the disadvantage is that this may make the legs or feet feel uncomfortable. Various ways of easing this position are shown in the photographs accompanying exercise 23, floor instep, in lesson 4 (page 77). Alternatively, the exercise may be performed effectively sitting on a chair or sitting with the legs folded. If sitting on the floor, I recommend placing a cushion or rolled mat under the bottom as I am doing, so that the body is slightly tipped forward; this makes it possible to hold yourself straight with much less effort.

Sit in any position that makes holding your spine straight comfortable. You will be distracted by sensations in the back or hips if you are not completely comfortable—and that will mean that you cannot attend to the sensations in the neck.

Sitting up, let your neck bend forwards until the weight of the head gives you a stretch in the back of the neck. In some people this stretch will be felt in the middle of the back as well. Rest in this position for a few breaths. This may be a sufficient stretch. If you want a stronger sensation, reach the arms up and place a couple of fingers of both hands behind the highest part of the head. Very slowly let the weight of the arms be felt on the muscles of the back of the neck. For many people this is sufficient stretch; to make it stronger, clasp the hands together and let the full weight of the arms be felt.

A **C–R stretch** makes this an extremely effective exercise indeed and helps many people with tension headaches and stiff necks. While holding the head in the stretch position, gently press the head back against the hands. As before, *do not let the head move during this contraction.* Press for a count of three (recall that small muscles seem to need less contraction time to achieve a beneficial stretch), stop pressing and breathe in. The hands maintain the position of the head in relation to the body all the while. On a breath out, let the neck relax as much as you can and at the same time very carefully pull the head forwards so the chin moves closer to the chest. When you feel a sufficient stretch, hold the final position for a few breaths in and out.

Next, the natural inclination is to want to stretch the neck backwards, but many people do not like this movement. The next part of exercise 6 helps explain this reservation.

Once you have returned to the starting position, take in a breath, relax and let it out. Open the mouth as wide as you can. Holding the mouth in this position, slowly tilt the head backwards on the neck, and then tilt the neck backwards too. Doing it this way will probably feel more comfortable than it usually does. Once all the way back, very slowly close the teeth. When you are used to the stretch, slightly incline the chin to one side; this will stretch the muscles on the other side. Repeat for the second side.

When we close the teeth in the extended position, we are using the powerful clenching muscles of the jaw (*masseter* and *temporalis*, among others) to stretch the muscles of the front of the neck. When you stretch the head back with the mouth closed in the usual way, not only are the rear neck muscles having to move the head, they are also having to stretch the front neck muscles too. This additional effort can make the rear neck muscles spasm (any muscle asked to do work in the contracted end of their range of movement is likely to display this unfortunate effect—try pointing your foot hard for a moment), so knowing this we can considerably ease the discomfort of bending the neck back.

As soon as you let the head come forwards into the neutral position, slowly lower the chin to the chest once more for a second or two to relax the muscles at the back of the neck.

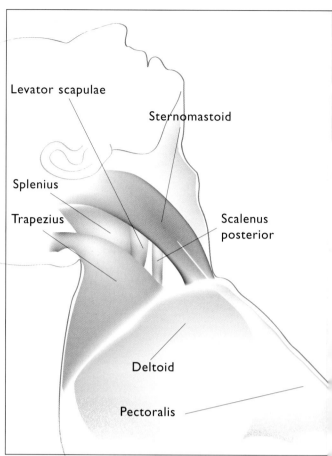

Muscles of the neck, side view, extended

Cues

let chin go to chest

place a couple of fingers behind head

allow weight of arms to stretch neck

C–R: press head softly to fingers

restretch: gently pull head forwards

pause

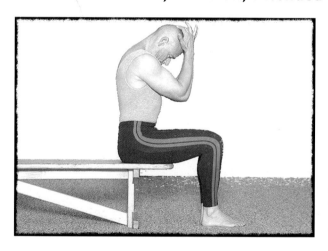

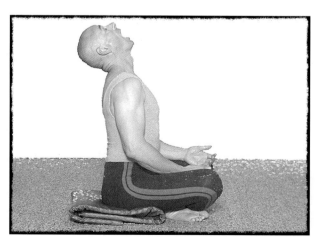

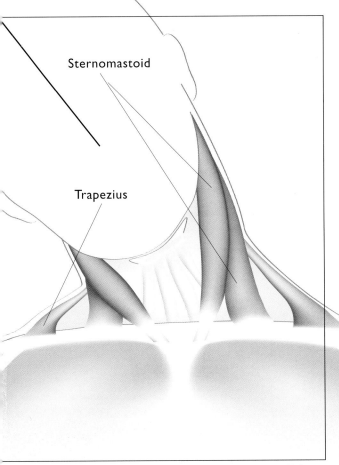

Sternomastoid

Trapezius

Muscles of the neck, in side-bend position

The neck muscles react to stress strongly and this may be because of the many ways these muscles are used in ordinary daily life to express fine shades of attitude and emotion. The position of the head on the neck and the relation between the neck and the shoulders—as everyone knows—very often says more about your state of mind than what you say. Hunching of the shoulders is a fundamental defensive and protective posture, for example, whereas shoulders carried low under a loose neck suggest a state of relaxed readiness. All negative emotions have characteristic, though different for every individual, postural signatures or patterns of holding tension that are displayed in these muscles.

We have found that stretching the neck muscles has an immediate effect on one's state of mind, compared with stretching other larger muscles such as *quadriceps* and hamstrings. Stretching larger muscles has a more diffuse effect on the body in terms of relaxation, whereas loosening the neck muscles seems to affect the way we feel directly.

This movement stretches all the muscles at the side of the neck in addition to muscles that span the neck and the shoulder. See the illustration for details. As there is tremendous variation in the flexibility of people's necks, we offer this stretch in a number of versions. Begin with the easiest, even if you are sure that you can use a stronger version. The sitting position and variations are the same as for the previous neck exercise.

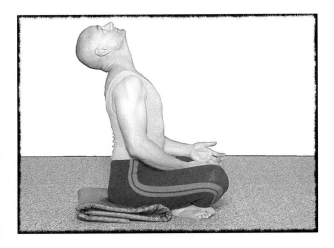

Cues

open mouth to take head backwards

incline head slowly to both sides

gently stretch head forwards to recover

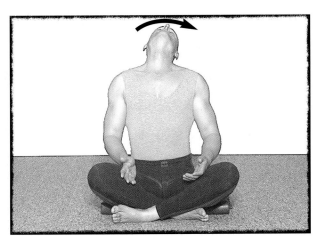

7. Neck side bend

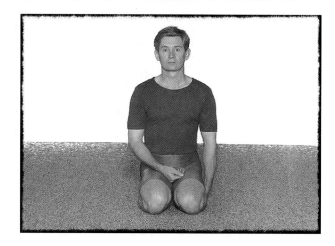

The simplest movement is to sit up straight and try to incline the head to one side, directly over the shoulder, and without lifting the shoulder up to the ear—the usual way everyone does this. Gary is demonstrating the positions. Any suitable seating position may be used and office chairs lend themselves particularly well to neck exercises. Consciously hold the opposite shoulder down (you will use the *latissimus dorsi* muscle under the arm to do this) and incline the head to the other side. You will feel a stretch along the side of the neck, from the ear to the shoulder you are holding down.

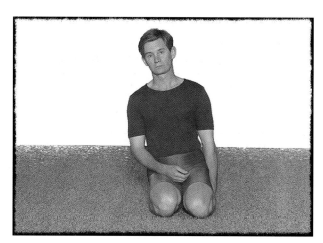

The stretch may be made stronger by restraining the shoulder you are stretching away from. Hold the shin of the leg you are sitting on, or your thigh if you are sitting cross-legged. If you are sitting on a chair, holding the base is effective, and is demonstrated opposite. Whichever holding position you are using, lean away from this hand until you feel a stretch in the muscles between the neck and the shoulder. This action pre-stretches the muscles involved. Now incline the head away, towards the other shoulder; this will immediately increase the stretch as you take the other end of the same muscles further away. Hold this new position for a few breaths in and out.

It is common to feel a strong stretch sensation in the arm used to hold the support. As the head is inclined away from the shoulder, the nerves of the neck and arm, the *brachial plexus*, are stretched as well as the muscles. People with overuse injuries will find this effective.

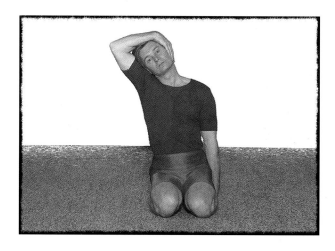

A **C–R stretch** is a most effective way to improve the range of movement. In the position just achieved, reach your free hand up to above the ear, as shown. *Do not increase the stretch at this point.* Rather, use this hand as a barrier against which to push the head gently for a few seconds; the head must not move while you do this. Stop pushing, take a breath in and, on a breath out relax the neck muscles and very softly pull the head slightly closer to the shoulder. Hold the final position for five breaths in and out. Repeat for the other side, and note which is the tighter. For most, stretching *away* from your dominant arm side is more difficult—the neck and arm muscles are usually more developed on this side, and generally this leaves them tighter. Stretch the tighter side again.

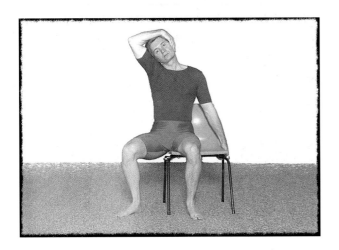

Cues

hold support to restrain shoulder

lean head directly to side

C–R: shrug shoulder; and

restretch: lean body further away,

C–R: press head to fingers

restretch: draw head gently to side

The final photograph shows the same exercise done in a chair—office workers will love this one. To get into this position, sit to one side of the chair, and hold the seat opposite the hip joint. If your arms are long in relation to your trunk length, you can sit with just one hip on the chair, and one leg out to the side for balance, as Gary is doing. The head is in the neutral position, directly over the shoulders.

Lean away from the hand holding the chair and you will feel the shoulder being pulled down and, perhaps, a stretch in the arm, too. Once in this position, lean the head directly to the side, away from the restraining hand. This may be a sufficient stretch; if not, place a couple of fingers on the head as shown, and gently take the head to the side.

A **C–R stretch** can be done, with two different contractions to great effect. The first **C–R** is to try to lift the shoulder of the hand holding the chair, the second is to gently press the head across to the hand holding the chair. You may restretch after each **C–R**, or after having done both. Be very gentle with yourself in the restretch phase; this is a strong stretch. The contractions need only be seconds long and the restretch will be three to five breaths.

Once finished, take the hand off the head, place it on the knee and use the arm to lift the body back to the start position. Do the other side, and note any differences.

To finish this lesson, return to the daily five and repeat them. When you are familiar with the sequence, it will take only seven or eight minutes to complete.

LESSON TWO: SHOULDERS

This lesson covers exercises for the three major shoulder muscles (front or *anterior deltoid*, side or *lateral deltoid*, and back or *posterior deltoid*). See the illustration for details. Good shoulder stretches will also affect the other major muscles that move the upper arm, including the large flat muscles on the front of the chest (the pectorals, or *pectoralis major* and *minor*) and the large muscles under the arms that give the upper body its characteristic 'V' shape when seen from behind, *latissimus dorsi*. Generally, we do not isolate the muscles of the shoulder, concentrating instead on movements that are chosen on the basis of complex *functions*. For example, an exercise that stretches the front *deltoid* will also stretch either the pectorals or the muscle at the front of the arm, *biceps brachii,* depending on the orientation of the arm to the shoulder. Both the pectorals and *biceps* can limit movement of the upper arm at the shoulder, so it is efficient to use large-scale movements that stretch these muscles in addition to the shoulder muscles. The muscle that is the limiting factor in the complex movement will be more stressed and will adapt the faster, without the need to identify which one is actually the limiting factor. This generalisation also applies to other soft-tissue limitations to movement, including the nerves that innervate the arm and any adhesions between the many layers of *fascia* that cover these structures.

To begin the session, do the daily five trunk exercises we learned in lesson 1. The first new exercise is a partner version of exercise 3.

8. Partner lying rotation

Alan (kneeling) and Pierre are showing how to do the exercise on this page, and Julie and Steve opposite. Begin this movement with your tighter side. Assuming that you are in the final position of exercise 3, lying rotation, ask your partner to kneel alongside you as shown. Look at the first photograph. Note that one of your partner's knees will be on the floor next to the armpit of your extended arm, and the other is placed in such a way as to be a brace for the elbow of the hand that will be placed on your hip.

Ask your partner to lean weight through a relaxed hand onto the shoulder of the extended arm, and to place the other hand *behind* the hip of the leg you are taking towards

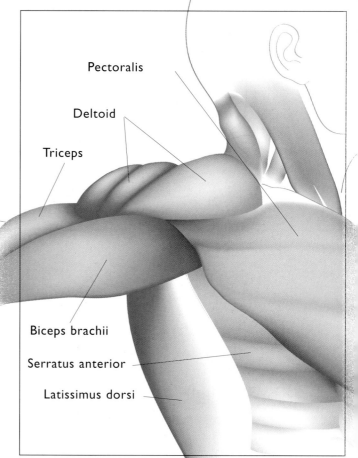

Pectoralis

Deltoid

Triceps

Biceps brachii

Serratus anterior

Latissimus dorsi

Muscles of arm and chest, arm lifted behin

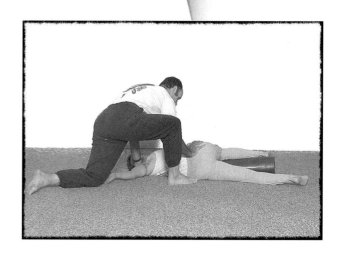

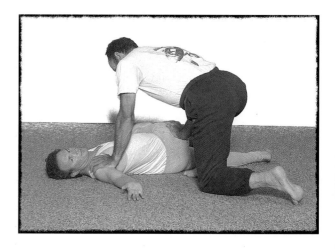

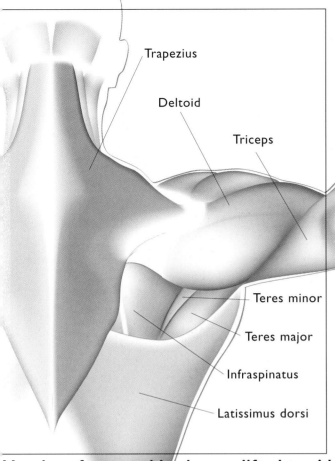

Trapezius

Deltoid

Triceps

Teres minor

Teres major

Infraspinatus

Latissimus dorsi

Muscles of arm and back, arm lifted to side

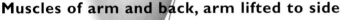

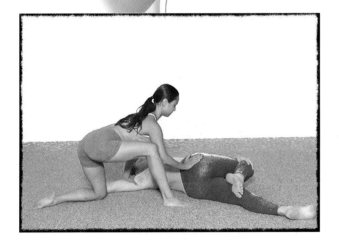

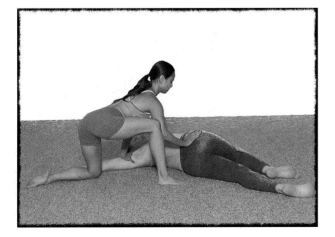

the floor. In a moment, you will be pushing your hip against their hand so it needs the support of the knee to be a secure barrier to this movement. You will find it most comfortable if your partner leans weight through a straight arm, rather than *pressing* your shoulder onto the floor. Your partner may lean on your upper arm if that feels better, or place a cushion or a mat between their hand and your arm for comfort.

Once in position, ask your partner to hold you stable; then gently push your top hip back against their hand for a few breaths; this is a **C–R stretch**. You do not need to push hard—if your partner cannot hold you in position you *are* pushing too hard; we have not found that a stronger effort produces a better stretch. If anything, the opposite is true because, if you do push hard, many other muscles must become involved to stabilise the action. After pushing back gently for a while, stop pushing, breathe in, and, on a breath out, slowly take your knee closer to the floor until you feel the desired stretch. Make sure that this second stretching action is slow; you may need a few breaths in and out before you reach the new end point. Ask your partner to hold you in this new position for five to ten breaths, and then stretch the other side. You may stretch the first side a second time if there is a big difference between the tightness of the sides. The stretch should be felt in the muscles between the hip of the leg you are taking to the side, and in the spine, and all the way up the back to the shoulder blades. If your front arm or chest muscles are tight, you will feel this exercise in these places too and this will be a good warm-up for exercise 10, below.

Cues

take leg to floor, as far as you can

partner places hand behind hip

C–R: press back to partner

restretch: take knee further to floor

9. Arm across body

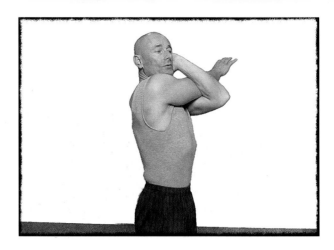

The standing version of this exercise is gentle and the floor version is a much stronger stretch. If you are large or muscular, do the standing version first; if you are slender, do the floor version, as you may feel no stretch using the standing version.

Look at the first photograph. Extend one arm out to the side, parallel with the floor. Swing the arm at a moderate pace across the body and catch it in the crook of the elbow of the other arm. You will need to swing the arm to get it into this position; if you move it too slowly you may not be able to bring it close enough to hold. Once held, use the arm, shoulder and back muscles of the second arm to draw the arm onto the front of your *neck*; if you bring the arm onto the chest there may be no stretch at all. If you can, you may hold the back of your neck as a way of holding the stretch for a while without much effort.

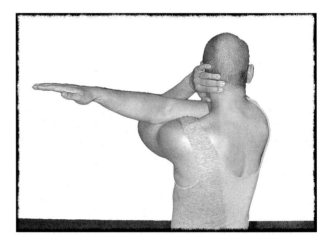

A **C–R stretch** can be achieved by pressing the straight arm away from you gently while holding it for a few seconds. Stop pressing, relax and breathe in and, on a breath out, increase the stretch by pulling the arm closer to the front of the neck. Hold for four or five breaths in and out and repeat for the other side. You should feel the effect at the back of the shoulder, and perhaps across the back, and you may feel a small compression sensation in the joint itself.

The lying version is much stronger, as the weight of the upper body stretches the involved muscles. Some people may feel a strong compression sensation in the shoulder itself if the exercise is too strong for their present level of flexibility. Look at the photographs on the facing page.

Begin by lying face down on the floor and bringing one arm into the position we used to begin the last stretch. Support yourself on the other arm and lift the shoulder of the first arm clear of the floor. This is the starting position. Bring the leg into position alongside you as shown. Make sure you bring the correct leg into position; not doing so is the most common mistake in this exercise. When in position, very gradually lower the shoulder to the floor—the leg out to the side will twist the body enough to strongly stretch the shoulder of the arm underneath you. Make sure that the arm is across the front of the neck; if you are lying with your chest on the arm there will be little stretch.

Cues

clasp arm to throat
hold back of neck
C–R: press arm to forearm
restretch: draw arm closer

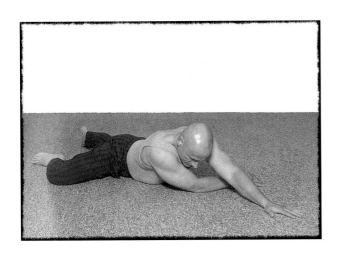

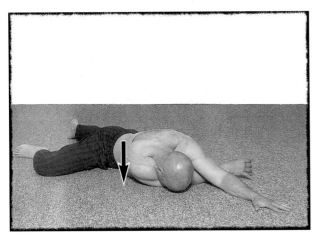

Adding a **C–R stretch** can be useful too; simply press the arm under you into the floor (the shoulder may yet be off the ground at this point) for a few seconds, breathe in and, on a breath out, relax and slowly lower the shoulder closer to the floor. Remain in the final position for three to five breaths in and out. The stretch can be made stronger still by lowering the armpit of the outstretched arm onto the arm under you, as indicated by the arrow in the last photograph.

Some people feel their hands going numb in this position; this is probably due to the blood supply being cut off to the arm (in a few cases it might be compression of the nerves that innervate the arm, the *brachial plexus*). If this happens, come out of the stretch and swing the arm around for a short while. Stretch the other arm.

Cues

draw same-side leg to side and
lie with arm across throat

lower chest to floor

C–R: press arm into floor

restretch: lower body closer to floor

10. Partner front arm

This exercise is by far the most effective stretch for the muscle that fills the space between the crook of the elbow and the shoulder, *biceps brachii*, or usually *biceps* for short. (Another *biceps* muscle, *biceps femoris*, is located in an analogous position at the back of the leg, between knee and bottom.) We usually teach the partner version first in the classes. Once you know what the stretch should feel like and precisely how the location of the effect can be changed by simple alterations of pose, you will be in a good position to do the stretch by yourself. The standing version of the stretch may be conveniently used in the gym while training the arms or chest, or on location any time you feel a need to stretch this muscle. Experience shows that this muscle is frequently very tight indeed. In fact, general tightness of the *biceps* muscle and irritation of the tendon of the long head of *biceps* (where it passes along the *intertubercular groove*) sometimes masquerades as a *rotator cuff* injury. Two specific rotator cuff stretches are offered later (see exercises 59 and 60) and using these three exercises together can often identify the true cause of common shoulder soreness.

The exercise will focus its main effect on either the pectoral and front *deltoid* muscle or the *biceps* muscle of the arm being stretched, depending on the angle of the arm in relation to the floor and which surface of the forearm is placed against the wall. Look at the first photograph in the series; Olivia is helping me. Face the wall directly, and place your arm against it, with the thumb up. Your partner can hold it there by pressing the upper arm onto the wall.

Now rotate the whole body using the feet so that your other shoulder comes away from the wall (you are pivoting around the shoulder held against the wall) and bring your other hand up to the position shown to hold yourself there. Do not lean forwards as you rotate the body—this is the most common way people avoid the stretch. If desired, your partner may lightly cup the shoulder to help you hold it in position, as shown in the second photograph. You should feel the stretch in the front of the chest on the side of the arm that is extended against the wall and also in that shoulder. Some will feel it in the *biceps*, too. Try the arm a little higher or lower to vary the effect. These variations will need to be only small. The most common mistake observed in the classes is that a student will not have the fingers roughly in line with the top of the head.

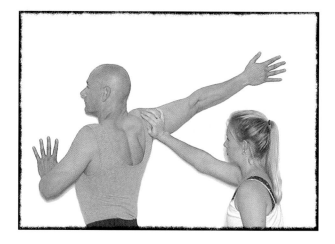

Cues

thumb up; hand level with top of head

bring other shoulder away from wall

C–R: press hand into wall

slowly bring other shoulder
away from wall

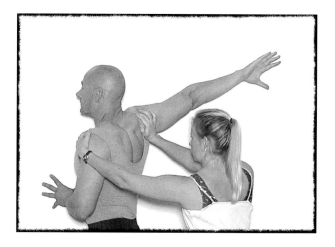

Cues

thumb down to stretch *biceps*

bring other shoulder away from wall

C–R: press back of wrist into wall

slowly bring other shoulder
away from wall

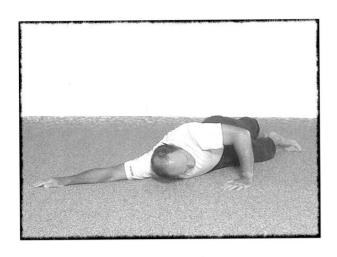

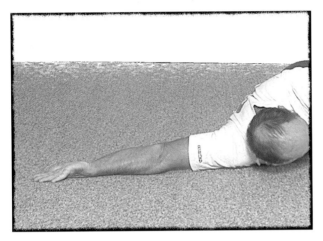

Cues

make sure arm is at correct angle

use other arm to lift shoulder

C–R: press arm into floor

restretch: roll top shoulder further back

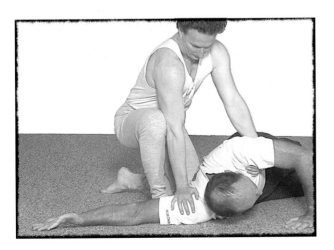

A **C–R stretch** makes this very effective indeed. While you are held in position, press your palm and arm into the wall gently for five seconds or so. Use a long, slow, pushing action, increasing the effort slightly as you do. Stop pressing, take a breath in and, on a breath out, very slowly rotate the other shoulder further away from the wall. It is essential that you be in control of the final stretch position, so do not let your partner move your shoulder. Ask them to follow you as you move the shoulder further from the wall, and to hold you in the new position. Being held allows you to concentrate on the sensations in your arm, to attend to your breathing, and to let the muscles you are stretching relax properly. Even though you will think that you are relaxed in any new end position, always take another deliberate breath in, and let yourself relax once more. You will always be able to take yourself a little further. Stretch the other arm, and note any left–right differences. The effect of this version will mainly be felt in the chest and shoulder and, to some extent, in the arm.

The next version will be felt almost completely in the *biceps* muscle of the upper arm and, in some people, will also be felt in two other arm muscles, *brachialis* and *brachioradialis*. To begin, stand facing the wall as before (second photo, facing page). This time, when you place the arm against the wall, roll the arm and shoulder over so that your thumb points down to the floor. In all respects other than the orientation of the forearm the exercise is the same as just described. When doing the **C–R stretch**, try to press the back of the wrist into the wall using the *biceps* and other arm muscles rather than the chest and shoulder muscles. So doing will emphasise the effects on the *biceps*. As with the first version, small alterations in arm angle can change the location of the major effect.

The final sequence of photographs (Alan, assisted by Pierre) shows the same exercise being done on the floor. I suggest you try the wall version first, to ensure that the form is correct. Most people have the arm too low (below the level of the head, if you are doing the exercise standing) and lose some of the *biceps* effect as a result. Once you are familiar with where the stretch is supposed to be felt, doing the exercise on the floor makes it very easy to hold the final position. Gravity is working in your favour, especially if you drop the top leg over behind you, as Alan is doing in the top photograph. A partner may assist as shown—Pierre is simply holding Alan in his final position, making the **C–R** contraction and the restretch final position easier to hold.

11. Partner arms up behind back

This is another chest, shoulders and *biceps* combination movement. If your shoulders are tight, you may hold a strap between your hands to allow them to separate (up to shoulder width) to make early attempts easier, as I am showing in the top photograph. This is also an excellent stretch for the nerves that innervate the arm (the *brachial plexus*). If you have any shoulder, arm or forearm problem where the nerves might be suspected of playing a causal role (such as overuse injuries), this exercise may be helpful. The exercise may be done standing, kneeling or sitting, depending on the relative heights of you and your partner.

Olivia and I are showing the easiest version of the exercise. I have wrapped a thick cotton strap around both hands and wrists to allow separation between the hands, which makes the movement much easier to do. All directions below relating to **C–R stretches** apply to this assisted version, too. Once you can get the arms horizontal in this version (while standing with the trunk vertical!) you may try the next version.

This exercise can be done on your own, too, by clasping your hands together behind you, or using a strap as described, bending forwards, and placing them on a suitable support. The stretch is effected by lowering yourself; the **C–R stretch** is done as usual (described below), and the final stretch is achieved by lowering yourself further. If using a strap, you may experiment with rolling the forearms inwards or outwards to vary the final stretch effects.

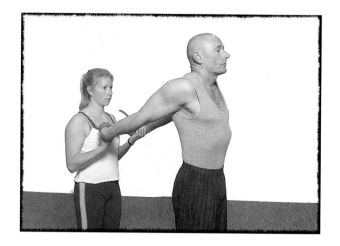

Cues

use strap if necessary
roll shoulders back to begin
partner elevates arms slowly
C–R: press hands to floor
restretch: partner slowly lifts arms

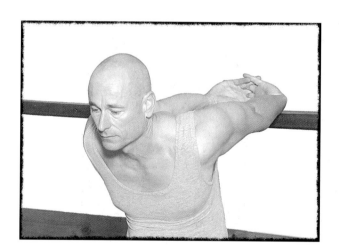

Cues

fingers together or use strap
roll shoulders back to begin
lower body to stretch
C–R: press hands into support
restretch: lower body further

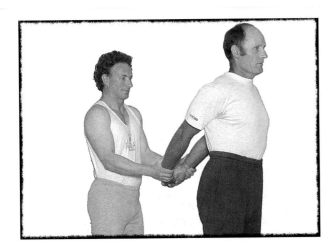

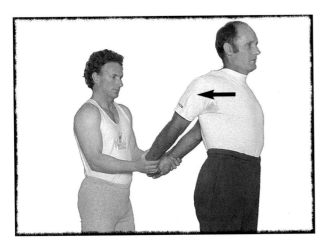

Alan and Pierre are showing the intermediate exercise from the standing position but, if you kneel as shown in the last photograph, the task of holding the arms in the final position is made easier. The choice of start position depends on your respective heights. Clasp your hands behind your back, or use a strap as suggested. Alan is demonstrating the essential backwards roll of the shoulders *before* the arms are lifted up behind (second photograph). Ask your partner to take the arms up behind you as far as feels comfortable. The closer your hands are to each other, the more intense the stretch in the arms and shoulders will be. When you feel a sufficient stretch, stop. Do not sacrifice movement at the shoulder joint for the sake of height of the arms behind you; the most common error in this pose is to allow the upper back to bend forwards.

To loosen the muscles, a **C–R stretch** is required. Ask your partner to hold you in position and press your hands down in the direction of the floor. As always, the arms must not move during the contraction; if they do, either you are not getting enough support or you are pushing too hard. In this exercise, a longer push is beneficial, so count to '10' to yourself. Stop pressing, breathe in (this is a good opportunity to fully straighten your upper back by lifting the chest!) and, on a breath out, ask your partner to very slowly lift your arms up until the stretch is strong enough.

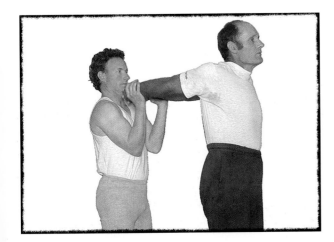

Alternatively, if you want to control the extent of the final position more directly, you can ask your partner to hold you in the contraction position and you can increase the stretch yourself by letting your legs bend, lowering your body until the desired stretch is felt. As before, do not let the trunk bend forwards to achieve this; it is better to do the exercise in good form.

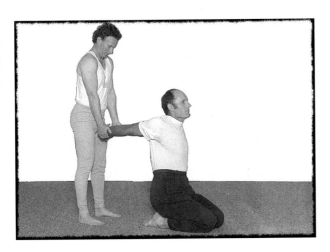

Cues

roll shoulders back to begin
partner lifts arms
C–R: press hands to floor
restretch: partner slowly elevates arms

12. Partner arm up behind shoulder blade

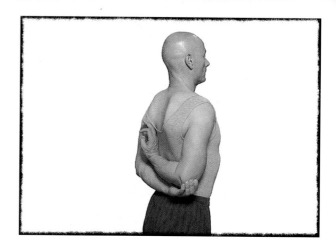

In our experience, the next compound shoulder movement reveals the most noticeable reduction in shoulder flexibility in the normal person as they become older and is most dramatically observed on the dominant arm side. For this reason, choose your dominant arm to begin, so that it may be given an extra stretch once the other is done. This movement stretches the external rotators of the shoulder joint (*infraspinatus* and *teres minor*) in addition to the front and middle *deltoid* so, if you find that getting into the first position is difficult, you may wish to stretch these muscles now (see exercise 60, shoulder external rotation).

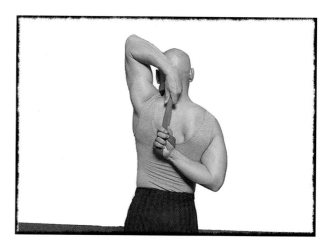

Place the back of your hand up between your shoulder blades. Now try to reach behind you to grasp the elbow of this arm; if you cannot, you may ask your partner to stand to one side as shown and grasp the elbow for you. Julie is assisting Steve in the third photograph in this way. If you are on your own, you can use a strap to get into position: make a loop in the strap, lower it behind you as shown and put the wrist of the first hand through it. By gently pulling on the strap, you will be able to get the arm into position. The elbow of the held arm will be protruding past your side, and you can lean against the elbow to tighten the position and to provide a barrier against which to push in the next part of the exercise if you are on your own.

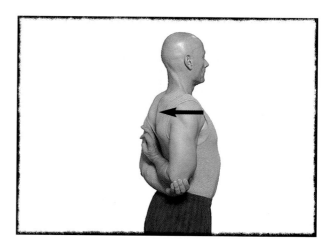

If you do not have a strap handy, you can lean the bottom arm's elbow against a wall (by leaning *away* from the wall first) or against a support, as shown (top photo facing page). No matter which approach you use, the first stretch movement is to pull the shoulder being stretched directly *backwards*, as indicated by the arrow in the second photograph. This movement, mainly initiated by the rhomboid muscles, draws the scapula onto the rib cage and significantly increases the stretch sensation. This may be a sufficient stretch.

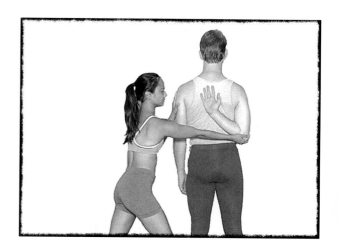

A **C–R stretch** will loosen all the muscles limiting the movement. Either by pressing the elbow directly out to the side against your partner's support, or pressing it against some other barrier (a wall or bar), contract the shoulder muscles for a count of five. Without moving, relax the shoulder, breathe in and, on a breath out, very cautiously press your body towards the barrier to move the elbow closer to the trunk. Hold the new position for five breaths in and

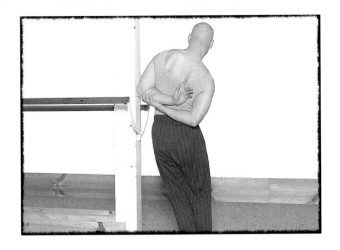

Cues

draw arm and shoulder behind body

lean on point of elbow if necessary

pull stretched shoulder back

C–R: press elbow directly to side

restretch: pull elbow across
and pull shoulder back

out. The stretch in this shoulder can be intensified by using the muscles of the back to slowly pull the stretched shoulder *backwards* once more while holding the position. Usually this action increases the stretch effect in the very front of the shoulder.

To relieve the ache in the front of the shoulder that everyone seems to feel after doing this exercise, relax the arm concerned and lift it above your head from your side. Let it drop and make a few circles, and the arm will feel normal. The end position of this exercise is usually much improved with a second try so, after doing your non-dominant arm, restretch the first shoulder. Was there a big difference between the shoulder movements? We have found that left–right arm and shoulder comparisons of flexibility reveal significant differences in most people. Many minor shoulder and arm problems can be solved by simply making the body more symmetrical in this regard.

Another way of making the shoulder feel completely loose and relaxed is to repeat exercise 10, partner front arm, immediately. These exercises in combination have improved many shoulder problems. From a more general perspective, because both exercises stretch the muscles that pull the shoulder joint and arm forwards, they are the best way to improve slumping or rounded shoulders. If this is your problem, combine these exercises with exercise 14, wall middle and upper back backward bend, or exercise 27, partner backward bend over support.

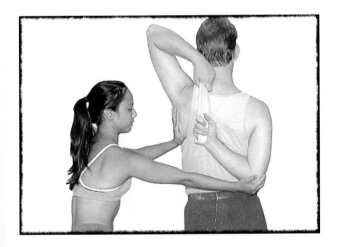

Cues

partner helps you get into position

draw shoulder back to increase stretch

C–R: press elbow to side

restretch: ask partner to move elbow

13. Arm behind head

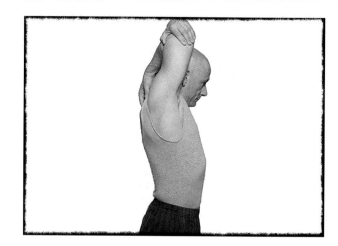

This exercise stretches the widest muscle of the back, *latissimus dorsi*. It also stretches *triceps* (the muscle of the back of the upper arm) strongly if the elbow joint is closed during its execution. Place the palm of one hand between the shoulder blades, from above. Now reach your other arm across, hold the elbow as I am showing, and gently pull the elbow across behind your head. Look at your position: if the stretched arm is not approximately in line with your body as seen from the side, use the neck muscles to press the arm back. You will see your chest lift as you do this, and the action will increase the stretch in the muscles under the arm. A wall can be used to similar effect, by standing away from it enough to lean the point of this elbow on it. By straightening the back and leaning on the elbow, it will be moved backwards in line with the rest of the body. This version requires no effort from the neck muscles, and may be preferred.

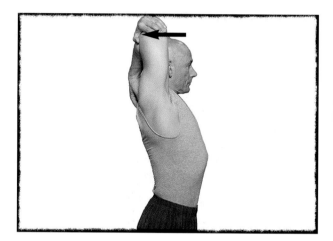

By now, the **C–R stretch** should suggest itself to you: by pressing the held elbow directly out to the side, *latissimus dorsi* will be activated and, accordingly, will experience the extra stretch. After pressing for a count of five, breathe in, relax and, on a breath out, bring the upper arm further behind your head. Have regard to the alignment of the upper arm in relation to the body in the new position; if it is forwards, press the arm back. Hold the final position for five breaths in and out. Compared with other shoulder movements, most people are quite flexible in this action.

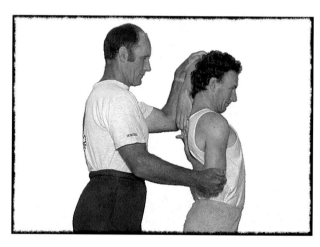

Cues

take folded arm behind head

use head to press arm backwards

C–R: press elbow to side

restretch: arm across further
press arm back with head

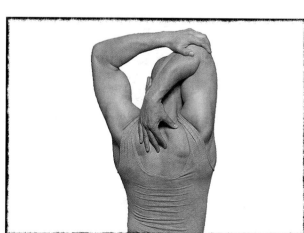

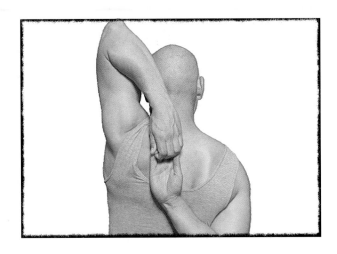

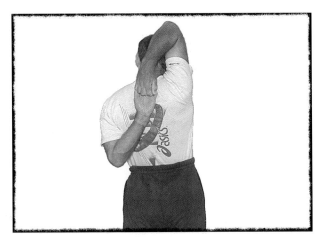

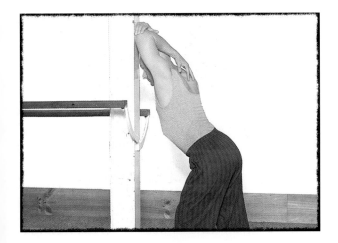

Exercises 12 and 13 may be combined if you are loose enough, either by using a strap as shown above (exercise 12), or linking the finger tips together. As you become more flexible, clasp the hands more closely together. Look at the shape *both* arms make with the body, and apply appropriate correction.

If the elbow of the arm behind your back is outside the line of the body, you need to concentrate on loosening the front and middle shoulder muscles using exercise 12. If the elbow of the top arm is *outside* the line of the shoulder, or the line of the arm is in front of the shoulder as would be seen from the side, you will need to concentrate on the *latissimus dorsi* component of the stretch by using exercise 13. Merely being able to clasp the hands behind you does not mean that the shoulders are adequately flexible—your proportions play a part, and some people can clasp their hands because the top arm demonstrates much better than average flexibility in this position. We are trying to achieve *all-round* flexibility rather than enhance the flexibility of a part already loose, so check your form carefully.

The final photograph shows Alan applying both corrections to Pierre; by placing his left elbow on Pierre's left shoulder, he can gently pull the top elbow back and, at the same time, he can help to move the bottom elbow closer to the centre-line of the body.

Petra is demonstrating a wrist-to-wrist grip in the final photograph, which flexible students may attempt. Use a fingertip-to-fingertip grip to begin, then use the fingers to bring the wrists closer together. Do not force this position.

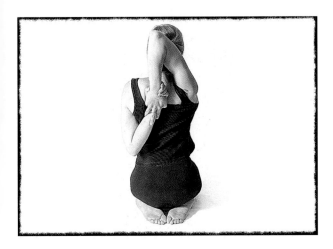

Cues

clasp fingers together

look at position of arms; adjust

use wall or partner to assist

14. Wall middle and upper back backward bend

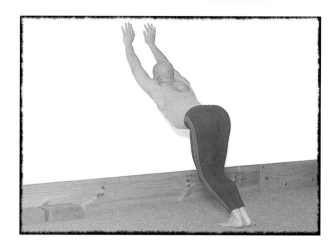

A forwards rounding of the upper back and a slumping of the shoulders are frequent accompaniments to ageing. These effects are mainly due to gravity and our incomplete efforts to keep ourselves upright against it. Sedentary occupations where one spends hours of each day hunched over paperwork and keyboards only worsens this tendency. As the shape of the body changes, a number of structural and functional alterations occur. Chief among these are a shortening of key muscles in the shoulders and the front side of the trunk, and changes to the shape of the whole spine. The most unfortunate aspect of these changes is that they are no longer confined to middle age and beyond. The next exercise directly stretches the muscles that shorten as one's posture alters: the chest muscles (*pectoralis major* and *minor*), front shoulder muscle (*anterior deltoid*), the muscles between the ribs (*intercostales*) and the muscle at the front of the upper arm (*biceps brachii*). Various ligaments, tendons and intrinsic muscles of the spine are affected too.

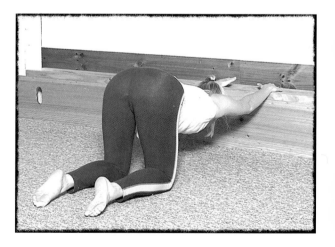

Look at the first photograph. Stand away from a wall as I am doing—the exact distance will have to be found by experiment. The further away from the wall you are, the stronger the stretch will be, so err on the side of caution the first time. Extend the arms above the head at about shoulder width. Some people will feel a compression in the shoulder joint and often this can be alleviated by changing the hand spacing, either closer together or further apart. Place your hands on the wall and bend your legs slightly. Lean onto the wall while extending the arms off the body as far as you can. Gravity will pull the body down, and you will find the trunk bending backwards as it is suspended between hands and hips. You will need to relax completely in this position to be stretched; if the effect is too intense, begin again but stand a little closer to the wall. In the second photograph Eldon is helping me by applying a very light force between my shoulder blades with his forearm.

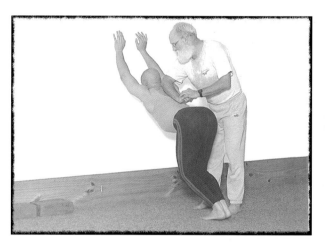

In the last two photographs, Olivia is demonstrating a kneeling version of the exercise, which is far more gentle and can be used if either of the wall versions is too strong. Because significantly less force is experienced on the shoulders, you will need to make a conscious effort to relax to make this an effective stretch. A gentle **C–R stretch** can be achieved by pressing the hands onto the support. A

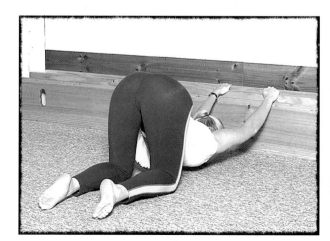

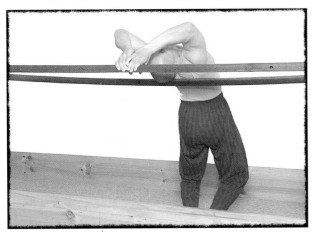

Cues (left page)

extend straight arms off body

lean into support so back bends

C–R: pull hands down wall

restretch: lean further into wall

Cues (below)

C–R: press hands up to ceiling

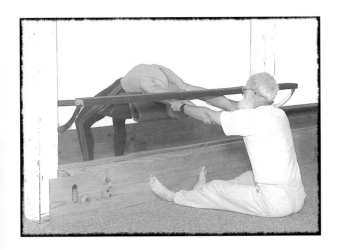

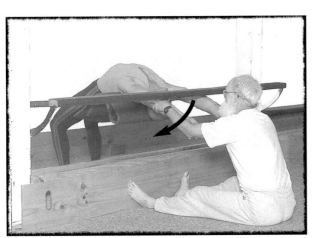

partner floor version of this stretch is shown in lesson 5, exercise 35.

In the standing version, a surprisingly effective **C–R stretch** can be effected by trying to *pull* the hands down the wall once in the final position. Friction will hold the hands in position, and all of the muscles mentioned will contract in the action. After pulling for a count of 10 or so, take in a deep breath (this will help to expand the whole rib cage), relax the upper body completely except for the effort required to extend the arms and, on a breath out, let the body sink further into the pose. Try to breathe more deeply than usual in the final position, and hold it for 10 breaths in and out if you can.

I am showing a very intense version of the stretch on this page that concentrates the effect high up in the back (at about the level of the middle of the shoulder blades) by leaning over a narrow support, padded if required. Effective in either partner or solo versions, this is the best exercise to use to reduce a 'scholarly stoop', or that premature forward curving of the upper back so often seen in middle-aged people. To use this most effectively, you need to place the least flexible part of the middle or upper back on the support. The **C–R stretch** involves gently pressing the arms in the direction of the ceiling; the restretch requires either the hips to be lowered (solo) or the partner helping to take the arms closer to the floor. Try to relax in the final position.

The following is the first of the repeated exercises. As the lessons progress, we will see more of these. The page number shows where the exercise will be found, and in many cases the **Cues** are repeated too.

Exercise 7, Floor neck side bend

Refer back to lesson 1 for details of how to do this exercise, and ensure that the key points are observed.

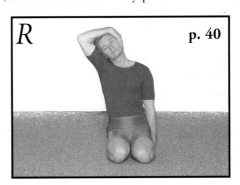

R   p. 40

15. Floor neck rotation

This seemingly simple movement stretches all of the major and many of the minor muscles of the neck. The movement also exemplifies the general principle that one's achievable flexibility depends more on one's daily pattern of movement than on any bony or muscular limitation. Daily life activities generate a neuromuscular mapping of these patterns which constitute a major fraction of the brain's activity. The outer edges of these maps are real constraints on our flexibility and this is what we experience when we feel that we cannot go any further in a movement.

Sit in any comfortable way that lets you hold the upper body straight without too much effort—cross legged on the floor is fine, but use a cushion under your bottom to tip the body forwards slightly. An office chair is good, as is sitting on folded legs. Without inclining the head forwards or backwards and without tilting it to the side, slowly turn your head as far as you can in one direction until it will not go any further. Pause and count to three; now turn the head further. Everyone can. Now do the same on the other side and feel which side is tighter. Briefly turn once more to whichever side you first turned, to relax the opposite muscles.

When you turn your head to the right, you are contracting the left *sternomastoid* to achieve the movement; looking to the left uses the right *sternomastoid*. What stops you turning your head in the first instance is a reflex contraction of the muscles that produce the *opposite* movement. The point in your range of movement at which these contractions are triggered is precisely that end point of the range of movement you use in daily life. Resetting these points (up to physiological limits) is just a matter of gently imposing new ranges of movements. Even very flexible people demonstrate this effect.

For most people, turning to the side of the dominant arm is more difficult because you are using your non-dominant *sternomastoid* to look towards your dominant side. Ask yourself which shoulder you look over when you back your car out of the driveway—this will be the looser side. The most often repeated patterns are dominant. This applies equally to patterns functional and dysfunctional.

Cues

turn head to side as far as possible

after pause, slowly turn further

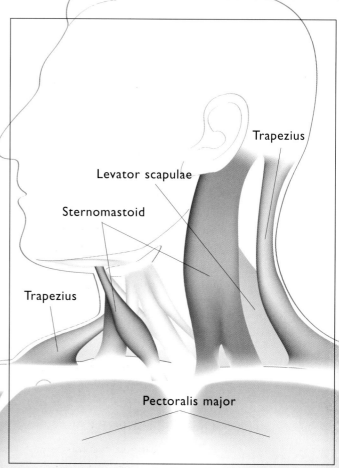

Muscles of the neck, head rotated

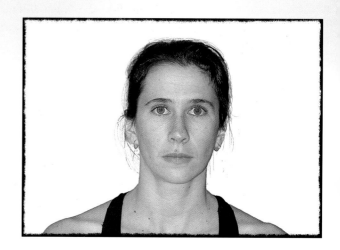

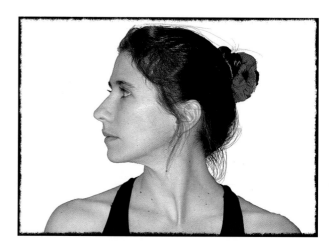

LESSON THREE: CALF AND HAMSTRINGS

If you were attending a *Posture & Flexibility* class, today's lesson would be the last time we would take you through the daily five in a formal way. Our classes are structured so that the first 15 minutes is spent doing your own warm-up movements, and many people include the daily five in this period. We encourage students to practise exercises for their tightest areas, but many do not—most begin by repeating favoured movements, and this means ones that feel good to do. You may well care to do the same. Be guided by how you feel on the day. Do not be surprised, however, to find that, when a problem area feels as though nothing you do will loosen it, later in the session you have a breakthrough in stretching that part—this has been reported to us too often to be ignored. In this lesson we are going to begin what most regard as *real* stretching: loosening the muscles at the back of the legs.

Not a day goes by where one does not read in the sporting press of a top athlete out of action with a pulled hamstring. What does this term mean and why do superbly conditioned athletes seem so prone to this problem? One reason, certainly, is a lack of flexibility or suppleness in these major muscles, and another is strength imbalances between opposing pairs of muscles that control the movements involved in the particular activity (*agonist* and *antagonist* groups). We have found that the **C–R approach** can go a long way to addressing strength imbalances and a very long way in addressing simple tightness—common among top athletes, you may be surprised to learn.

The common term hamstrings describes the large muscles that span the bottom bones we sit on (the *ischial tuberosities*) and the lower leg, as illustrated on pages 60 and 61. Because these three muscles cross the hip joint as well as the knee, they can either extend the upper leg with respect to the trunk or flex the knee joint, or any balance of action between these two functions. Electromyograph studies have shown that fast running requires part of the hamstrings to be contracting to produce forward movement while another part lengthens to allow straightening of the knee. In some cases, the hamstring muscle pulls itself apart during explosive movement if insufficiently strong or too tight.

We begin this lesson with a very simple but effective floor combination of back and stomach muscle strengthening movements. The first exercise is a mild whole-spine movement which has the benefit of increasing awareness of one's posture and the second exercise affects mainly *rectus abdominis*, the muscle comprising the enviable 'six-pack'—always admired but too seldom seen. Cosmetic dimensions aside, this muscle (along with the obliques and associated others) form a necessary muscular girdle to strengthen the whole trunk.

16. *Floor face down arm and leg lifts, and abdominal curls*

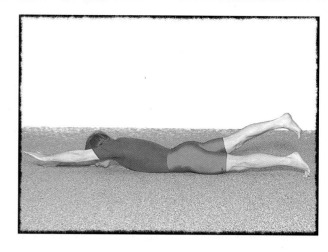

The key to body weight strengthening movements, where the resistance of the movement is largely fixed, is to perform the movements slowly—slowly enough such that momentum can play no role in the movement. In the first of these two exercises, lifting the arm and leg more quickly than recommended certainly will get them higher off the ground, but so doing will defeat the purpose completely. You need to move with deliberation so as to *maximise* the sensations. Concentrate on the feeling of doing the movement rather than on how many repetitions you can do. Postural muscles respond quickly to this approach and, as you lift your limbs, the entire body is extended.

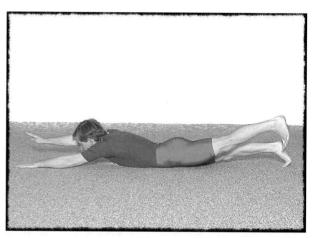

Lie face down as Gary is doing. You may put a low cushion or mat under your forehead, or turn the head to one side for a few repetitions and turn it to the other for the remainder so that the muscles of the neck and upper back are evenly stressed. Lift one arm and the opposite leg together, as high off the floor as you can. *Do this slowly*, and feel how a great number of muscles is coordinated in this simple-looking movement. Lower the limbs to the floor, let the body relax, and lift the complementary pair of limbs. The first time you try the exercise, do just eight to ten on each side. When you become stronger and your capacity to exert your strength in this new movement improves, you can increase the resistance with light weights in the hands, and weights on the ankles. Variations include lifting the arm and leg on the same side together, and both arms and legs together. This last version is the most difficult in terms of effort, but the first version teaches your body how to exert its strength symmetrically, the important consideration in this movement.

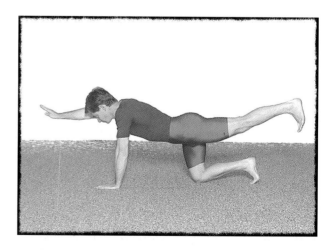

Gary is demonstrating two versions of the exercise; one done while lying as described above, and one done on all fours. This latter version involves more torsion around the long axis of the body because the trunk is freer to move in rotation; accordingly, it is more difficult than the lying version. Movements should be slow in this version too.

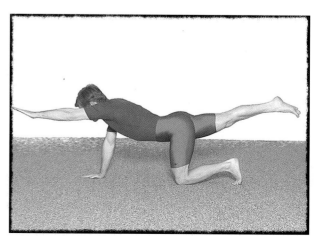

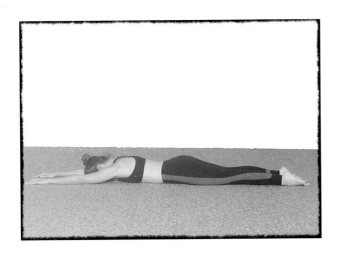

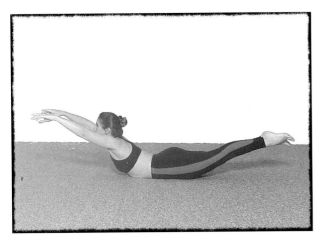

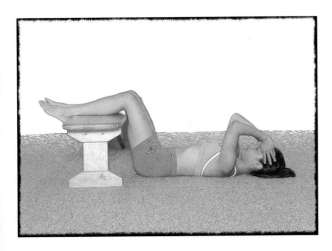

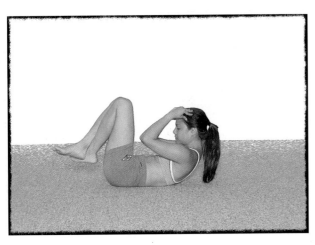

The top two photographs of Jennifer show arms and legs lifted together; this is closer to a pure extension movement of the spine because the trunk cannot rotate. Breathing will be difficult in the extended position due to the pressure of your body's weight on the abdomen. Jennifer is lifting her arms as high as she can, to maximise involvement of the middle and upper back muscles.

The next exercise, demonstrated by Julie, will provide a pleasant stretch to counter the tightening effects of the last one. As an aside, the conventional sit-up, in which the trunk is lifted from the floor to complete the movement, can hurt the lower back because another pair of muscles (the hip flexors) come into play as soon as the lower back starts to leave the floor. This criticism applies to the many variations of this basic movement too, including touching the elbow to the opposite side's knee. The exercise shown here has no such drawbacks, and may even be done by people with back problems.

Look at the third photograph. Placing the lower legs on a chair makes keeping good form even easier, but the exercise may be done on the floor just as effectively. Julie has placed her fingers next to her temples; deliberately, she avoids using her arms to hold her head and, in this way, she can strengthen the essential front neck muscles too. Once in position, breathe in. On a breath out, very slowly curl the entire trunk, starting with the neck, in one smooth movement. Curl up slowly as high as you can *without lifting the body off the floor.* If you are doing the exercise correctly, the lower back will be increasingly pressed onto the floor. This demonstrates the lumbar-curve-flattening action characteristic of contractions in this muscle group. Hold the top position of the movement for a count of two. Lower yourself while breathing in, let the head touch the floor for an instant, and begin again.

When you can do 10 slow repetitions, these muscles will be quite strong. The resistance of the movement may be increased by holding a weight against the forehead (a book will do to start). You may feel the main effects of this exercise in the muscles in the front of the neck in the first few weeks and, if the neck tires before the abdominal muscles, you may use the arms to help lift the head for the last repetitions. If you feel the effects in the *back* of the neck, you need to lift the head and neck proportionately faster than you are now doing—the back of the neck can feel sore if the neck bends backwards at all in the movement. If the back of the neck is left feeling tight by doing this exercise, do exercise 6, chin to chest, immediately afterwards.

Did you notice that curling the trunk stretched the lower and middle back muscles that were tightened during the previous exercise? These paired movements are complementary and any unwanted effects of the former are released by the latter. Do the exercises in the order suggested.

17. Partner floor single leg forward bend

We begin the lesson with a test of your hamstring flexibility. The forward bend over one leg—if done in good form with the back held straight between hips and shoulders—is both an excellent stretch for all the muscles at the back of the legs (hamstring and calf muscles) and a modest strengthening exercise. The movement also helps you become aware of the shape that your body makes in various positions and, in time, this increase in awareness helps both posture and flexibility. The following exercises in this lesson are what we call the *partial poses;* they will help you identify which of the many muscles involved in this basic movement are limiting forward bending and, at the same time, teach you the most effective exercises to target these tight areas. At the end of the lesson we will do this exercise again, to see if you have improved.

Look at the illustrations. The three hamstring muscles (*semimembranosus,* the innermost muscle, *semitendinosus,* slightly further to the outside, and *biceps femoris,* the outermost hamstring muscle) have interesting anatomy. They span both the hip and the knee joints, and the shorter head of *biceps femoris* is attached to the *femur,* the bone of the upper leg, for about half its length. This means that even if the knee if flexed during the movement, one part of the hamstring group is being stretched; when the leg is straight and moved towards the head all parts of the group are stretched. The arrangement of the muscles, where they arise on the skeleton (the *origin*), and the place they attach (the *insertion*), all determine their functions and how they might be worked. This description simplifies great complexity and, the capacity to bend easily at the hip owes much to factors that are not easily seen in the muscle and bone picture just presented. We will cover some of these other factors below.

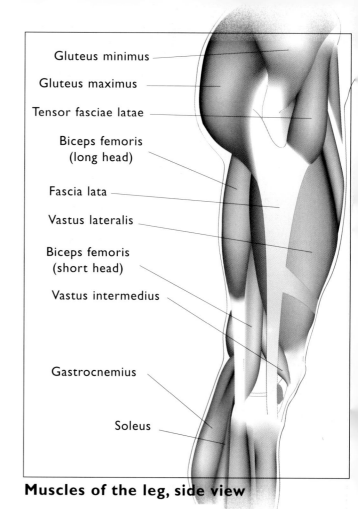

Muscles of the leg, side view

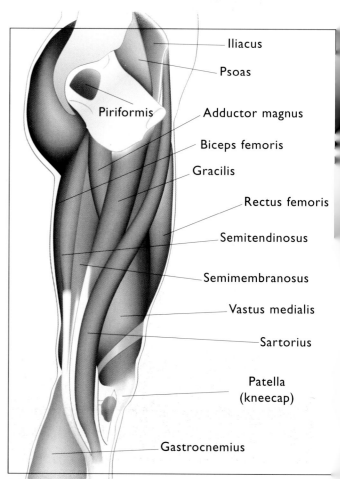

Muscles of the leg, inside view

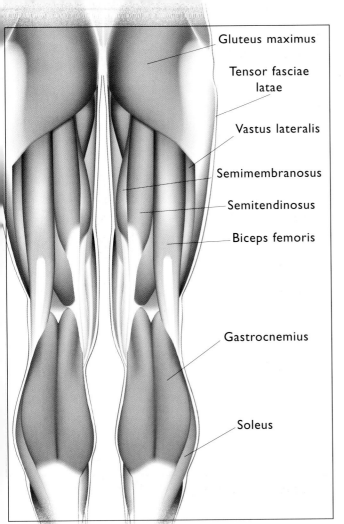

- Gluteus maximus
- Tensor fasciae latae
- Vastus lateralis
- Semimembranosus
- Semitendinosus
- Biceps femoris
- Gastrocnemius
- Soleus

Muscles of the legs, from behind

Look at the photograph. You will need a strap to hold your foot and, if you are not particularly flexible, a cushion or a mat under your bottom will help concentrate the stretch in the back of the leg. Loop the strap around one foot, and reach down the strap as far as you can without bending the back. A mirror is helpful, or better yet, a partner who can tell you where your back is bending. To get an idea of your flexibility, reach down the strap a little, and breathe in, straightening the back at the same time, until you feel a stretch down the back of the leg, somewhere in between the bottom bone and the top of the lower leg (this sensation often feels like it is in the calf muscle). When you have gone as far as you can, note how far down the strap you are able to reach. You may of course be able to hold your foot; if so, check to see that your back is still straight.

It will come as a surprise to some to learn that the calf muscles can limit movement at the hip. Look at the illustration overleaf: the underlying calf muscle, *soleus*, shares the Achilles tendon with the other calf muscle, *gastrocnemius*. *Soleus* arises from the bones of the lower leg, the *tibia* and *fibula*, whereas *gastrocnemius* arises from the end of the *femur*. For this reason, we will need two exercises to stretch both muscles. The branches of the *sciatic* nerve, the longest in the body, passes through both muscles and a number of researchers have claimed that it is restrictions to its gliding through the calf muscles that can limit movement of the trunk at the hip joint: if the nerve branches cannot slide they is placed under tension and signal pain or discomfort. When you try exercise 17, note where you feel the main effects of the stretch, and look at the angle your foot makes with the leg. If your foot is strongly pointed (rather than being close to, or in the neutral position) and you feel the main effect in the calf muscles, suspect that they might be the limiting factor in forward bending.

If you feel that the main effect is in the hamstring muscles themselves, make a mental note. If you feel the effect in the hip of the leg being stretched, make a note of that, too; we will stretch these muscles later in exercise 22, lying hip.

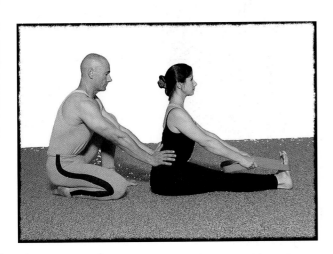

Cues

hold strap or foot;
trunk must be straight

partner supports lower back

18. *Floor folded leg calf (soleus)*

Tightness in *soleus* is not a significant limiter of flexion at the hip. However, stretching *soleus* is a good warm-up for stretching *gastrocnemius* and, because the knee is flexed, the position allows you to stretch the ankle joint more directly. You will feel the stretch deep in the calf muscle as well as in the arch of the foot itself, and you may feel a slight compression sensation in the front of the ankle joint.

Kneel as Gary is showing. If you cannot fold the other leg, you may put it in any comfortable position. The key to this exercise is to have the knee directly over the foot, and to ensure that the ankle does not roll inwards (*pronation*). Misalignment will render the exercise ineffective so, if the ankle does want to roll in, press harder on the *little-toe* side of the foot, and only go as far into the stretch as you can while still maintaining the recommended shape.

Place the elbow on the leg, just behind the knee as shown. By leaning your body's weight through the elbow, the ankle will flex. If you are tight, or you need more weight on the knee to make the stretch effective, reach your other arm out and grasp a stable support. By pulling on this arm, the stretch will be increased.

A **C–R stretch** is achieved by pressing the ball of the foot gently into the floor once in the final position for a count of six to ten. Keep holding yourself in position, take a breath in, relax, and press the knee further in the stretch direction. Hold the final position for at least 10 breaths in and out—the Achilles tendon is the thickest in the body and responds to a decent stretch. Check the shape the foot and lower leg make with each other, and ensure that the ankle is not pronating in the final position.

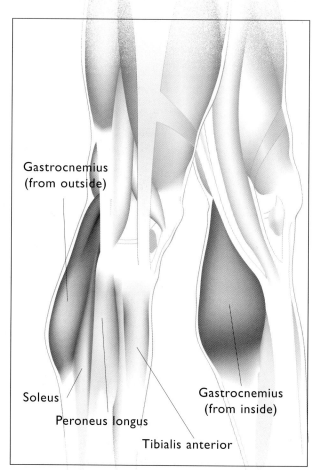

Gastrocnemius
(from outside)

Soleus

Peroneus longus

Gastrocnemius
(from inside)

Tibialis anterior

Muscles of the lower leg

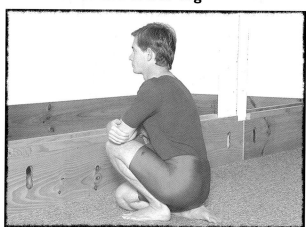

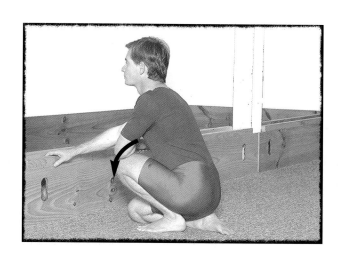

Cues

hold support; elbow behind knee

ensure arch is maintained

C–R: press ball of foot into floor

restretch: lean weight onto knee

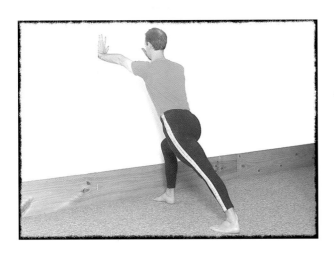

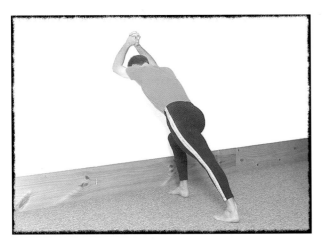

19. Wall standing calf (gastrocnemius)

Gastrocnemius can limit hip movement when the leg is straight. This exercise is our version of the popular runners' stretch you can see being done everywhere. Look at the photograph; Kevin is demonstrating the recommended position.

Take a long pace back behind you with one leg, and lean into the wall, gently pressing the leg straight by tightening the thigh muscle (this action is sometimes described as pulling the kneecap up). You may support yourself on either your elbows or hands. As you lean into the wall, again ensure that your foot is not turned out to the side (in other words, the knee needs to track directly over the foot) and that the ankle does not roll inwards (or pronate). Pressing more weight on the little toe side of the foot will help maintain alignment. The other leg may be bent and placed between the first foot and the wall for security, or you may place it on the back of the straight leg, which will give the strongest stretch, because more of the body's weight is being applied. Take the hips and body towards the wall, keeping the heel firmly on the ground. You will feel a strong stretch in the calf muscle, and behind the knee.

A **C–R stretch** is effected by pressing the ball of the foot into the floor, but without lifting the heel, for a count from 10 to 15. *Gastrocnemius* shares the Achilles tendon with *soleus*; this, together with the fact that we carry the body's weight around on these muscles, usually means that they are both strong and tight. We recommend a longer contraction in calf muscle exercises than in many of the other exercises and a longer time spent in the final position, as experience shows that this produces a desirable stretch effect. Hold the final position for 10 breaths in and out, and you may find that a second **C–R** will allow you to move even closer to the wall. Stretch the other leg.

The last frame shows how a partner may assist: I am pressing Kevin's heel down to the floor so that he can concentrate on maintaining the arch in his foot and leaning towards the wall. **C–R stretches** for *gastrocnemius* are particularly effective when assisted in this way.

Cues

with foot under knee, lean onto wall

maintain arch shape

press leg straight

C–R: press ball of foot into floor

restretch: lean further into wall

partner can hold heel on floor

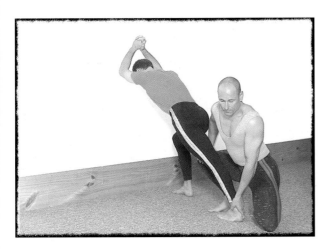

20. Floor single leg calf

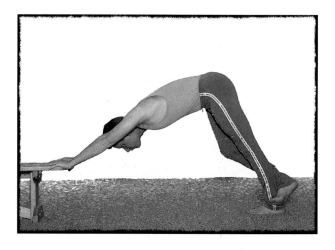

This is the strongest of the calf muscle exercises, even though less of the body's weight is experienced than in the wall version, above. Exercise 20 gives the strongest stretch (in terms of how the stretch *feels*) because the hips, as well as the ankle, are flexed. A number of versions are shown, allowing you to choose a version that suits your pattern of flexibility.

Steve is demonstrating a version that everyone will be able to do. He is leaning against the end of a bench, the other end of which is against a wall. The support you use must be completely stable. Stand far enough away from the support so that, when you reach your hands down to it, the heel of the leg you are stretching just stays on the ground. Once you have the right distance worked out, with one foot in front for support, bend at the waist until you can place your hands on the support. This will already be a stretch for the calf muscles. The support leg may be moved to behind the leg being stretched if you like, as Steve is demonstrating in the photograph. Like exercise 19, wall standing calf, putting the support leg in this position increases the stretch effect.

A **C–R stretch** may be done in this first position, to loosen the leg and prepare it for the next step. Once in a reasonable stretch position, straighten your back (tell yourself to lift the chest or to arch the back) and bend forwards from the *hips* until your arms and body are in the same line, or close to it, as shown. This second movement will dramatically demonstrate the functional relationship between calf and hamstring flexibility.

Your hips will move backwards in relation to the back foot when you bend at the hips, and this will reduce the stretch on the calf muscle—even though the stretch sensation down the back of the leg increases. After you get used to the new stretch, you can increase the effect in the calf muscle by coming out of the stretch slightly, moving the foot further back (but still keeping the heel on the floor) and bending at the hips once again. A **C–R stretch**, achieved by pressing the ball of the foot into the floor, can be done at any stage in the movement to release the tension in the back of the leg.

Cues

lean on support; foot under knee
lean forward to stretch calf
C–R: press ball of foot into floor
restretch: lean further forwards, and
lower body closer to floor (bend forward at hips)

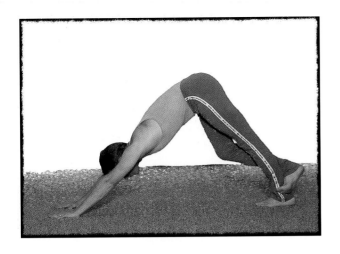

Cues

keep heel on floor

hold back straight, and
pull body towards floor

C–R: press ball of foot into floor

restretch: arch back and
pull body closer to floor

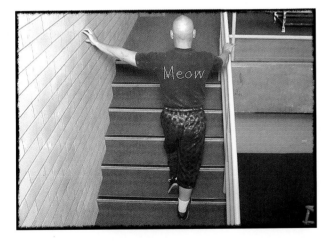

Cues

with straight leg, hang heel from support

C–R: take some weight on calf muscle

restretch: let heel hang further down

If your hands and feet grip the floor adequately and you have the flexibility, try the next version Steve is showing in the photograph at the top of this page. If your foot slips, try placing the heel against the join between the wall and the floor. If your hands slip, turn around and place the fingers against the join. The **C–R stretch** to be applied is the same as for the preceding versions. If neither of these strategies is effective (if you still feel that the unsupported limb is in danger of slipping) we will show you a partner-assisted version later, in exercise 70, partner floor single leg.

Runners often hang a heel from a road curb or the like while standing waiting for traffic lights to change; the **C–R** technique can be used to make this stretch more effective. Once in the stretch position I am demonstrating in the second photograph (assuming that you have the whole body's weight hanging from one foot), gently try to lift yourself up from the bottom position. The operative word is *try*; take just enough weight on the calf muscle to be able to feel it doing work *without* allowing the heel to lift, for a count of five to ten. Stop lifting and, on a breath out, let the calf muscle relax completely and let the heel sink further down. This stretch is much stronger for the calf muscles than the wall version described in exercise 19, wall standing calf, because the whole weight of the body is felt in the stretch. A set of steps works well.

21. Buttock and hip flexor

This is a personal favourite and a wonderful warm-up movement. Everyone will be able to do it in one form or another—we always use it on our *Overcome neck & back pain* workshops. As you are supporting your weight entirely on your arms, you can allow as gentle or as strong a stretch as you wish and, depending on where the stretch most affects you, you will gain insight into your tight areas. It is a compound movement, stretching both legs—but in different places.

Have a support handy, if you think that you may not be able to reach the floor. Begin on all fours and, supporting your weight on both hands and one knee, swing the other foot *out* and around, and place it on the floor with a bent knee. The foot needs to be in front of the knee (the knee is stable in this position, but not if behind the line of the foot). Once in position, reach the other leg out further behind you by making small, sliding movements of the knee back as far as you can, and rest there for a moment. Draw the ball of the foot under the ankle, and let it take some weight, as I am showing in the first photograph, opposite. Take in a breath and, as you breath, out try to straighten the back leg *without letting the hips rise*. Most people cannot straighten the back leg—it is the straightening action that provides the stretch.

For some, the main effects will be felt in the back of the front leg: the buttock muscles (*gluteus maximus* and some of the smaller muscles), the adductors (the muscles on the inside of the thigh that pull the leg in to the centre-line of the body) and part of the hamstrings. For others, the main effect will be felt in the front of the back leg: the hip flexors (*iliacus* and *psoas*) and those parts of the front thigh muscles closest to the hip joint (*rectus femoris* and other parts of *quadriceps*). See the illustration for details of the *quadriceps* group, see page 75 for details of the hip flexors, and page 60 for details of the muscles at the back and inside of the leg.

A **C–R stretch** can be used here, too. To loosen the muscles at the back of the front leg, gently press the foot straight down into the floor—not so hard that the hips lift; contractions must not produce movement if they are to yield the maximum stretch effect. After a breath in, relax and, on a breath out, let your arms bend until the desired stretch is felt. If you have trouble keeping the back straight, try gently pulling back on the hands first; this action

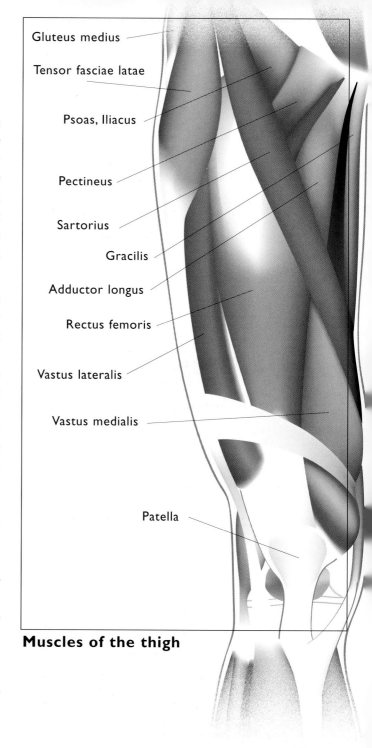

Gluteus medius
Tensor fasciae latae
Psoas, Iliacus
Pectineus
Sartorius
Gracilis
Adductor longus
Rectus femoris
Vastus lateralis
Vastus medialis
Patella

Muscles of the thigh

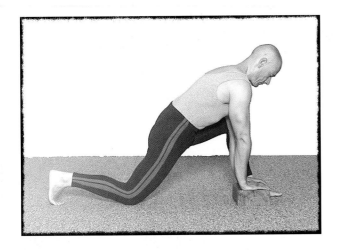

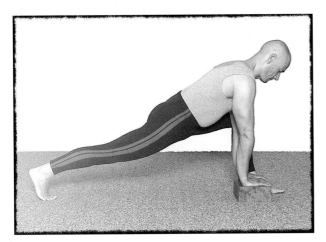

engages the muscles under the arms and will straighten the back. Simply straightening the back will intensify the stretch in the back of the front leg. Once you are used to this, you may increase it further by bending the arms as described— but only as far as you can hold the back straight.

If the main effect in exercise 21 is felt in the front of the *back* leg, make a note. This sensation suggests that the *quadriceps* and the hip flexors are likely to be tight. We will be concentrating on this area in the next lesson. In the meantime, the back-straightening action described above will stretch you more intensely here than in the back of the leg if these are the tighter muscles. We are often asked why someone feels a stretch in one place when it is supposed to be a stretch for another muscle entirely. The reason is that, in compound movements, you will feel the stretch most strongly in whichever of the muscles is the tightest in the chain of muscles involved in the movement.

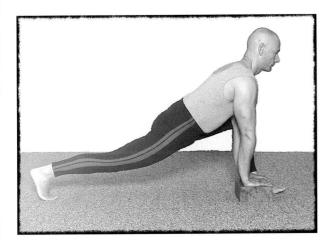

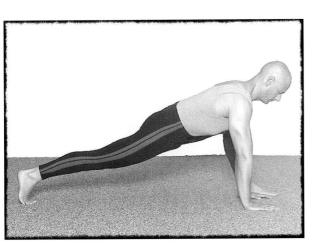

Cues

use support if necessary
support weight on hands
press back leg straight
pull back gently on hands
C–R: press front foot into floor
restretch: lower hips; restraighten back

22. Lying hip (piriformis)

Exercise 5, seated hip, in lesson 1 provided the first of the piriformis stretches. This relatively small muscle deep in the hip is one of the four external hip rotators. Hip pain can be caused by *piriformis* pressing the sciatic nerve against part of the pelvis (see the illustration this page). In 20-37 per cent of the population, however, part of the sciatic nerve passes through this muscle (see the illustration opposite). In such cases, if *piriformis* is tight, sufficient pressure may be applied to this part of the nerve as to affect the flow of information. In mild cases, either condition contributes to stiffness of the hip and an inability to bend forward at the hips but, in severe cases, *piriformis syndrome* can cause symptoms indistinguishable from disc-induced *sciatica* pain.

Exercise 22 shows a movement that stretches the same muscle, but from a different angle, and that applies the stretching tension to its other end. If we think about muscles simplistically (for example, thinking about them as being analogous to elastic bands) we will mistakenly conclude that pulling on one end of a muscle will produce the same stretch within the muscle as will pulling on the other end. For many reasons this is not the case: in any particular position, muscles may hold tension only at one location within them (the familiar trigger point is one example); muscles pull over bony promontories in many cases; joint position determines the angle of pull; and muscles contain tendons within them. All these factors contribute to uneven distribution of tension. Accordingly, different versions of an exercise produce different stretch sensations and effects. Additionally, there is considerable variation in the normal population as to the precise locations of origins and insertions in relation to joints. The one stretching exercise is unlikely to affect everyone the same way and we need to provide variations on basic movements to ensure that all can benefit. One advantage of exercise 22 is that, because you are lying on the floor and drawing the leg towards you, there is no strain on the back.

Lie face up as Olivia is demonstrating, with the legs bent. Place one ankle on the thigh of the other, near the knee. We want the knee of the first leg to be as far outside the line of the body as possible so, if your lower leg bones are short, place as little of the foot on the thigh as is practicable. Reach through the legs and hold the folded leg as shown; hold only

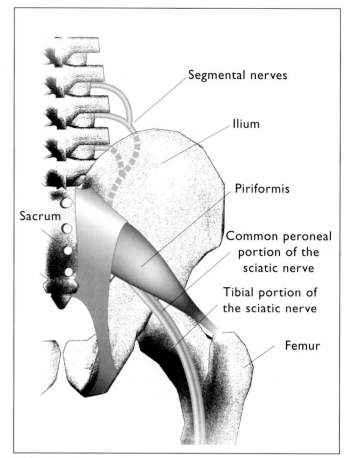

Sciatic nerve passes under *piriformis*

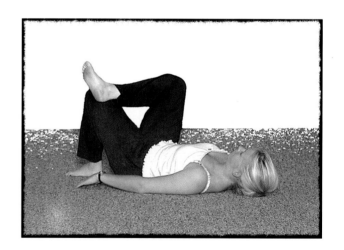

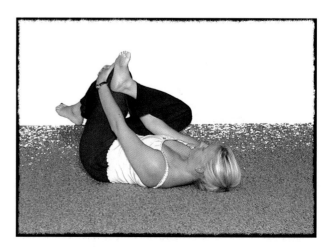

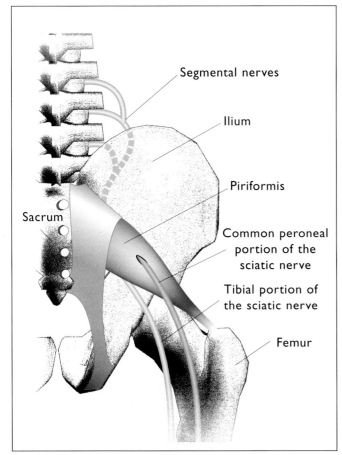

Part of sciatic nerve pierces *piriformis*

Labels on the diagram:
- Segmental nerves
- Ilium
- Piriformis
- Common peroneal portion of the sciatic nerve
- Tibial portion of the sciatic nerve
- Femur
- Sacrum

the back of the thigh rather than the knee if you cannot reach this far, or use a strap around the leg.

For proportional or flexibility reasons, you may find that even holding the back of the thigh means the hips and the head and shoulders will be lifted off the floor. This is not an effective position for the stretch, so use a pillow under the head to enable you to relax in the first position. Pull the folded leg towards your armpit; this will stretch the hip of the other leg. Keep your back *and hips* on the floor.

The **C–R stretch** is done by pressing the foot that is on the thigh directly *into* the leg. You will feel the hip muscles being activated. Press for a count of five, stop pushing and breathe in. On a breath out, relax the hip and slowly pull the folded leg closer into the armpit. Hold the final position for five breaths in and out.

Experiment with small variations in foot positions and, if you wish, you can push the knee of the leg that is on the thigh further out to the side with the closest elbow, as Olivia is showing in the top photograph in the left column on this page.

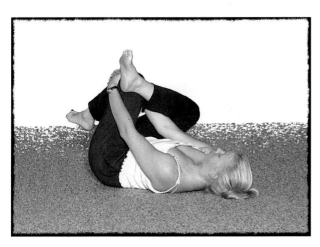

Cues
lie face up, with foot on thigh
hold back of leg, or knee
C–R: press closest foot into thigh
restretch: pull held leg closer

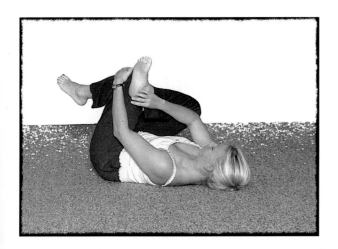

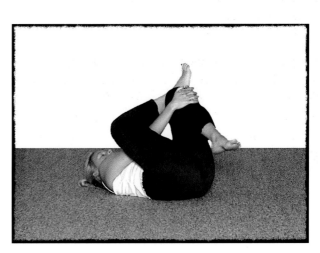

Exercise 8, Partner lying rotation, revisited

The first movement of exercise 3, lying rotation, is to pull the knee to the armpit with both hands (see page 42). The first way to increase the intensity of this movement is to use a **C–R stretch**. Press the knee away from you in the stretch position for a count of five and restretch after a breath out, as usual. Hold the end position for a full six to eight breaths.

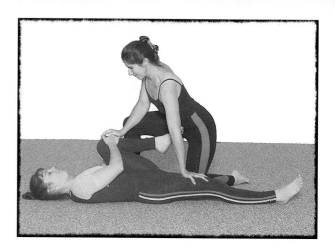

A partner can make this a much more impressive stretch. Your partner kneels by your side, as Jennifer is demonstrating with Sharon. Make sure they position themselves as shown, as we have found this to be the most stable position. While restraining the thigh of the straight leg (do not lean weight on the kneecap), your partner leans gently on the thigh you are holding. This alone will increase the stretch. To improve the position, use the **C–R stretch** technique: press the held leg back against the resistance of your arms and your partner's weight for a count of six to eight. The knee must not be allowed to move. Take in a deliberate deep breath, relax the thigh and, as you slowly breathe out, pull your knee towards you. You must do the restretch action yourself.

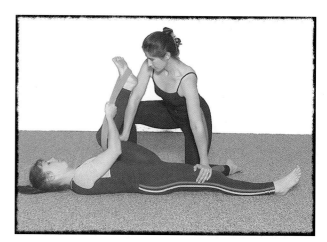

The stretch may be made more effective again by opening out the knee angle to around 90 degrees. So doing involves the hamstring muscles (and, in some people, the adductors) in the stretch too. In this variation, your partner will lean on the back of the leg and you will hold the foot from the inside; if you cannot reach without lifting your head and shoulders off the floor, use a strap to hold the foot, as shown. The final frame shows a version for looser students: Sharon has opened the knee angle to about 135 degrees, and Jennifer is supporting the back of her knee. This variation increases the stretch in the hamstrings: the greater the knee angle, the stronger the hamstring effect.

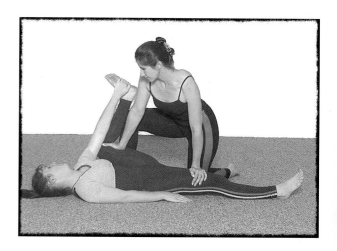

The **C–R stretch** is achieved by pressing your foot into your hand, and the back of the leg into your partner's hand. The partner's lower leg can stop your thigh from going too far outside the line of your body. Recall from exercise 3 that some people feel an uncomfortable compression in the inside of the hip doing this stretch; if this is the case, let the leg go further outside the line of the body and ask your partner to reposition their lower leg to hold you in this new position. Hold the final stretch position for 10 breaths in and out.

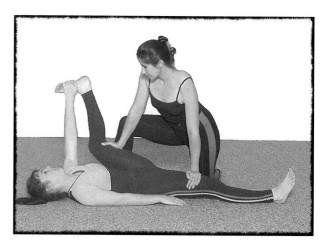

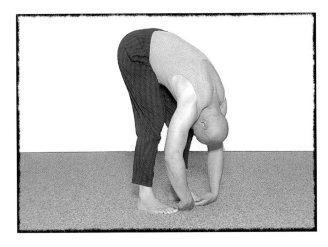

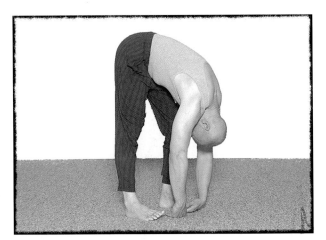

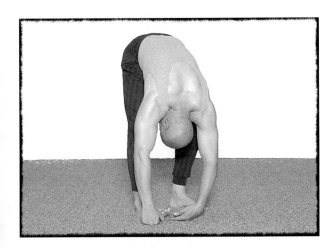

Standing alternate leg forward bend warm-up

This is the first of our warm-up exercises. We decided not to give them numbers, because they are loose versions of more formal exercises. It is worth noting, however, that you can get a fantastic stretch by doing *only* the warm-ups—and because they are less strict in form, you can often stretch areas in the body that are not usually stretched using orthodox flexibility moves. Another way of thinking about warm-up movements is that they are transitions between the idealised positions of the formal exercises; accordingly, because the positions you find yourself in are slightly different and because the warm-ups are often done dynamically (stretching while moving slowly), they have a quality all of their own. In most cases, the movements are done with the body as relaxed as possible, in contrast to the exercises where one part of the body is doing work in order to stretch another, so the stretch effect is more diffused.

If you cannot put your fingertips on the floor, you may use a support or hold onto your ankles. The secret to this series of movements being used as a warm-up is in being able to lean on your arms while bending forwards at the hips. Start by letting the chin go towards the chest, and let the upper body slump forwards. As you go further forwards, let the knees bend enough to take the stretch away from the hamstrings. Hang over like this for a few breaths, leaning on your arms. Now move around to one side, directly over one leg and, while continuing to lean, straighten the *other* leg. Rotate the shoulders from side to side. Bend the straight leg, move across to it, and straighten the first one. Again rotate the shoulders from side to side. Repeat this sequence until the lower back and hips feel loose.

In the next sequence, straighten one leg *before* bending over it and repeat the sequence; this time the leg that you will be bending over will be straight—and so will give far more of a hamstring stretch instead of an upper leg/hip stretch. You will get a better stretch if the weight of the upper body is supported, if you are not particularly flexible.

Finally, try to straighten one leg at a time; then try to straighten both legs at the same time. Small back-straightening movements can be used throughout; as you try to straighten the back the stretch will be made stronger in the hamstrings and hips. Bend the legs to come back to the standing position. Alternatively, you may stand on your hands as shown in the last frame, and add a slight pulling action to increase the intensity of all the movements.

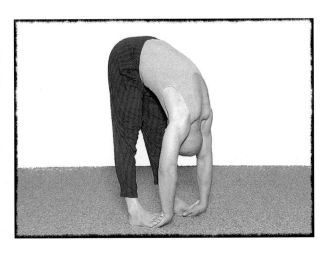

Exercise 17, Partner floor single leg forward bend, revisited

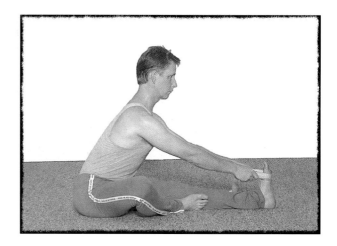

Now we will be able to see how doing partial, contributing poses can lead to a significant improvement in a complex pose. Use a strap if you need to, and see how much closer to your feet your hands are now. In the repeat of this exercise (page 60), I want to show you how to get the most out of it.

Lean forward over the straight leg as Steve is demonstrating and reach down the strap as far as you can, while trying to keep the back straight. 'Keeping the back straight' is not a direction for aesthetics (although it does look good); it is to ensure that the bending movement occurs from the *hips* and not the lower or middle back. This is where a partner can help; ask your partner to look at your back and place their hands on the roundest part. Where you feel their hands is precisely where you need to exert a stronger straightening effort. Julie is assisting Steve by placing her hands just above his lower back which, as shown in the second frame, is where he is beginning to bend.

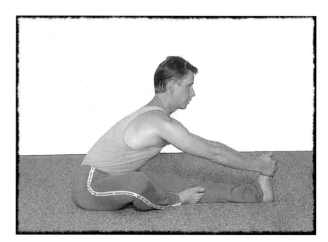

The **C–R stretch** version of this pose is very effective (it may be done on your own as well). Using your partner's guidance to hold your back straight, make a separate effort to lift your chest up; this will be a straightening effort in the middle and upper back. Holding onto the strap with both hands, try to *pull your hands away from your feet*. If doing this with a partner, pull away from your feet as well as press back to their hands. When you press back or pull back, do not permit any trunk movement—the body stays still.

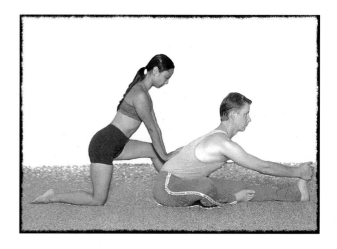

Pressing without a resultant movement is called an *isometric* contraction, and is a feature of most of our stretches. Experience has shown that any movement in this phase reduces the final stretch effect. Another important point is that, in a compound movement, often a large number of muscles can produce the main contraction. In exercise 17, for example, if you do not hold the lower part of your back absolutely straight, the main contraction effort can be made using the large muscles that run up the spine, *erector spinae*, rather than using the hamstrings to move the body in relation to the feet. Of course, the spine muscles must work too, to hold the body straight, but the feeling of the contraction—the main place you need to be aware is doing the pulling—needs to be in the hamstrings in order that they experience the stretch effect. In every case in the class

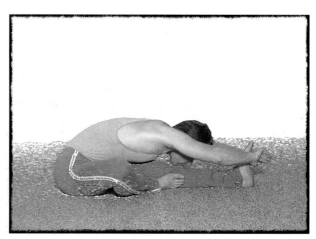

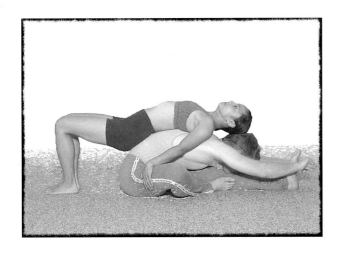

Cues

hold foot or strap

hold trunk straight; lift chest

partner supports roundest part of back

C–R: try to pull hands from feet

restretch: go closer to leg; back straight

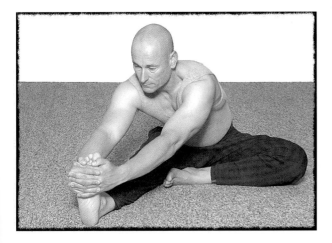

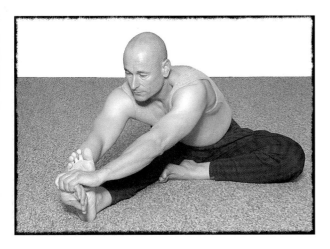

situation, when a student cannot feel the contraction effort in the hamstrings, their lower back is not straight. Better still, the back should be slightly bent backwards.

After pushing or pulling for a count of 10 or so (these are big muscles and benefit from a long contraction), breathe in and relax. Reach further down the strap or hold your foot and, on a breath out, slowly pull yourself *along* your leg, trying to hold the back straight. When you have gone as far as you can, ask your partner to again place their hands on the roundest part of your back and use this prompt to straighten the back again. The stretch sensation in the hamstring muscles of the straight leg will be much stronger now. Hold the final position for 10 breaths; try to breathe slowly. On each breath out, let the hamstring muscles relax, and imagine their lengthening.

Various support positions are shown. If your upper body is closer to your leg than approximately 45 degrees, you will benefit from your partner lying along your body, back to back, as Julie is doing for Steve in the top photograph. This is very comfortable and their weight is stable. This helps you to relax. Make sure that you can support this person's weight without straining—to make sure, take one hand off the strap and place it on the ground in a support position as they lower themselves onto you. Once in position, they can take some of their weight on their own hands or lie on you with their full weight. Perhaps surprisingly, it is much easier to relax with someone's weight on you than it is when they support you with their hands. The reason is that someone's weight is a far more stable force than the muscular effort of pressing with the arms. When you have stretched one leg sufficiently, change legs and stretch the other side. Make a note of the tighter side and next time you stretch begin with that side.

I am showing two different hand positions in the last two photographs; try both to see which is easier to hold for long periods. Let the back bend when reaching for these more difficult positions and straighten your back on a breath in to increase the hamstring effect. You will notice that in all suggested holding positions, whether using a strap or not, the arms are *straight*; if the arms are bent in the restretch position, they will straighten as you relax, and much of the potential hamstring effect will be lost.

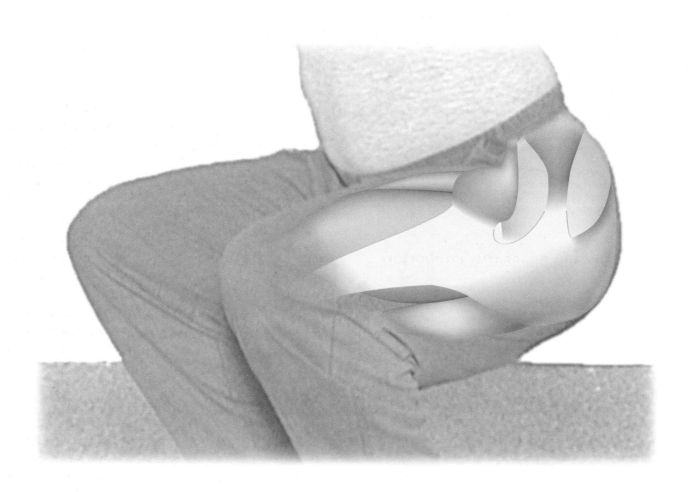

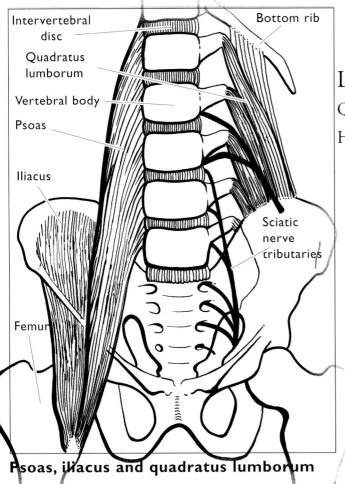

Intervertebral disc

Quadratus lumborum

Vertebral body

Psoas

Iliacus

Femur

Bottom rib

Sciatic nerve tributaries

Psoas, iliacus and quadratus lumborum

LESSON FOUR: HIP FLEXORS, QUADRICEPS, TRUNK BACKWARDS AND HAMSTRINGS

This lesson concentrates on the muscles that draw the legs forwards and backwards. The hip flexors, *ilio-psoas* and part of *quadriceps*, pull the thigh forwards; additionally, *quadriceps* extends the leg at the knee. The hamstrings pull the leg back and also pull the heel to the bottom by flexing the knee. The illustration accompanying this lesson shows the details of the hip flexors. These muscles have particular significance for low back pain, as one end of *psoas* attaches directly to the front of the bones that protrude from the vertebrae (the *anterior* surfaces of the *transverse processes*). If these muscles are tight, they will increase the lumbar spine's forward curve (*lordosis*) which affects the biomechanics of the entire spine. A schematic of the possible effects will be found on page 108. The hip flexors are difficult to stretch for this reason, as most exercises extend the spine rather than stretch *ilio-psoas*. Athletes, dancers and gymnasts will find it useful to know that it is far more efficient to stretch the muscles limiting the *back* leg in front splits than to overemphasise hamstring flexibility—if you can loosen the muscles of the back leg, you will be able to sit in front splits with far less hyperextension than may be the case currently. This additional flexibility will let you sit in this position with your hips far closer to square, as well.

Free squats warm-up, partner or solo

This delightful series of movements will rapidly warm-up the required muscles, and make your legs stronger as well. Start by squatting down with the legs in a shoulder width or narrower stance and keeping your heels on the ground. If you cannot keep your heels on the floor, it is because your ankles are tight: the knees cannot move far enough forwards to allow you to balance over your centre of gravity, so you lift your heels to tip your weight further forwards. All this means at this stage is that you need to concentrate on exercises 18, floor folded leg calf, and 19, wall standing calf. If you cannot keep your heels on the floor, you may use a board under them—this will tip your centre of gravity far enough forwards to be able to balance.

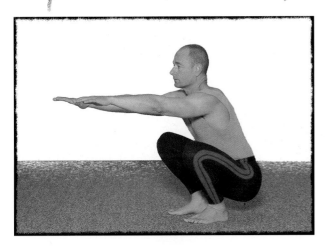

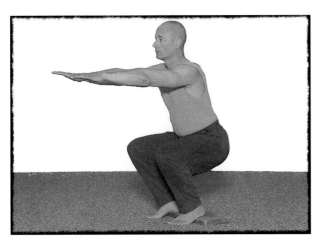

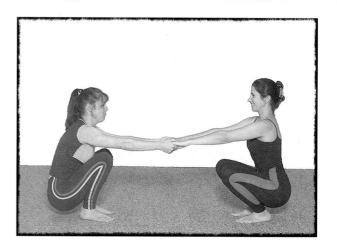

Alternatively, you can find something to hold on to while doing the movement; the third photograph shows Sharon doing the exercise while holding onto a bar, using her fingertips for balance—if you hold on with your hands, your arms will do most of the work!

If you have a partner to assist, you can do the exercise together, as Sharon and Jennifer are showing in the top two photographs. By holding hands, you can keep the body more upright and this makes it possible for everyone to do the movements with the heels on the floor.

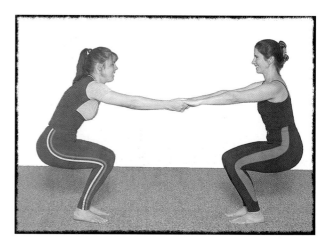

Whichever approach you use, squat up and down relatively slowly and rhythmically. If doing the exercise on your own, you can use your arms for counter balance, by extending them out in front of you at shoulder height, as I am showing in the first photograph on the previous page. For a few of the repetitions, stay down in the bottom position; even this will be a stretch for some people, especially if you let yourself relax in this position. We would normally do 20 repetitions or so, especially if the room is cold.

Once you have finished, move over to a painted, smooth wall—a brick wall will make the exercise too easy, due to the much greater friction. Put your back up against the wall, and, by bending your legs, let your back slide down until the thighs are parallel to the floor with the lower legs vertical, as shown by Olivia in the last photograph. Keep your arms by your sides or fingers linked behind the head. It looks easy—and feels easy at first, but quickly becomes difficult. Start by holding yourself in this position for 30 seconds, then 45 seconds, then a minute on subsequent attempts in later workouts. Do not be worried if your legs start to shake; this means only that they are working hard.

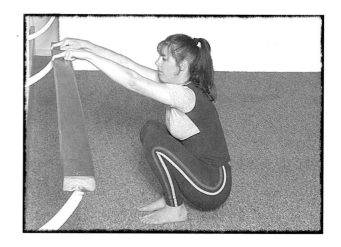

Olivia is smiling, because she had been holding this position for about two minutes by the time I got around to taking this shot!

Cues

keep heels on floor

make movements rhythmic and graceful

breathe in before squatting

breathe out as you rise

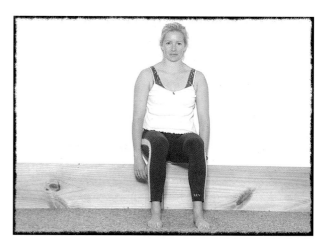

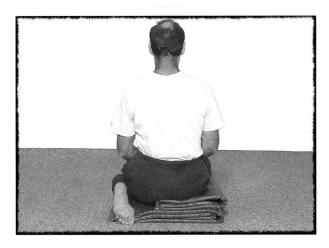

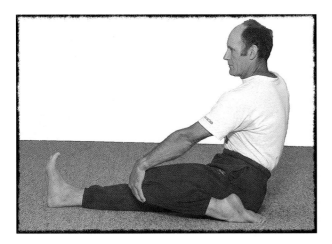

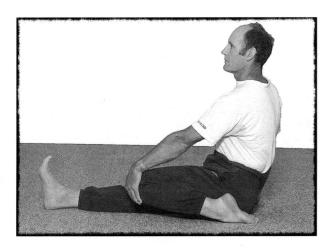

Cues

ensure hips are level

lean weight onto hip of folded leg

lift knee to stretch instep

C–R: try to pull toes to knee

restretch: lift held knee higher

23. Floor instep

This is the best stretch for a painful condition called shin splints, a common affliction of athletes who train on hard surfaces. Exercise 23 is the complementary movement to exercises 18, floor folded leg calf, and 19, wall standing calf. Alan is demonstrating the positions.

To make this little stretch effective, you will need to be able to sit with one leg folded beside you, with the hips level and both parts of the bottom on the floor. This will itself be too strong a stretch in the beginning for some people, so try the movements and use mats to adjust your position as necessary, referring to the photographs. The general rule is that if you cannot sit with both buttocks on the floor, you will need to prop up the hip of the straight leg. If this gives you too much stretch in the instep, you will need to let the toes and part of the instep hang over the edge of a mat. If there is too much stretch in the front thigh muscle of the folded leg, you will need to place a mat in between that buttock and the heel to increase the knee angle, which will reduce the stretch in *quadriceps*. The foot needs to be pointing straight back behind you, not angled across behind you, the first position you are likely to adopt.

Once in position, the instep can be further stretched by reaching over to the knee, grasping it and, *while leaning weight over to the same hip*, lift the knee off the floor. If you are leaning weight on the correct hip (instead of leaning away, as most people do, to avoid the stretch) you will feel a strong stretch in the instep. Some people will feel a strong stretch in the front shin muscle too (*tibialis anterior*).

The **C–R stretch** is performed by gently trying to pull the toes of the foot to the knee; in other words, when in position try to press the toes back down into the floor while holding the knee for a count of five to eight. Stop pressing, take a breath in, relax the toes, instep and shin muscles, and, on a breath out, very slowly lift the knee a little further. You will need to make a conscious effort to relax the instep to get the best end position; you will need to consciously *make* your shin muscles and small feet muscles let go. Sometimes a second brief contraction can help you do this. Hold the end position for five breaths in and out, or longer if you feel it is doing you good. Note your required seating position; we will need the same seating position for exercise 26, seated/lying single leg *quadriceps*, below.

24. Standing quadriceps

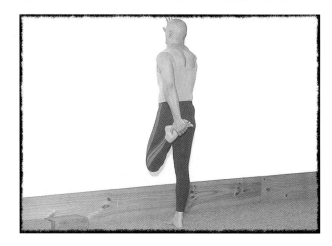

This useful stretch can be done anywhere, but it needs to be done carefully if you want to get the effect in *quadriceps*. When most people do this stretch, they avoid the full possible effect by letting the spine be pulled further into extension (*hyperextension*). I am showing the solo movement and Eldon is assisting.

Stand opposite a support and grasp the ankle as shown. If you are tight in this area, sometimes it is better *not* to pull the foot all the way back to the buttock to begin. Rather, tighten your abdominal muscles by slightly curling the trunk forwards and use the bottom muscles on the side you are stretching to pull the upper leg back in line with the body first. Once you get it in line (or close to it), pull the foot as close to the bottom as possible.

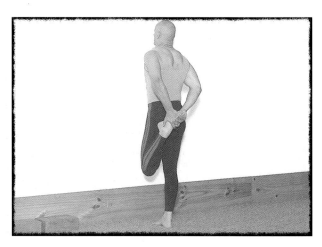

It is necessary to tighten the abdominal muscles *before* you pull the leg back, otherwise drawing the leg back or pulling the foot to the bottom will only tip the pelvis forwards, increasing the lumbar curve. Every increment of pelvic tilt decreases the effectiveness of the stretch, as far as *quadriceps* is concerned. One of our standard principles is that good form in a stretch often requires that one group of muscles is tightened to hold another part in position so that a second action may stretch it properly.

A **C–R stretch** may be achieved if desired. Two contractions are possible here (a partner can help you by holding the knee and buttock as Eldon is showing, but the exercise can be done by yourself too). The first **C–R** requires that, once in the stretch position, you try to straighten the leg for a count of five. This activates *quadriceps* strongly. After a breath in, pull the foot closer to the bottom. A second **C–R** is to pull the knee of the folded leg forwards while you or (better) your partner holds it there. Activating the leg in this way uses the muscles in the middle and top of the thigh, whereas the first **C–R** affects mainly the muscles close to the knee. Do both for the best effect. *Quadriceps* is a large muscle, and it can take a long stretch. I regard the standing stretch as a useful warm-up for the lying version, which is much easier to hold for long periods of time, or an effective, quick movement to do before some aerobic activity.

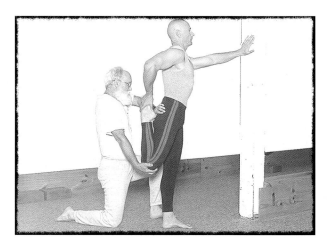

Cues

pull heel to bottom, then

take folded leg back

C–Rs: try to straighten leg;
try to pull folded leg forwards

restretch: heel closer to bottom;
folded leg further back

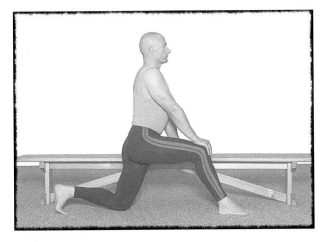

25. *Standing suspended hip flexor*

The *ilio-psoas* pair, *rectus femoris* and *sartorius* all act to draw the leg forwards in different leg and hip positions. The next exercise will stretch these muscles effectively. It may be done without a support if your balance is good, but a better stretch will be achieved by using a support in the beginning. Stronger versions using a partner will be described below (exercises 39, partner hip flexor, and 41, partner standing suspended hip flexor).

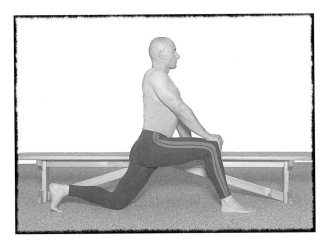

Take a big pace forwards so that the feet are well apart and stand alongside a support, with the leg that is behind you closest to the support (we will call this the back leg). Place your hand on your knee and hold the support with the other. Now let the back leg bend, and let the hips sink to the floor until the knee of the back leg is on the floor as shown. Using the waist muscles, rotate the hip of the *back* leg forwards until the hips are square (at 90 degrees) to the line of the legs. Ensure that your trunk is vertical or close to it, with the supporting arm on the leg held straight. Press the hand on the knee down firmly; this will tighten the abdominal muscles. This is the first position.

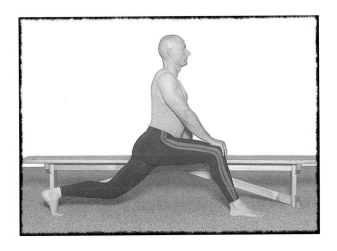

To stretch *quadriceps* and the hip flexors of the back leg, slowly straighten the back leg *without letting the hips rise any higher off the floor*. The operative word here will be *try*, because, if you do maintain the height of the hips at the start position, only very flexible people will be able to get the back leg fully straight. For many, the action of trying to straighten the leg will provide a strong stretch; hold this position for five to ten breaths in and out.

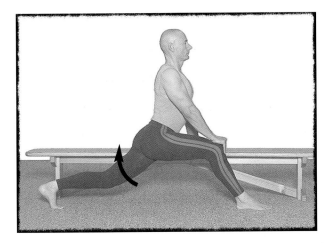

Cues

back leg behind as far as possible
lower hips to floor
try to straighten back leg
C–R: try to drag back leg forwards
restretch: restraighten back leg

To make the effect stronger, use a **C–R stretch**. While holding the leg straight (or as straight as you can) use the muscles of the front of the hip to *try* to drag the whole back leg forwards for a count of eight to ten. This will need to be a gentle contraction, because only your own strength is available to hold you in the contraction position—nothing must move as you try to pull the leg forwards. Stop pulling, take in a breath, check your trunk is vertical and, on a breath out, let the back leg bend once more and let the hips sink lower to the floor. Tighten the abdominal muscles once more, rotate the hips square and, without letting the hips rise, try to straighten the back leg. Hold the final position for a ten-breath cycle. You should feel a very strong stretch in the top of the back leg, in close to the hip joint.

The major form faults are failing to keep the hips square, failing to keep the trunk vertical, and failing to tighten the abdominal muscles to maintain the normal curve of the lower spine.

Some flexible individuals who are not strong enough in the abdominal muscles to maintain trunk straightness or the desirable curve in the lower lumbar spine may use an alternative correction. Once in the deep position, use the buttock muscles of the back leg to *tuck the bottom under* before trying to restraighten the back leg after the **C–R**. Tucking the bottom under is always effective in isolating the hip flexors. We call this tucking action a positive thrust, in contrast to a negative one which moves the hips in the opposite direction, and which was described in exercise 5, seated hip. Once again we are using one group of muscles to position a part of the body so that it can be stretched efficiently.

Cues (right)

from push-up position
lower body to floor

in lowest position, straighten legs

suspended between hands and feet,
lean back slowly

open mouth, take head back, close teeth

breathe deeply

curl up to finish

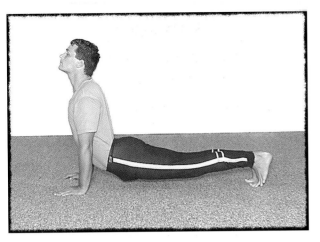

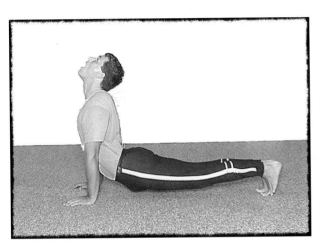

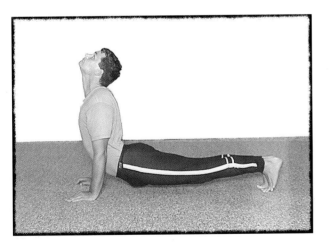

Exercise 2, Backward bend from floor, suspended variation

Re-read the directions for exercise 2, if necessary, and do the exercise. Because we have stretched the *quadriceps* and the hip flexors, expect that your backward bend will be better this time around. This is because both these muscle groups limit extension of the spine in the full-stretch position.

After doing exercise 2, we will now do a suspended version of the same movement. For reasons of proportion (lengths of respective body segments) this version will give some people a better stretch than exercise 2. Mark is demonstrating.

Start in the end position of the familiar push-up exercise: arms directly under shoulders, legs straight and the whole body aligned between shoulders and feet. Keeping the arms straight, take a breath in and, as you breathe out, slowly let the hips start sinking towards the floor, letting the whole body (apart from the arms!) relax. You will sink down until the front of the thighs just touches the floor. At this point straighten the legs, and relax into the stretch. This will be enough stretch for many people.

To increase the stretch, very cautiously pull back on the hands; because they are fixed on the floor by body weight your back will bend further backwards instead. Provided this action does not tighten the back muscles in an unpleasant way, hold the position. To make the stretch stronger still, open the mouth wide (recall exercise 6, chin to chest), incline the head backwards slowly as far as it will go, and then bring the teeth together. Finally, pull the shoulders back as far as you can. Try to breathe as normally as you can, and maintain the final position for five to ten breath cycles.

Come out of the pose and use either the knees clasped to the chest position shown at the end of exercise 2, or the position shown in the last frame in this sequence. Let the whole body relax for a few breaths in and out.

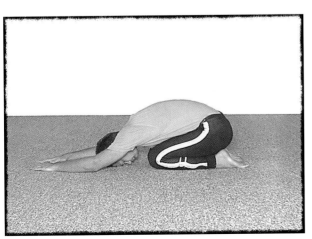

Exercise 1, Floor clasped feet middle and upper back, revisited

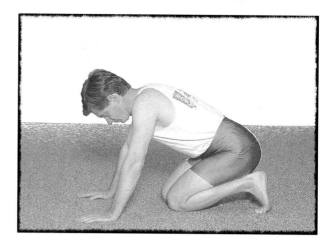

Review the instructions for exercise 1. We are going to add two contractions to exercise 1 (described on page 25) and show you a second version of the exercise, which might suit some people better, for reasons of proportion.

Once in the final position of exercise 1, two **C–R stretches** will enhance the effectiveness of this exercise significantly. The first contraction requires you to try to *shrug* your shoulders, by trying to pull your hands away from your feet—but you are holding tight, so the muscles between the neck and the shoulders contract instead. Hold this contraction for a count of five. Stop shrugging, relax and take in a breath. On a long breath out, push the hips forwards once again to restretch. In the final position, breathe as normally as you can and hold the position for five breaths or so.

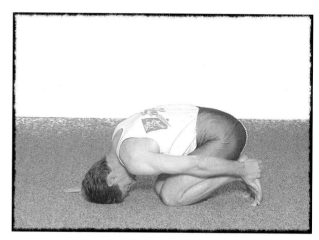

The second **C–R stretch** contraction is a bit harder to understand. Once in the final position, try to pull your shoulder blades *together* behind your back (this tightens the *rhomboideus* muscles). Restretch in the same manner as above, and hold the new final position for another five breaths.

The second version of exercise 1 is similar to the one you know, except that the feet are held *outside* the legs. Gary is showing the suggested form in the movement. Your knees will need to be closer together so the arms do not bind against them, and the feet apart so you can hold them. In all other respects, including getting into and out of the stretch, the exercise is the same as exercise 1. Try both versions, and see which one you prefer. Your proportions influence where the focus of the stretch will be felt.

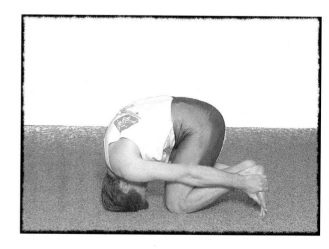

The same two **C–R stretches** can be used in this version of the exercise, too. You may care to try lesson 1's version first and do this version second. Try to feel the difference in stretch focus between the two versions.

Cues

hold feet from inside or outside

push hips forward

C–Rs: pull shoulder blades together; shrug shoulders strongly

restretch: push hips further forwards

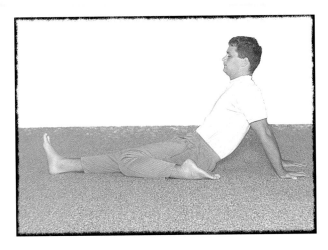

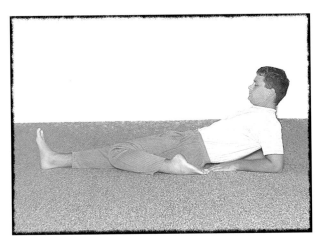

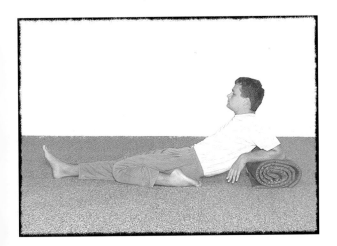

Cues

ensure hips are level

tighten abdominal muscles

C–R: press foot into floor

restretch: retighten abdominals;
lower trunk closer to floor

26. Seated/lying single leg quadriceps

Because you will be fully supported in the final position of this pose, holding the position for 30 seconds to a minute will be possible. As mentioned above, *quadriceps* is a large muscle group and responds to a long stretch. Mark is showing the positions.

Use whichever of the seating positions you needed to do exercise 23, floor instep, above. To stretch quadriceps safely, the foot needs to point directly out behind you—if you have the foot turned out to the side (so often seen in aerobics classes, because the students are wearing shoes and their insteps are not supple enough to sit in the recommended position) you will be placing a potentially dangerous rotation stress on the knee, especially on the inside (*medial*) ligaments. Once in position (the start position of exercise 23 above), tighten the abdominal muscles, tighten the buttock muscles to tuck the bottom under a little (this alone can give quite a strong stretch) and lean back onto your arms, or to stretch further, onto your elbows. *Do not let the back hyperextend*—not only might this hurt the lower back in this position, but hyperextension helps to avoid the stretch. If anything, curl the trunk forwards before leaning back and you will improve the stretch. Permit me to labour a point: the purpose of a stretching exercise is not to make a particular shape—it is to provide a stretch in a particular place. If you can do this in a less dramatic (and hence safer) position, it is to be preferred. If you stretch properly, progress is assured. Injury will stop your progress completely.

One **C–R stretch** is offered here, as we are doing the solo version. Once in the stretch position, take a few breaths in and out to get used to it. Now try to straighten the folded leg by pressing the foot next to you into the floor for a count of eight to ten. Stop pressing, relax, take a breath in and, on a breath out, tighten the abdominal muscles again, lowering yourself further. Use a mat under your shoulders to get closer to the floor or, if you can, lie down completely on the floor. Again, the lower back must not be allowed to hyperextend.

To keep the hips level, you can bring the other leg up to your hip and hold it (Gary is demonstrating this addition in the second photograph); now you can put extra pressure on the hip of the thigh being stretched. Change legs, and, as always, compare left with right. Start your stretching with the tighter thigh next time.

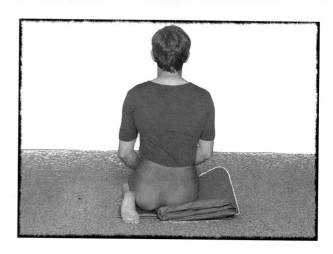

The final frame in the photograph column shows Mark doing a two-leg version that we do not recommend unless you are flexible enough to do it without a strong bend in the lower back (*hyperextension*). One can see this exercise being done badly everywhere—we strongly suggest that a better stretch can be achieved by doing one leg at a time. A much more intense exercise is demonstrated in chapter three (exercise 86, the ultimate *quadriceps* stretch). Remember, it is the combined tension of both the thigh muscles *and* the hip flexors that extend the lower back if attempting the two-leg version—so if you want to really stretch these muscles, partial poses doing one leg at a time are the way to go.

Exercise 14, Wall middle and upper back backward bend

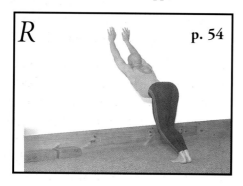

p. 54

Do this exercise from lesson 2 again; this will complete the series of stretches for the front of the body (23, 24, 25, and 2). Do not be surprised if you can get considerably closer to the wall this time, having stretched these other muscle groups, all of which limit your backward bending capacity.

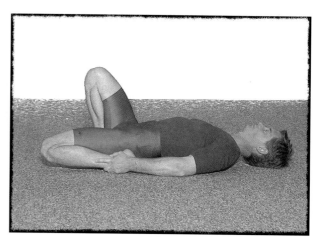

Cues

ensure hips are level

tighten abdominals before leaning back

C–R: press instep into floor

restretch: retighten abdominals and lean further back

hold foot of support leg for stability

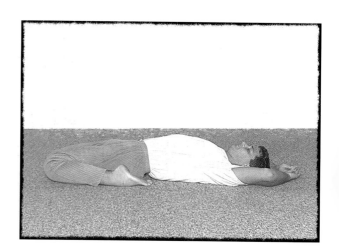

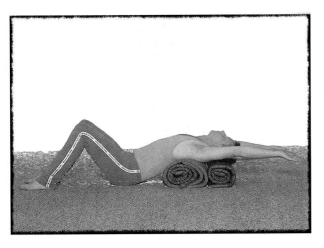

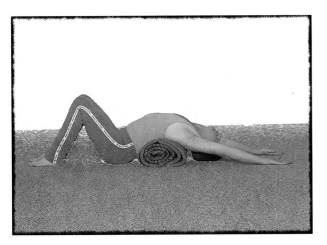

Cues

lie face up over support

use support for head if necessary

extend arms from body

C–R: raise the head slightly

restretch: let yourself relax over support

partner can extend and press on arms

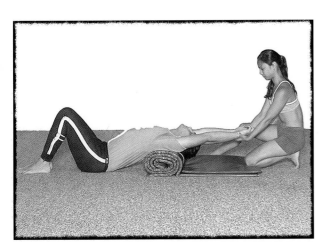

27. Partner backward bend over support

This apparently simple exercise exemplifies our approach, and is a wonderful backwards bend for the entire trunk. Its advantage over the many backwards bends from various disciplines is that the body's weight is *supported*. This allows an exploration of the sensations of lengthening and opening all of the muscles and joints on the front of the body that no other backward bend can emulate. It also allows you to add small rolling movements side to side which stretch many small muscles that are left untouched in standard exercises. We use a 'low-tech' tool: large metal drums split lengthways. A little ingenuity will allow you to come up with substitutes; if you have nothing readily available you may use your partner (shown last in this sequence, overleaf). If you are doing these lessons at home, you can use the end of a couch (make sure that it will not tip over), tightly rolled mats (we tie ours to keep them tight), or a narrow padded bench. One of my teachers in California uses old electrical cable reels. The radius of the support will be chosen according to the length of your trunk and your degree of flexibility. You need to feel comfortable in the stretch—you cannot relax otherwise—so cover the support with something soft.

This exercise can be done on your own; simply drape yourself over the support making sure that the back of the head rests on something too (you can add an extra support if necessary as Steve is showing in the first photograph)—then raise your arms up over your head and press them away from you. This will be a good stretch by itself. Stay in this position for at least 10 breath cycles, then roll a small amount to one side, and relax in that position for a while. Repeat for the other side. A gentle solo **C–R stretch** can be done: raise the head and slightly tighten the abdominal muscles as though you were going to sit up. Relax and restretch.

Recall my observations regarding backward bending made in an earlier lesson. You may expect the muscles (on the inside of the curve you are making with your body) to tighten as you go further into the stretch. Accordingly, when you *roll* sideways off the support, get down onto the floor and immediately do exercise 1, or one of the other recovery poses described for exercise 2, in lesson 1. This will stretch the middle back muscles that will have tightened doing the exercise. Julie is assisting Mark in the bottom photograph, by gently drawing his arms towards her.

The least-intense partner version over a higher support is shown first. Steve is sitting on a bench, so only his upper and middle back is being bent, useful for those with lower back problems. Julie has lowered Steve's head for him. Steve then stretches his arms out. This is the first position.

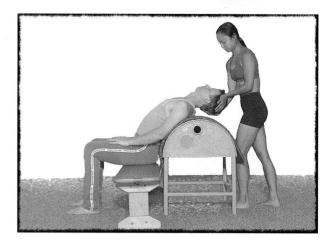

If you have a partner handy, you can increase the intensity of this stretch, as Julie is demonstrating in the second frame. Once in the final position of the solo stretch, your partner takes hold of your wrists (we find the trapeze grip the best where you hold each other's wrists) and to begin draws the arms directly out from the shoulders. This increases the stretch by expanding the rib cage and lifting the chest. Now the partner slowly takes the arms down to the floor while maintaining the elongating pull until you have a strong enough stretch. Breathe deeply in this position—breathing will be more difficult than usual, because the chest is fully open. Simply making the effort to breathe deeply in this position will strengthen the diaphragm.

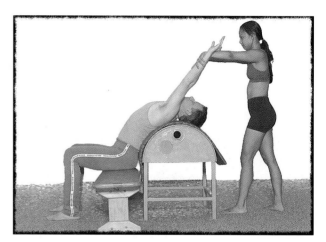

The **C–R stretch** requires you to gently press your hands up towards the ceiling. This will use all the muscles that shorten as we age (described in exercise 14, wall middle and upper back backward bend). Stop pressing, breathe in and, on a breath out, ask your partner to gently take the arms further towards the floor. Hold the final position for 10 breaths. Once you are finished, roll across the support to come out of the stretch and immediately do one of the recovery poses.

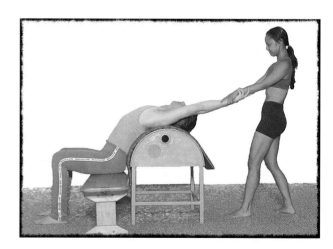

It may be that having someone press on your arms in this position makes you feel a strong compression in the shoulder joint itself—so much so that you are unable to relax sufficiently in the stretch. An alternative support position that requires you to fold your arms about 90 degrees at the elbows and hold the palms together is shown on the facing page in the second photograph.

In the top photograph, opposite, Mark is demonstrating a more intense solo stretch over a smaller-radius support. Small sideways stretches can be added to the backward bend by rolling to each side in turn. Do this slowly to maximise the effects.

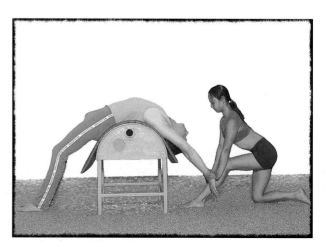

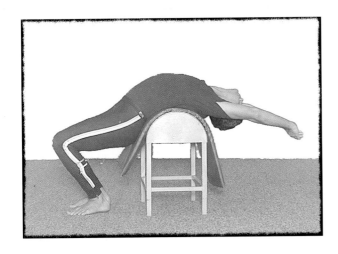

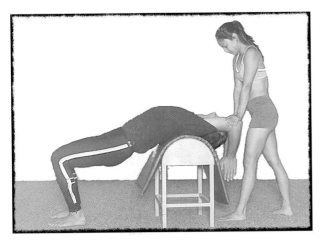

Cues

relax back over support; extend arms

partner takes arms further

C–R: press hands to ceiling

restretch: partner extends arms and
gently presses arms to floor, or
you lower hips towards floor

do forward bend to finish

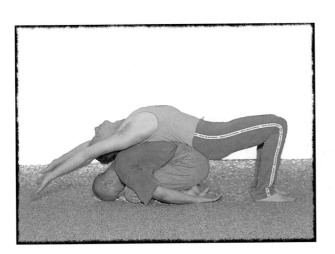

Mark and Julie are demonstrating the alternative, bent-arm support position in the second photograph. Your partner will press the elbows in until the upper arms are near your head, and then will press the elbows *down* in the direction of the floor. The **C–R stretch** requires you to press your elbows, rather than your hands, to your partner. This arm position will relieve a considerable amount of compression from the shoulders. In terms of effect, this variation will stretch the upper chest more than the standard version. Both are excellent.

Consider for a moment the effect of different starting positions on the support. If you have your shoulders on the highest part of the support (you can position your hips off the support by holding them away with the legs, if you wish) and you do the exercise as described, the major effect will be in the upper back and chest. If you try the stretch this way, the final effect can be made more intense by slowly letting your hips drop down onto the support once your partner has taken the arms down as far as possible. In this way, you control the final intensity completely.

If you have the middle of the back over the highest part of the support, the entire thoracic spine will be bent backwards, with consequently less effect in the shoulders; this is Steve's position in the bottom photograph opposite. Try a number of positions, and feel the different effects. All versions will have the anti-gravity effects described in exercise 14; they are stronger in exercise 27 because the **C–R stretch** is easier to apply (gravity is helping your end position), making it easy to hold and, finally, you will stay in the position longer, as it allows you to relax.

The last frame on this page shows how the exercise may be done if you do not have support handy, but you do have a willing partner; Steve and I are demonstrating. The partner's position is a lovely lower-back stretch, assuming that your partner is flexible enough to get into the support position. The partner's chest and ribs will be pressing on their thighs, so unless you are very different sizes, no strain will be felt in the back. Let common sense be the guide, of course. The partner adopts the position, then, making sure that you lower your weight slowly, stretch back over their body. If you have a second partner the **C–R stretch** can be done, but the partner will be finding it difficult to breathe, so it is probably better to limit the use of this technique to simple backward bends.

Exercise 4, Standing side bend, hanging version

To the standing side bend we already know, I wish to add a hanging version. Positioned in various ways, this variation is an excellent stretch for *tensor fasciae latae*, the oblique group of waist muscles, and *gluteus minimus* and *medius*. This version is considerably stronger than one from the daily five, so give yourself sufficient rest before doing it again.

The hanging version requires a strong support. A vertical bar is good, but a protruding room corner or door frame will do just as well. Stand less than arm's length away from the bar (the closer you stand to the support, the stronger the effect, so do not stand too close the first time you try) and grasp it firmly. Let the hips move directly to the side in line with the shoulders. Once you have gone as far as you can, extend the other arm up and across the head. Straighten it if you can; this will intensify the stretch considerably. You may bend the leg closest to the support if that makes the stretch more effective. All of the effects will be felt in the side of the body you are stretching away from, and in the lower back muscles on the same side. A **C–R stretch** can be done by pressing the outside foot gently directly away from the bar (the *opposite* movement, in effect). This action will involve the adductors of the hip. Stop pressing, relax and on a breath out, slowly try to increase the movement of the hips away from the bar or, alternatively, press the upper arm away from the body more strongly. The former will stretch the *adductors* more, the latter will stretch the muscles above the waist more.

To stretch *tensor fasciae latae*, roll the inside hip *forwards* while maintaining the lean. The **C–R stretch** should come instinctively now: once in the new position, use *tensor fasciae latae* to press the outside foot away and also slightly in front of you (of course, it will not move because you have all your weight on it), and restretch.

To stretch *gluteus minumus* and *medius*, roll the inside hip *backwards* until you can feel these muscles, above and behind the hip joint. The **C–R** is to push the foot away and slightly *behind* you. Breathe and restretch. This latter movement can use some forward bending at the hip to intensify the effects, if you wish—in other words, let the hips move *back* slightly as you lean to the side. Repeat for the other side. These are surprisingly intense stretches, so err on the side of caution the first few times you attempt them.

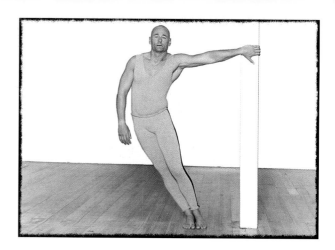

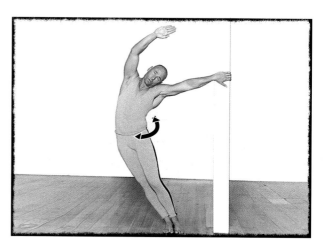

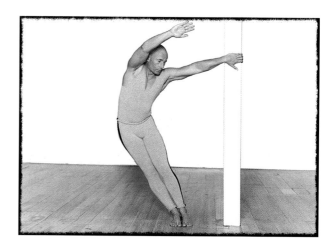

Cues

stand inside arm's length from support

let body hang from arm;
let hips go to side

rotate hips forwards and backwards

C–R: press foot away to the side

restretch: let yourself hang further

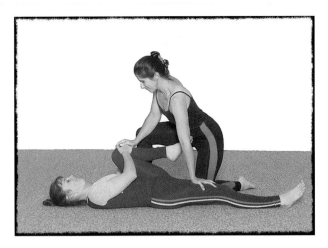

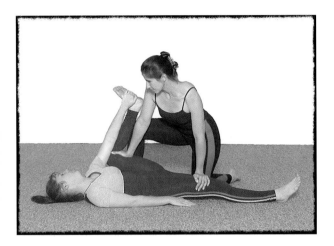

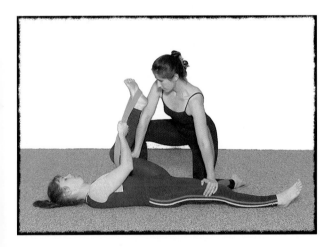

Cues

pull thigh to armpit with flexed knee

partner helps you try to straighten leg

C–R: try to pull heel to bottom

restretch: partner gently applies
straightening effort to heel

28. Partner lying hamstring, knee flexed

The hamstring stretch we are going to do from this position feels completely different from most hamstring movements because we are going to work into the stretch from a strongly flexed *hip* position to the straight leg (extended knee) position. Most hamstring stretches start with an extended knee and that is what is familiar to your body. Achieving the stretch this new way stresses the proprioceptors and stretch receptors in an unusual way, and an immediate improvement in hamstring flexibility will be the result.

Look at the third photograph in lesson 3's extension of exercise 8, page 70, showing the lying hip stretch with the knee opened at 90 degrees. After all we have done this session you will not need to warm-up for this, so get into your best position. Your hip flexibility may require the use of a strap. Sharon is being stretched; Jennifer is assisting.

Your partner will be in position as shown. You may use a **C–R stretch** to help you get into a strong first position. You hold the back of your leg as close to the side of your body as you can with both arms (first frame), or hold the foot if you are sufficiently flexible (next frame). The last photograph shows how to use a strap if these positions are too strong. Your partner supports the lower leg and the other hand holds the thigh of the extended leg. Press the back of the thigh against your partner's support (or press your foot into your hand) for a count of 10 and, on a breath out, take the thigh closer to the floor.

A second stretch may be done. While your partner holds the thigh as close to your body as possible, slowly try to straighten the leg. This action will provide a strong stretch to the bulk of the hamstring muscles. Hold the position you get to for 10 breaths. On no account let the leg you are holding move away from the side of your body.

The **C–R stretch** used here requires that you try to pull your foot back to your bottom by flexing at the knee. Your partner will need to change their support position (shown overleaf), so that the foot is held completely still against your contractions. Hold the contraction for a count of eight to twelve. Stop pulling, both you and your partner stay still, take in a deep breath and relax the back of the active leg and, on a breath out, ask your partner to move the leg closer to being straight, very slowly. The object here is to get a strong stretch, *so do not let the thigh you are holding move at all.* The final effect, in time, will be much stronger if you can do this. Even if you move the foot only a little with respect to the knee, the stretch will be intense. You need to move particularly slowly in this last extension movement, because you are now working in an unfamiliar range of movement. You are trying to *let* the muscles stretch—and if you try to do this quickly the stretch receptors will fire and all extra movement will cease. Make sure you are breathing deeply and slowly. Hold the end position for at least 10 breaths in and out. We have seen even flexible people improve their end position (as assessed by a standard hamstring stretch) by 15 degrees with a single iteration of this exercise. Do not cheat yourself in the movement. Olivia is assisting me to do the exercise in the photograph on this page and I am clasping my thigh tightly by wrapping my arms around the back of the leg. This assistance position is good if there is a great disparity in your respective sizes.

This exercise can also be done on your own (not shown), but is more difficult. Assume the held-foot 90-degree lower-leg position, keep the thigh as close to you as possible, and use your hand to open the knee angle until you feel the required stretch. The **C–R stretch** is to pull the foot back to the bottom against the resistance of your hand for the suggested time. When you do the restretch, use the strength of your arm together with the *quadriceps* of the same leg to try to straighten the leg. Do not sacrifice thigh position to get the leg straighter: a better stretch will be felt with the thigh still held in the end position of exercise 8, close to the body.

Exercise 8, Partner lying rotation

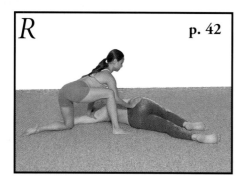

p. 42

Finish today's lesson with the rotation part of exercise 8; if you are working solo, remember that you can use the leg of a table or similar to hold the shoulder on the floor while you take the other knee to the floor.

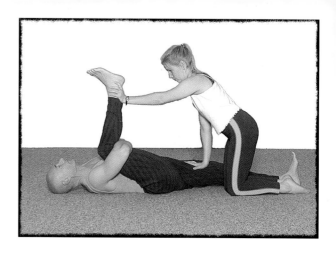

Cues

do not lose thigh position
as you try to straighten leg

apply straightening effort slowly

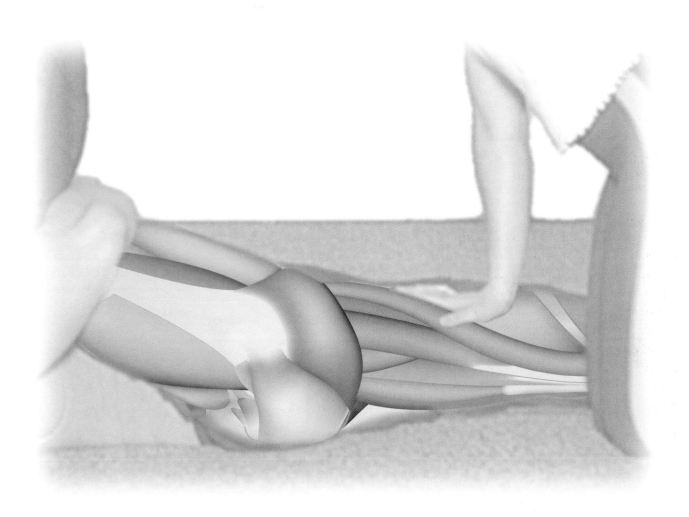

LESSON FIVE: LEGS APART AND ROTATION

The bulk of this lesson is devoted to the average person's tightest range of movement—getting the legs wide apart. Women seem to have an easier time making progress in the beginning, and anatomists point to the wider angle between the hip joints (as seen from above) as the reason. Some authorities claim that the maximum angle that men can achieve is around 160 degrees as opposed to 180 degrees for women. And a truism of the dance world has it that once you are an adult, the 'turnout' you take into the dance studio for your first class is the turnout you will have for the rest of your dance life. In our experience, none of these claims is true.

While women generally progress more quickly than men in this movement, the difference between individuals of the same sex is far greater than the supposed difference between the sexes. Because women do have better legs-apart flexibility than men—in the untrained individual—and everyone knows this, the ground is set for a self-perpetuating myth. Also, men are naturally stronger than women and we have already discussed the inverse relationship between the attributes of strength and flexibility. The right kind of training can develop dramatic flexibility, however, and if this is experienced in the context of sufficient supporting strength, the result is far better than simply being flexible. It is also true that most gymnasts, dancers, skaters and divers acquire their flexibility as children and reach maturity being able to demonstrate full flexibility. But we have taught many adults with no flexibility training in their past and they have demonstrated superior flexibility with three to five years' practice. The sooner we begin, the sooner that day will come!

The muscles that limit hip abduction are the adductors (*adductor magnus, adductor longus, adductor brevis, gracilis, pectineus*) and the three hamstring muscles in decreasing significance from *semitendinosus* to *biceps femoris*. Pure abduction (feet kept parallel as legs are taken apart; lower back straight) is a limited movement; for most people it ends when the legs are at about 90 degrees to each other. As one leg is taken to the side (see the top illustration and the top photograph), the abducted leg takes the pelvis with it and the pelvis is then abducted in relation to the vertical leg.

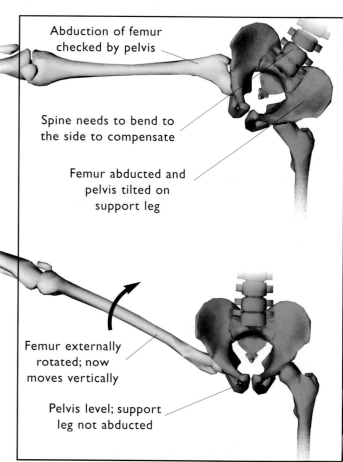

Abduction of femur checked by pelvis

Spine needs to bend to the side to compensate

Femur abducted and pelvis tilted on support leg

Femur externally rotated; now moves vertically

Pelvis level; support leg not abducted

How 'turnout' helps hip abduction

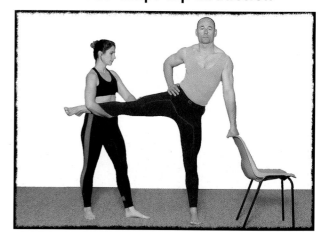

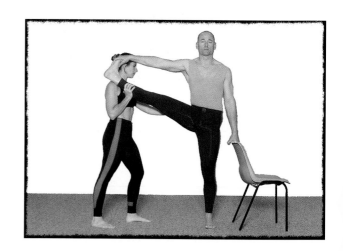

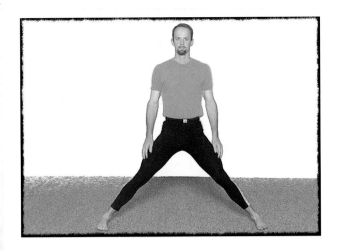

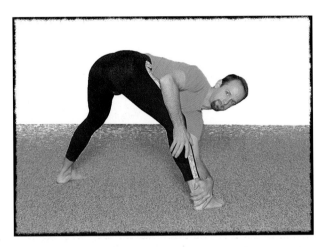

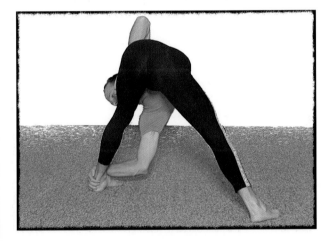

Cues

stretch forwards with bent legs

hold onto ankles for support

use gentle back and leg
straightening efforts

Pure abduction stops when one or more of three things has occurred: the adductor muscles have reached their limit of extensibility, the *pubofemoral* ligaments have reached their limit of movement, or the femoral neck is checked by the *acetabular rim* of the hip joint (see the illustration opposite). This last aspect is the reason dancers and gymnasts develop *turnout*—the capacity to externally rotate the *femur* in the hip joint for, when that happens, movement of the leg to the side is limited only by hamstring and adductor flexibility. In the second photograph, Jennifer has turned out my leg and, as a result, she can lift my leg up alongside my body easily—and notice that my hips are now close to level. One further physiological fact is of the greatest importance in getting the legs apart: the side-splits position is a combination of (i) adductor and hamstring flexibility if you can turn the leg out, together with (ii) hyperextension of the spine in order to loosen the *iliofemoral* ligaments. The lesson here is to work on turnout and lower spine backward bending to get the legs apart effortlessly. Many partial poses can help this task.

Another lesson to be learned at this point is that the direction from which you approach the legs-apart position is also significant. Your most limited legs-apart position is when you sit on the floor with your feet pointing up to the ceiling, as the hips are not turned out. And the protective mechanisms in the adductors seem to be particularly active in this position, probably because of the close relation between the femoral neck and the hip joint. An exercise we will do in lesson 10 (exercise 62, partner wall seated legs apart) will get us towards the side-splits position, but will go via the hamstrings; in other words, we will defeat the normal protective mechanisms and we will take maximal advantage of the turned-out position.

Standing legs apart warm-up, bent and straight legs

This sequence is done free in the middle of a room in this lesson, and a stronger version is described in lesson 10. It is similar in form to the standing alternate leg forward bend warm-up described in lesson 3, but with the legs spaced at various distances apart.

Start with the legs about two-and-a-half shoulder-widths apart, as Kevin is demonstrating in the first photograph. Bend the legs at the knees slightly and slowly fold the body

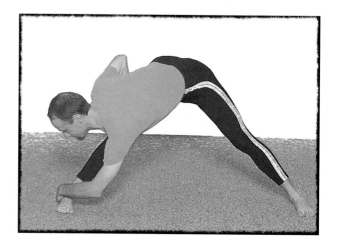

down in between the thighs. Hang there with the legs bent to stretch the bottom muscles (the 'glutes', as they are generally called) and to provide a gentle stretch for the hamstrings. You may support yourself by holding onto your lower legs or ankles, or you can rest the fingertips on the floor. Try rotating the shoulder with respect to the hips and feel the stretch in the side of the waist (first and second photographs) and do this on both sides.

Move across to one leg, position the body over it, and slowly straighten the other leg. Move back across to the straight leg now and feel the stretch on the inside and at the back of that straight leg. Let yourself hang in this position for a while. Bend this leg and straighten the other one, slowly move over to it, and stay there for a while. The back is allowed to assume its own shape during the preceding movements and the head also hangs down in a comfortable way. Move back to the position of where the body is between the legs. Reach across to the legs (or the ankles, if you are loose enough) and take a firm grasp. Now lift the head so that the spine is in a neutral shape and, by exerting the strength of the middle and lower back, slowly arch the back backwards as much as you can. As you do, you will feel the pelvis roll forwards, and the stretch in the adductors and the hamstrings will be increased significantly. Hold this position, breathing normally.

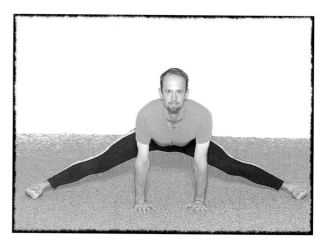

The next stage of the warm-up requires that you let the legs go further apart, keeping control. If you cannot support yourself on your hands, use a prop. Rest your upper body's weight on your hands, and let the feet slide apart. I suggest not letting them go wider than you can actually hang on to with arms outstretched—because you will be out of your normal range of movement and your capacity to control the movement will be reduced. If you have hold of the ankles, the movement will be safer. Once you have let the legs go further apart, repeat all the moves described above. To finish, take hold of the ankles, arch backwards to straighten the back and, very cautiously, pull yourself down to the floor between your legs. Gravity will help you hold the position and, because you are supporting your weight with the muscles you are stretching, the sensation will be intense. To come back to the standing position, bend the legs and, arching the back backwards once more, lead with the head and stand up.

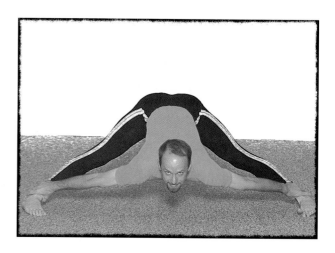

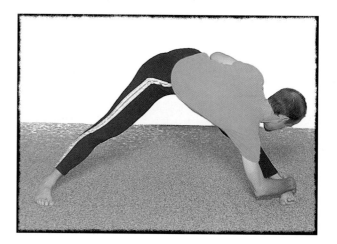

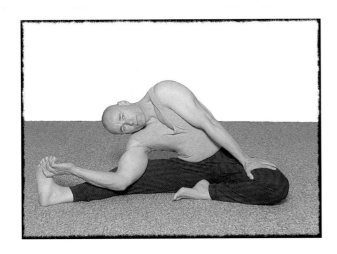

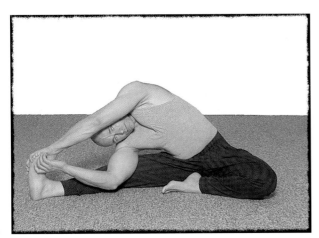

Cues (above)

hold foot or use strap
press bent elbow back against leg
roll top shoulder back
C–R: gently pull away from foot
restretch: pull trunk closer to leg

Cues (left)

widen legs and repeat sequence
hold ankles and straighten back
pull yourself forwards, first with bent legs, then with straight legs
support on arms and widen legs

Exercise 16, Floor abdominal curls

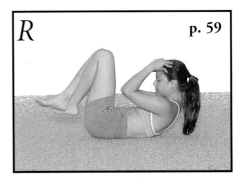

To further warm the body, do 10 to 15 slow abdominal curls.

29. Floor side bend over straight leg; other folded

In one sense I found the full benefits of this simple pose by accident. In the *Overcome neck & back pain* workshops, I realised that many people could not get their legs far enough apart to be able to bend the trunk sideways over one of the legs, so I tried the movement myself with one leg folded to remove the adductor restriction. I was surprised to find that as a *quadratus lumborum* stretch, this revised exercise had no equal and, in fact, was far more effective for stretching this deep muscle group than the standard legs-apart movement. We now use it in the *Posture & Flexibility* classes as a strong side bend for the waist, affecting *quadratus lumborum* primarily and *erector spinae* secondarily. The oblique group and *latissimus dorsi* are stretched too, increasingly as the top arm is taken towards the foot. The reason exercise 29 isolates *quadratus lumborum* so well is that folding one leg keeps that hip down on the floor—in the standard legs-apart exercises, the hip you are bending away from leaves the floor (in fact, the looser your hamstrings are, the more this occurs). This exercise is the best for a deep lower back stretch. If your hamstrings are not particularly flexible, you will find a strap useful. I have shown this in the middle of the room, but putting the straight leg up against a wall will provide you with both alignment and support.

Sit on the floor and (in contrast to a forward bend) put one leg out to the side as far as you can. Fold the other leg, as shown. Reach out and hold the big toe of the straight leg with a *palm up* grip (or loop a strap around it), pull gently on the hand so that the elbow bends, and put the elbow on the floor (or close to it) *inside* the leg. Press the elbow into the leg to bring the shoulder forwards. Using the bottom shoulder as a pivot, use the waist muscles to roll the top shoulder back (if you are using a wall, roll back until the shoulders are on the wall) and reach the top arm out towards the foot as far as you can. This combination side bend and rotation exposes the deep muscles between the hip and the spine to a strong stretch. If the stretch is felt strongly in the hamstring of the leg you are bending over, let the leg bend slightly at the knee: this will not reduce the effectiveness of the movement as a sideways bend for the spine.

If you are careful, a good **C–R stretch** can be done here in two ways depending on your end position. If you cannot hold the foot with the top arm, hold the foot (or the strap) with the other hand using a strong grip. Feel where the stretch is—if you are in the recommended position, the stretch will be between the hip from which you are stretching away and the waist and lower back on that same side. Holding yourself in position, gently try to pull your hand from the foot with these muscles for a count of five to ten. *Make this effort gentle.* Stop pulling, take a breath in and, on a slow breath out, use the hand holding the foot to bring you closer to the leg. This will be a strong stretch indeed the first time you do it, so do not exaggerate the movement. Hold the final position for a ten-breath cycle. Stretch the other side and, when you know which is the tighter, do this side again. This exercise can be effective for lower back pain.

The way the exercise is described, the movement is a strong sideways bend for the spine, but a great many positions can be achieved between the final position of this movement and that of exercise 17, partner floor single leg forward bend. Once you have gone as far to the side as possible, let the top shoulder roll *forwards* a little and lean to the side once more. The addition of some flexion of the spine that occurs as you roll the shoulder forwards will allow you to lean further to the side, exposing new areas to the stretch. Try three or four shoulder movements forwards—you will know when to come out of the final position because once the shoulder has rolled sufficiently forwards the stretch will disappear. If you try these variations, repeat all movements for the other side.

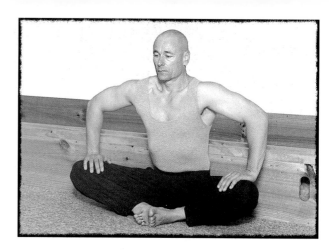

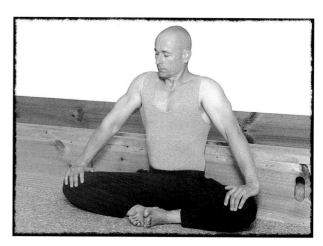

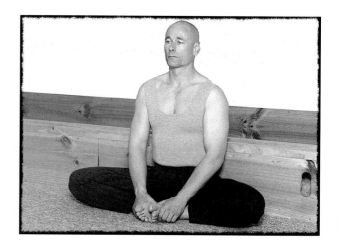

Cues

back against support
press knees to floor
C–R: lift knees against hands
restretch: press knees to floor

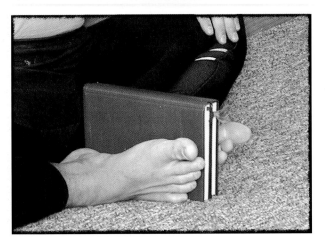

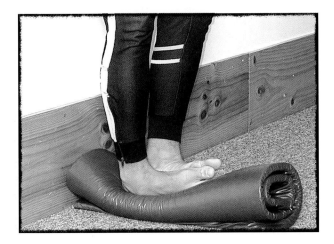

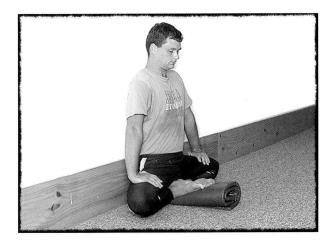

Cues

use object to widen foot position
use rolled mat to lift hips
C–R: lift knees to hands
restretch: press knees to floor

30. Wall seated knees apart

This is a standard in gymnastics, dance and yoga. The movement, in addition to stretching the adductors, is an effective stretch for the *pubofemoral ligaments*. Whereas the shoulder joint can become unstable if its ligaments are over-stretched, the hip joint is far more stable, and stretching these ligaments does not compromise the integrity of the joints. A partner version is shown later (exercise 61 partner wall seated knees apart).

In the dancers' version of this stretch, the knees are bounced up and down in the position shown in the first frame, on the facing page. This is adequate in a limbering class, as most of the dancers have perfect flexibility in this position, and the legs will go to the floor with ease. Bouncing the knees is an ineffective way to acquire this flexibility however. Using the **C–R** technique, your knees will be able to touch the floor in fairly short order.

Get into the position from above, rather than by trying to pull the feet close to you once you have sat down. To use this lowering technique, put the soles of the feet together a short distance from the wall (you do not want to sit *on* the feet), and carefully lower yourself to the floor. Get comfortable and place your hands on your knees, preferably with the arms straight, as I am showing in the photographs, opposite. Lift your shoulders up if necessary. If you cannot place your hands on your knees because the thighs are too high off the floor, hold your feet and press your elbows onto your thighs to achieve the stretch. Stay in this position until the muscles in between your legs relax a little.

A **C–R stretch** is very effective here, because the position is easy to hold, and supporting the contraction is simple. Holding the knees down with straight arms, lift the legs up to the hands reasonably strongly. The adductors are a large, strong group of muscles. Hold the contraction for a count of ten. Take a breath, stop lifting and, on a breath out, slowly press the knees down to the floor until you feel a sufficient stretch. Hold the final position for 10 breaths. To relieve the legs, let the stretch go, straighten the legs together out in front of you, and roll them in and out.

In the sequence on this page, Mark is demonstrating two assistance techniques. If you can get the legs to the floor easily (which is likely to be the case if the lower leg is relatively short compared with the upper leg, due to the reduced angle between the thighs as seen from above) you can make the stretch more effective by doing it in your shoes, or using a board or similar to increase the space between the feet. Doing the exercise this way widens the angle between the thighs. All **C–R stretch** directions for this variation remain the same.

If you can get the legs to the floor, but would like to go a little further, you may do the exercise with your bottom and your feet on a suitable support, as Mark is doing in the following two photographs, previous page. Fold a mat double or in three and sit on it. Now when you do the exercise the knees will be able to go lower than the hips and this affects the ligaments even more strongly. **C–R stretch** directions for this variation are the same, too. After doing this version, sitting on the floor with the legs in the final position will be no stretch at all. We will explore the next stage of the exercise in lesson 8.

31. Partner/solo kneeling knees apart

This exercise stretches the adductors in pure abduction *if* the lower back is held straight. Gravity works for you and your partner here too, making the final position effortless to hold. The stretch is intense, and seems to increase gradually once in the final position. It will help if you can organise your position so that the knees can slide apart easily—the movement is safe if you are sensible, as much of your weight will be supported by your arms and, if you feel the stretch is becoming too strong, you can use the arms to relieve the stretch instantly. I suggest a towel or similar under each knee and that you do the exercise on a shiny floor. Other approaches are to use a mat under each knee on a carpet floor, or to wear clothes that will slide on the floor of your exercise space. Julie is assisting Mark.

Get down on your hands and knees and spread the knees apart. Make sure that your hips are directly over your knees; most people will have the hips too far back. You want to stretch the hips in their *least* flexible position to affect the adductors precisely. To this end, ensure that you pull the stomach in, check that your lower back is straight (recall that hyperextension aids abduction). Have your partner kneel inside the line of your calf muscles, and ask them to use their knees to slowly spread your calf muscles apart. When you can go no further, hold the position for a few

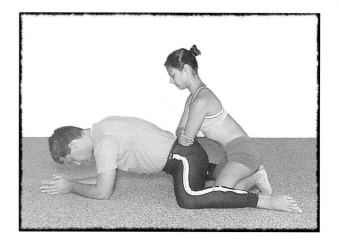

Cues

partner's weight directly above hips

keep lower back straight

C–R: squeeze knees together

restretch: let knees slide apart slowly

positions intensified if arms extended

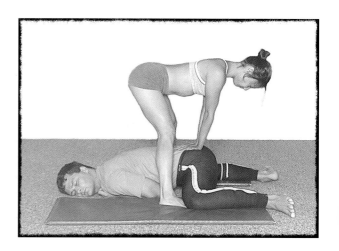

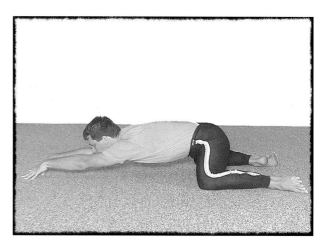

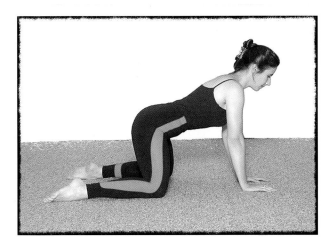

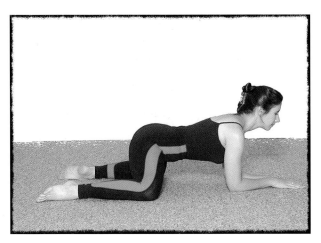

breaths. Ask your partner to place their hands midway between the buttocks, in line with the hip joints, and make sure that they do not place their weight too far towards the lumbar spine—in addition to being uncomfortable, weight there will only help the spine to hyperextend.

Now to the real stretch. The **C–R stretch** contraction to activate the adductors is simply to try to squeeze the knees together while your partner holds the hips down as described. Your partner will feel when you are contracting, as the hips will try to lift. If your partner is helping properly, this cannot happen. Contract the knees for a count of six to eight and then stop. Ask your partner to remove some of their assistance weight and, on a breath out, ask them to lean more weight, increasing the amount slowly until you feel enough stretch. Hold the final position for a ten-breath cycle. Your partner can lift you out of the end position by drawing your hips up away from the floor, or you can move the hips slowly forwards until you are in a lying position. Rest there for a moment to recover. A lower position is always possible with a second try so, after you help your partner, try again. Extending the arms in the final position makes the stretch stronger too.

This exercise can be done solo, as Jennifer is doing, but the effect is reduced. If you try it on your own, you can do a gentle contraction with your body's weight, the effect of which can be increased by extending your arms in the start position and resting your weight on your fingers instead of your elbows. Instead of doing the stretch only in the hips-above-knees position, you can develop a stronger stretch by first letting the hips go in front of the knees a little and getting into a stretch position and, once used to that, pushing your hips back to slightly *behind* the knees. This tightens the position considerably.

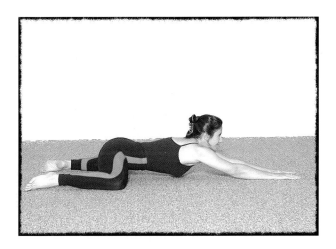

The last frame shows the slow, gentle way we suggest for getting out of the pose, by slowly drawing yourself forwards—the final position becomes intense, especially if you hold it for a while.

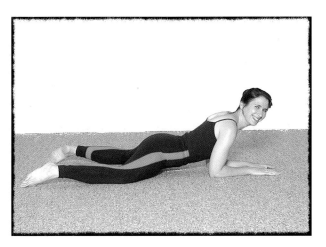

32. Partner/solo wall lying bent legs apart

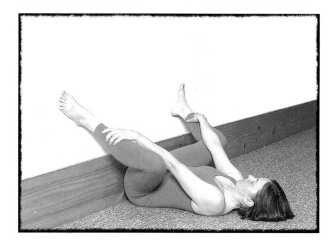

This can be an effective warm-up for the next exercise and is a good stretch for the adductors. Carol is lying on the floor, with her hips a little closer to the wall than her knees. She is pressing her knees to the floor. A **C–R stretch** is achieved by trying to squeeze the knees together against the resistance of the hands for a count of five to eight, then pressing the knees further apart on a breath out. A long stay in the final position (one to two minutes) is effective.

Carol and I are demonstrating the partner version, which is much stronger. In particular, the **C–R stretch** is easier to apply, and your partner can provide the restretching effect, too, if they are careful.

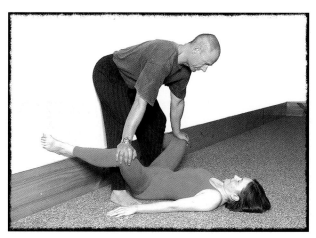

Notice that I am leaning on Carol's knees through straight arms; this kind of leaning force is tolerated far better than actively pushing with the arm muscles, as occurs when the arm is bent. When you lean, the weight of your body passes mainly through the bones and your partner will experience this as a stable force. When you push (in this example, you would use mainly the *triceps*, the muscles at the back of the upper arm) the muscles tire relatively quickly and they begin to shake. At first, this is imperceptible to you, but your partner's body can feel it and they will not be able to relax under this instability. In the class situation, we have tested the effects of these two ways of applying what may seem like identical force many times—and, even with eyes closed, the partner can distinguish easily between them. Always organise your assistance pressure as a leaning force.

In both the partner and solo versions, the stretch effect can be varied by trying the exercise with the hips closer to, or further away from, the wall. Make sure that the feet stay directly under the knees, or, putting it another way, the lower leg needs to be perpendicular to the wall no matter where the feet are placed. This will avoid strain on the knees.

Cues

feet on wall, under knees
ease knees apart (solo)
partner leans on knees
C–R: squeeze knees together
restretch: ask partner to press knees down to floor, gently

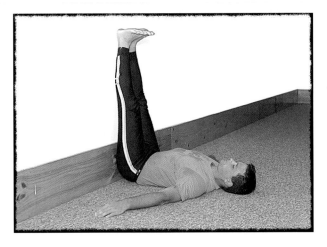

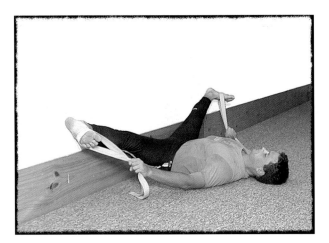

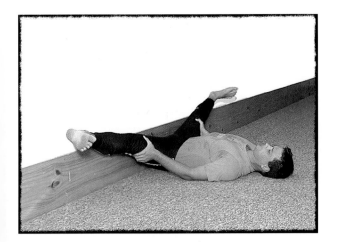

33. *Wall lying straight legs apart*

This is the easiest of the legs-apart stretches because you are lying throughout, and some people are surprised by its effectiveness. This is a useful solo exercise, too. Mark is demonstrating.

Lie with your legs reaching up the wall, and separate them. Straps may be used on each foot to increase the stretch, but most people find the weight of the legs alone is enough, providing you spend a few minutes in the position. Widen the leg position from time to time. Bring the legs together to rest for a moment, then repeat the stretch.

To make this a **C–R stretch**, hold the legs in the stretch position with your hands as you apply a light contraction for a count of ten. Stop, and, on a breath out, press the legs lower to the floor. Hold the end position for at least a minute. Many of our students hold the final position of this pose for five minutes or more—but I have often suspected that they are using this exercise as a rest instead of a stretch! Try it yourself and see what you think.

Cues

use straps if necessary

let legs go apart; let gravity work for you

C–R: try to bring legs together

restretch: gently widen legs

stay in final position for minutes

34. Wall seated straight legs apart

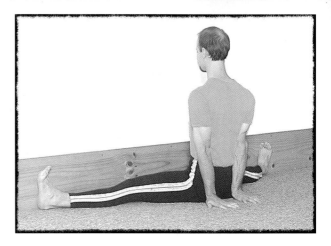

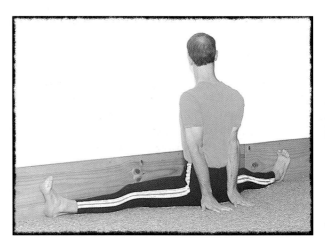

I prefer this movement to exercise 33 because I can apply more stretch effort and because the contractions can be done easily on your own. Look at the first photograph, where Kevin is demonstrating the start position.

Face the wall with the legs spread. Socks will help, as will a wall you can slide the feet apart on. Widen the legs and, with the hands on the floor behind you, push yourself slowly towards the wall until you cannot get the legs further apart. This is the start position, and you will need to hold it for half-a-minute to a minute to familiarise yourself with the sensations. You may feel the stretch anywhere from the groin to just below the knee, where a number of tendons join the bone (*gracilis* and *semitendinosus,* in particular).

The **C–R stretch** is obvious: while holding yourself in position with the hands behind the hips to stop yourself sliding away from the wall, try to draw the legs together, as if they could pass through the wall. Begin with a gentle contraction and, over a period of 10 seconds or so, slowly increase the effort. Do not increase the effort if this hurts the knees; this joint is not strong in relation to sideways (*lateral*) forces. Sometimes tightening the *quadriceps* at the same time as squeezing the legs together can overcome this sensation because tightening *quadriceps* locks the knee, tightens the ligaments, and makes the joint stronger against lateral forces. Relax, hold yourself in position, take in a deep breath and, on a breath out, carefully push the hips a little closer to the wall. Hold the final position for at least 10 breaths in and out.

Cues

feet point up
push hips to wall
C–R: squeeze legs together
restretch: use arms to push hips closer to wall
hold final position for minutes

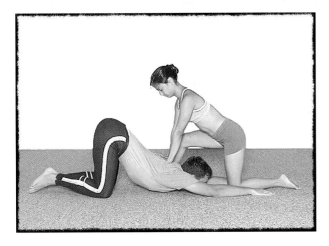

Cues

---

extend arms; let body go to floor

---

partner supports least flexible part

C–R: press hands into floor

---

restretch: partner gently helps
your chest move towards floor

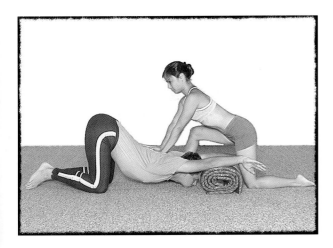

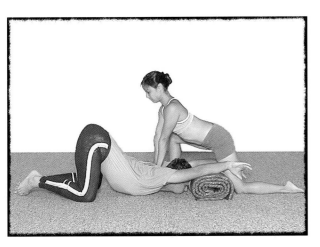

35. Partner floor middle and upper back bend

This technically simple exercise has many of the effects of exercise 14, wall middle and upper back backward bend, but for some people there will be less compression in the shoulders. The advantage of this stretch compared with exercise 14 is that your partner's assistance forces can be placed anywhere on the back, from high up between the shoulder blades (in which case the effects are felt in the upper back and the shoulders) all the way down to the lumbar spine. This pose has a tangible spine-lengthening effect and, when you stand up afterwards, you will feel and look taller.

The start position is on hands and knees. Position the hips over the knees (this is simply to get as much height in the hips as possible) and extend the arms out as far as you can. Lower the chest as close to the floor as possible. Stretch there for a moment; if you are already flexible, your own weight will straighten, then reverse, the normal forward curve in the middle back (*thoracic* spine). Ask your partner to kneel as shown and to locate the roundest part of your back. This will be the part of your spine that least wants to extend, and the part we will first concentrate upon. Ask you partner to lean their weight *at 90 degrees to the shape of that part of the back*, until you feel enough stretch.

The **C–R stretch** requires that you press your hands down into the floor with a moderate effort. This action will entail all the muscles that increase the forward curvature of the middle and upper back. Press for a count of ten, ask your partner to remove some weight (but to still keep you in position), relax and, on a long breath out, ask them to lean on you once more. Sink as low to the floor as you can.

If you are deep through the chest or flexible, your chest may contact the floor before enough extension is experienced. If so, roll a mat and place it under the elbows as shown. This will take some of the compression sensation from the shoulders for some people too, but the main usefulness lies in being able to experience a stronger bend backwards in the spine before anything touches the floor. It will remove the neck extension required as well, making it a more comfortable exercise for some.

Whichever arm position you use, the exercise can be altered in pleasing ways by asking your partner to change the lean contact position on your back. As they work their way along your back, their lean angle will need to alter also, so that it remains at roughly 90 degrees to the surface. If you have the time, small contractions can be done at any point in this movement. You will need to do exercise 1 to relax the muscles of the spine after you have come out of the final position. The top photograph shows a quick alternative recovery position: Mark is holding his knees and stretching by pulling gently on the arms and pushing the hips *back*. This will be detailed in exercise 43, folded legs clasped knees upper back, below. A second recovery movement is described here.

In any backward bending movement, it is normal (though undesirable) for the muscles on the *inside* of any curve being made by the body to tighten. If these happen to be back muscles, you may feel that there is a problem. A final way to release these muscles is shown.

Stand, put your hands together in front of you and let your chin move forwards as far as possible to your chest. Tighten the buttocks and make a small 'positive' thrust with the hips. Stop, and breathe in. On a breath out, while maintaining the position of the hips, slowly push the arms down the front of the body as far as you can, *without bending forwards at the waist*. It is essential to coordinate the movement with breathing out. This movement will round out the upper back, stretching the thoracic spine muscles as the last photograph shows and, when you stand up again, you will feel relaxed and taller than a moment ago. This minor exercise is useful for stretching many of the muscles across the upper back, too.

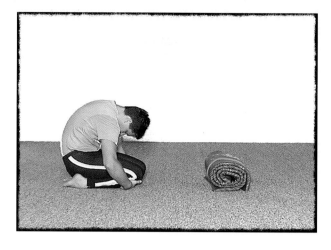

Cues (right)

bottom leg folded 90 degrees

lower trunk on bent arm

C–R: twist away from arm and leg

restretch: lower trunk closer to floor

Cues (this page, above)

chin to chest, and use arms to gently pull shoulders to thighs

Cues (this page, below)

chin to chest

push straight arms down body

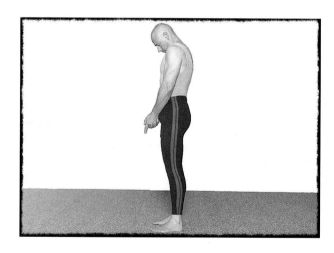

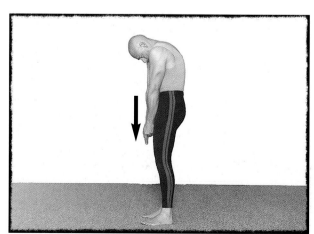

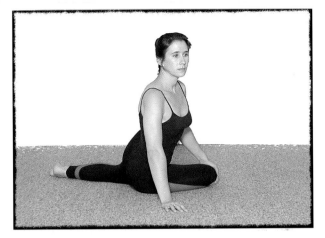

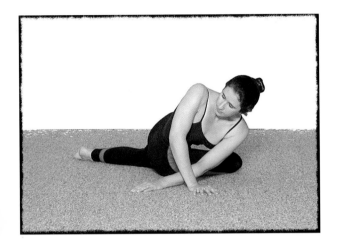

36. Partner/solo floor lying bottom leg folded rotation

This is a strong rotation movement in which the main locus of effect on the spine can be moved up and down by how you hold the shape of the spine. Too many muscles to mention are stretched in this movement and, in addition to the muscles, many layers of the *fascia* that separates muscle layers and that surrounds the abdominal cavity and the internal organs, are stretched too. Try this new exercise slowly and carefully; it is a very strong movement yet suitable for beginners and advanced students alike. The exercise is effective in solo and partner versions. The first solo version is shown by Jennifer.

Lie on your side, with the lowermost leg folded at about 90 degrees, as shown. Bend forwards, supporting yourself on one arm, bending it so that the palm bears down on the floor, with the elbow making a right angle as shown. Reach the other arm across in front of you and let the first arm bend, lowering the trunk towards the floor. This position may already be a good stretch. Using the supporting arm, lower your weight until your chest is near, or on, the floor. Slowly straighten your back, and feel the effect of the stretch change.

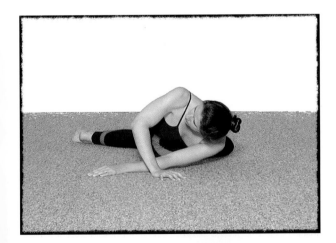

The **C–R stretch** here is to use the muscles of the waist to try to push the supporting arm into the floor (a counter-rotation) for a count of five to eight. Pause, relax, take in a breath (harder than usual, due to the restriction to rib cage movements imposed by the position) and, on a breath out, push the *top* shoulder further away from the floor. Hold the end position for five to ten breaths in and out. If you can, reach the other arm through under yourself too, as far as you can. This will tighten the stretch further. If you are very flexible, you may be able to get the back of the front shoulder on the ground.

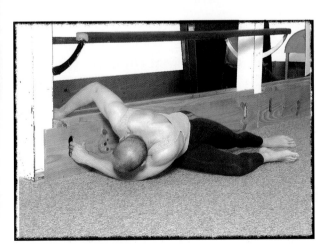

Alternatively, you can reach through to a suitable support, as I am demonstrating, hang from the bottom arm and push back with the top arm. The **C–R stretch** is to try to pull back from the support while holding yourself in position. Once in position, you may experiment by curling the trunk forwards slightly and adjusting the stretch, or by arching the back backwards. These slight movements change the focus of the stretch. After a rest, do the other side. Some people will feel the effect of this stretch in the hip muscles of the

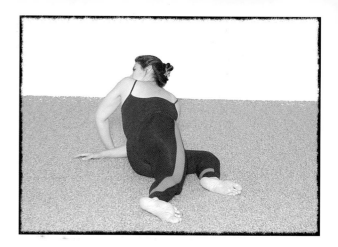

lower leg too. If this is what you feel, you can feel an excellent stretch by trying to emphasise moving the top hip across further in the stretch direction, even if the chest is quite a way off the floor.

Jennifer and Julie are demonstrating the easiest of the partner versions in the third photograph. The partner version can be applied in intensities varying from gentle to strong. In the **C–R** contraction, Jennifer pushes her shoulder back to Julie and, in the restretch, Julie helps her move her arm further though under her body.

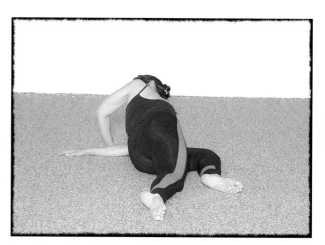

Pay attention to the details of the support positions of the intermediate version, shown on the facing page. The forearms need to be touching; otherwise the shoulders of the person being stretched will rotate away as the spine bends to the side away from the stretch. Julie is bracing Jennifer's elbow with her hand in the second photograph, in addition to providing foot support for the forearm, and is using her other hand to draw the arm under her body. The **C–R stretch** requires you to try to pull the arm gently back, away from your partner. Contract for a count of five to eight and, on a long breath out, ask your partner to slowly increase the pull on the arm until the desired stretch is felt. Remain in the final position for five breaths.

To finish the lesson, repeat the following exercises from lessons 1 and 2. Begin all exercises with your tighter side, do the looser side, and finish with the tighter side once more if there is a large variation in the comparative flexibilities.

Exercise 12, Partner arm up behind shoulder blade

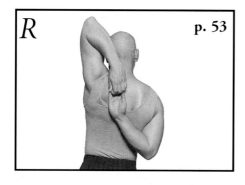

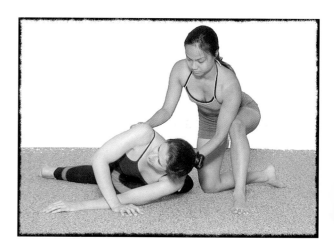

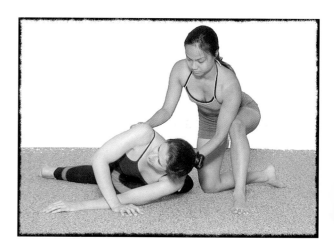

I am demonstrating the solo, compound version of this exercise but any of the variations may be used. The purpose of the movement is to feel the right sort of stretch effect in the muscles you need to stretch, rather than making a particular shape with your body.

Cues

partner helps bottom shoulder through

partner helps top shoulder back

C–R: rotate back against partner

restretch: partner helps improve position

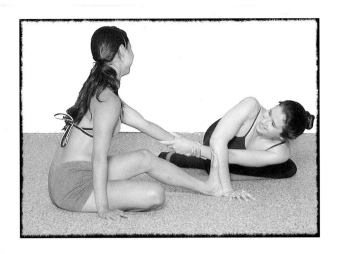

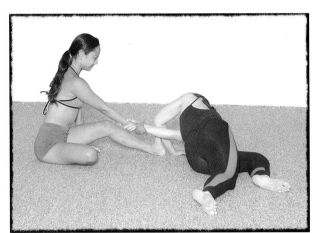

Cues

partner's foot against your forearm

hands held in trapeze grip

C–R: pull back against support

restretch: partner draws arm through

Exercise 7, Neck side bend

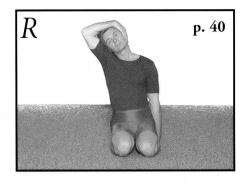

R   p. 40

Exercise 11, Partner arms up behind back

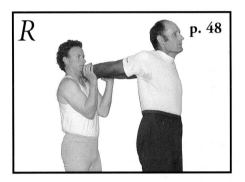

R   p. 48

Exercise 9, Arm across body; do either the standing or lying version

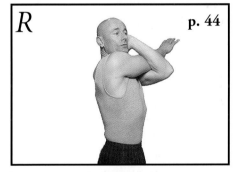

R   p. 44

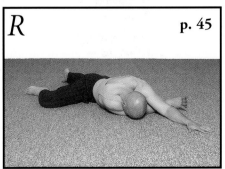

R   p. 45

LESSON SIX: HIP FLEXORS, BACK BEND AND ROTATION

Most of the exercises in this lesson contribute to bending the body backwards. Experience has shown that the hip flexors are a tight muscle group in most people and particularly among athletes. Keeping the hip flexors loose will help the spine to attain a shape that requires the least amount of energy to support, and general movement will become more graceful. The illustration shows the effects tight hip flexors have on the shape of all parts of the spine.

37. Abdominal curls over support

This is a much stronger version of exercise 16, the floor abdominal curl. We feel that this version is a must for recreational athletes (squash, tennis, and golf players, in particular) because their sporting activities require the strength of the abdominal muscles to be exerted in ranges of movement outside those of normal daily life. No single abdominal exercise can work these muscles through their entire range, so we will need to use at least two; one to work them in the range from from normal-to-contracted (exercise 16), and another to work them from stretched-to-normal length (exercise 37).

To work the abdominal muscles in the stretched-to-normal range, we need some kind of support. A curved surface is best. In the beginning, I prefer to work from a stable surface to develop the necessary coordination but, later, working on an unstable surface can be to your advantage, because ancillary muscles are required to stabilise the trunk to enable the abdominal muscles to contract effectively. As a functional group, these are often called stabiliser muscles. To begin, you may use the curved end of a heavy couch, mats tightly rolled and tied to the required radius, or even a bench over which you put additional padding—any surface over which you can stretch backwards. Jennifer is demonstrating the movement over one of our drums.

Start by letting yourself go backwards over the support. Aim to have the lower ribs over the highest part of the support. Let yourself relax backwards to stretch the muscles. Now place your fingers next to your temples and begin to curl the body forwards *slowly* (recall that momentum will defeat this exercise entirely). The head will move first, followed by the

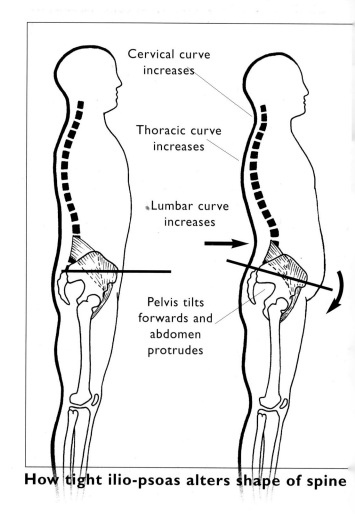

How tight ilio-psoas alters shape of spine

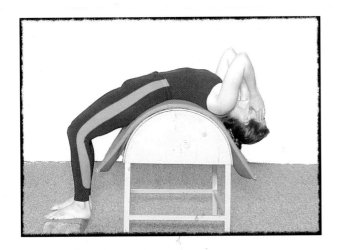

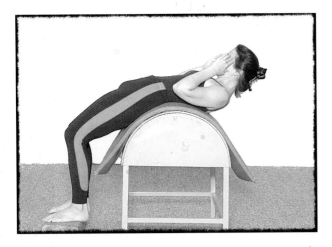

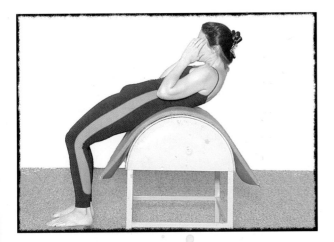

neck, then the chest and ribs and, last, the ribs will be drawn to the pubic bone. You naturally will find yourself breathing out in this phase. You will feel the lower back being pressed increasingly firmly onto the surface of the support. Once you have curled the body to an approximately straight, or slightly curved forwards position, stop and count to two. As you slowly lower yourself to the starting position, breathe in while the ribs are stretched open. Try to do 10 slow repetitions, then roll sideways off the support. This will do for today but, as the muscles become conditioned, you will move from the support to the floor, where you will immediately do 10 repetitions of exercise 16, floor abdominal curl. In this way, you will be doing a long set comprising the two different movements.

Do not do too many repetitions of exercise 37 the first time. Much of the soreness you will feel the next day is simply from working the abdominal muscles in an unfamiliar range and you do not want to compound that with the soreness of going all out. Take your time.

As before with exercise 16, you may find that the neck muscles tire first, whereas the abdominal muscles have done hardly any work. If this happens to you, do the exercise as described and, as soon as the neck muscles fatigue, use your hands to help yourself lift the head in the first part of the movement —but do not let them do all the work. In this way, the neck muscles will strengthen and, as a result, your abdominal workouts will become more intense.

Cues

stretch back over support; relax

lift head on breath out

slowly curl trunk

keep lower back on support

breathe in as you go backwards

38. Lying rotations

Like exercise 37, this exercise has both stretching and strengthening components too. It strengthens all the trunk muscles, including the oblique group and *quadratus lumborum*, and it also teaches you how to coordinate the nervous and muscular systems to a specific task, which is related to maintaining a strong and efficient posture. A moment's reflection will reveal that most activities require the body to transfer the strength of the legs to the arms or vice versa, and this can only occur through a strong trunk. Unfortunately, the majority of personal training programs only prescribe a few sit-up movements for this area of the body and generally these are done at the end of a workout when you are already tired, and so they are not particularly effective. This exercise is an excellent warm-up for the trunk in addition to being an effective strengthening movement, and the only equipment required is your own body.

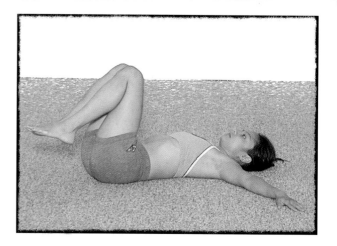

The exercise is shown in three stages. Lie down and flex the hips and knees as Julie is showing. Crossing the ankles will help to keep the legs together. Have your arms out to the sides, *palms facing the floor*; this will help you keep the shoulders flat. Now lift the knees about halfway to the chest (thighs about 45 degrees to the floor) and slowly lower the legs to one side so that the knees end up *pointing at one of your hands*. This direction is essential, for the same reason we tuck the opposite hip under the body in exercise 3, the lying rotation: *to keep the spine straight as seen from above.* This will distribute the rotation task over much of the spine, whereas if you lower the legs out to the side (so that the thighs make a 90 degree angle with the trunk) most of the rotation will be experienced in the lumbar vertebrae, which may be uncomfortable. This would also limit the stretching and strengthening effect of the exercise to one part of the spine but, if done as suggested, you would feel the effects up into the middle and upper back.

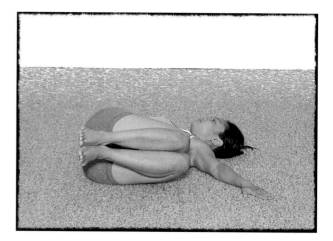

Once the legs are just touching the floor, pause for a count of two (do not rest the legs on the floor) and breathe in. On a breath out, slowly lift the knees until they are back over the centre-line of the body. Breathe in again and, as you lower the legs to the other side, breathe out. Repeat eight to ten times.

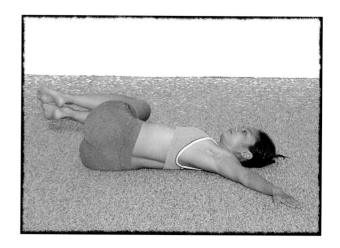

Cues

press hands on floor

lower legs to side

ensure knees point to hand

on breath out; slowly lift legs

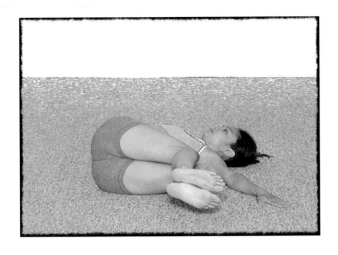

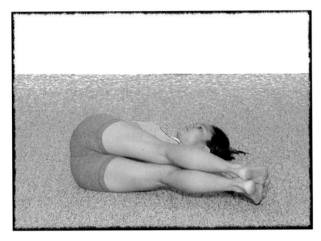

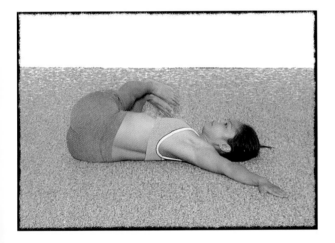

Once you can do 15 repetitions of the legs-folded version, you may increase the resistance by extending the legs until the knees make a 90 degree angle, as shown in the top photograph on this page. This increases the apparent weight of the legs considerably. Next time you try the movement, use this new leg position. For safe and rapid strength increases, the resistance you use should permit a minimum of six and a maximum of 15 repetitions. Adjust the resistance to fit these limits.

The last two frames show the most difficult version, in which the legs are straight. Be aware that this requires a strong trunk, so do not be in too much of a hurry to use this form. Most people will cheat shamelessly in this version of the movement by jerking their legs off the floor with a sudden action. This is not only potentially dangerous (demanding exertion from muscles in an extreme extended range of movement is far and away the most common cause of muscle pulls), but you will forfeit the strengthening aspect almost entirely. For this exercise to be effective, the lifting action must be smooth and continuous, and should look effortless. This will take a while.

Note if there is a tighter or weaker side in the movement and, if you prefer, you can do all repetitions for that side as one set first. Do as many repetitions as you can for this side and, on a second set, only do that many for the looser or stronger side. The general rule is that, because the weaker or stronger side is stressed more strongly, it will adapt more quickly. In this way any flexibility or strength imbalances will be redressed, in time.

Cues

press hands on floor

extend legs to increase resistance

lower legs to side

slowly lift from floor

breathe in as legs cross centre-line

Exercise 4, Side bend; standing or hanging versions

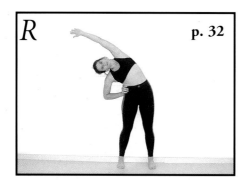

Cues (standing)

ensure bottom hand supports

extend top arm

roll top shoulder forwards

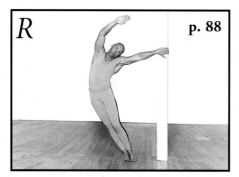

Cues (hanging)

stand inside line of shoulder

let hips move to side

reach out top arm

roll hips to move stretch

Try either of these movements again and see how much further you can go now that the trunk is warmed up. Do not forget to support yourself fully on one hand if doing the standing version.

Exercise 27, Backward bend over support

This movement, too, will be improved for the same reason.

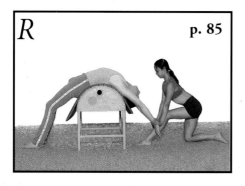

Cues

let yourself be stretched

extend arms off body

partner presses hands to floor

C–R: press hands to ceiling

restretch: partner eases hands to floor

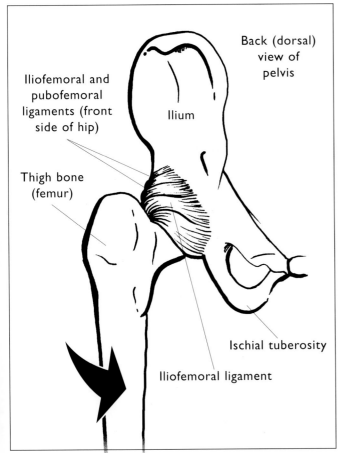

Iliofemoral and pubofemoral ligaments (front side of hip)

Back (dorsal) view of pelvis

Ilium

Thigh bone (femur)

Ischial tuberosity

Iliofemoral ligament

As leg extends, hip joint ligaments tighten around neck of femur

39. Partner hip flexor

Technically, and from the perspective of required strength, this precise hip flexor stretch is difficult. Few other exercises will target this problem area as effectively, however, so it is worth a try. The essence of good form is a vertical trunk and square hips, with the abdominal brace applied (or bottom tucked under). This is because the body is expert at avoiding stress or discomfort—and failing to observe any of these requirements will render the exercise ineffective.

As mentioned above, a number of constraints must be observed. In the chain of muscles that limit movements of the leg backwards in relation to the trunk, the hip flexors (*ilio-psoas*) are primary, and a number of the thigh muscles (*rectus femoris, sartorius* and other muscles with lesser influence) are secondary. Recall that fibres of *ilio-psoas* attach to the spine itself, as high as the 12th thoracic vertebra. Rarely mentioned, however, are the powerful ligaments of the hip joint itself: two on the front side of the hip (the *iliofemoral and pubofemoral* ligaments) and one behind (the *ischiofemoral* ligament). It is significant that in the standing position these ligaments are already wound around the hip joint and are under moderate tension; conversely, in the on-all-fours position, all three ligaments are relaxed. When the leg is extended (taken backwards past the standing position), these ligaments are tightly wound around the hip, with the *iliofemoral* ligament under the greatest tension. See the illustration. Accordingly, if we desire increased extension at the hip (essential for sitting in the front-splits position, for example) we will need to position the body so as to stress this area accurately. The body avoids stretching this region by three mechanisms: by inclining the trunk forwards to the legs (hence bringing one end of *ilio-psoas* closer to the femur and losing the stretch); by allowing the hip of the back leg to rotate away from the stretch (hence transferring the stretch to the adductors if enough rotation occurs); or by allowing the spine to hyperextend (in this case, the pelvis is allowed to roll forwards, and a potential stretching force bends the spine backwards instead of stretching the desired areas). None of these ploys is exclusive, and one often sees all three being used at once.

Kneel on the floor next to a support as shown, with the legs a little apart for lateral stability, as Jennifer is demonstrating. Your back leg is next to the support and that side's arm is holding the support; your foot will need to be a little in front of the front leg's knee and your hand on the knee ready to apply the abdominal brace. Your partner will be kneeling behind you in a low position, so that they may provide a counter-rotation for your hips. Look at the first photograph carefully. The partner holds the hip bone of the front leg, and places the other hand *under* the buttock on the back leg, as Olivia is doing. This latter direction is not for reasons of propriety; if you support the back of the hip at waist level, for example, your counter-rotating force will only make the back bend backwards more strongly, which we want to avoid. If you apply your force *under* the hip joint, all this effort will be transferred to the joint itself and the back leg will extend. Ask your partner to rotate your hips at least square and, if you are flexible, over square.

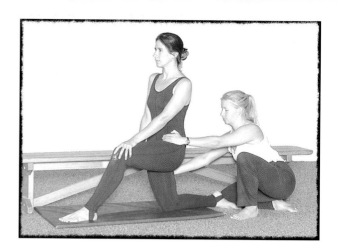

Ensure that your trunk is vertical and that the supporting arm on the front leg is straight, and is held that way throughout. To avoid the lower back bending backwards, either apply the abdominal brace by pressing this arm firmly down on the knee (you will feel the abdominal muscles tighten) or use the buttocks to tuck your bottom under (a 'positive' thrust). Either technique should result in a stretch sensation being produced in the front of the hip.

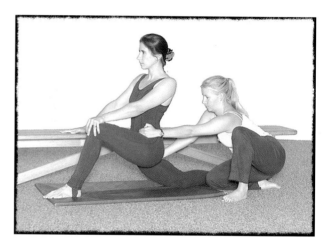

Now your partner leans on you while maintaining the rotation of the hips, so that you travel forwards with respect to the back leg. This is the start position and is already a good stretch. To alter your present pattern of flexibility, a **C–R stretch** will be necessary. The contraction is produced by *trying to drag the back knee forwards* while your partner holds you in position. If done properly, this will produce contraction sensations in the front of the hip. Of course, the leg does not actually move and the contraction is the same as always: done properly, it produces a sensation in the desired muscle, but no movement. Hold this contraction for a count of 10 and then stop.

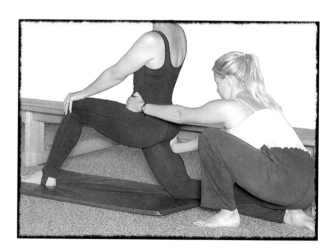

Your partner keeps you in position while you breathe in. On a breath out, check whether either brace is still being applied and ask your partner to lean more weight on the back leg's hip, maintaining the counter-rotation all the while. Let your hips move forwards further (thus taking the back leg further into extension) and hold the end position for a ten-breath

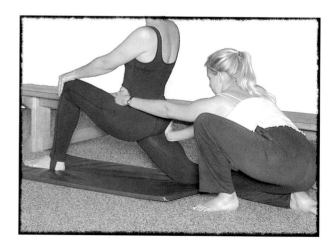

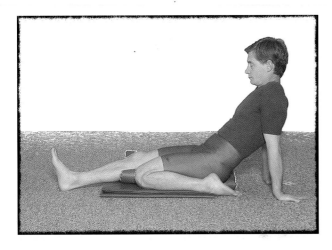

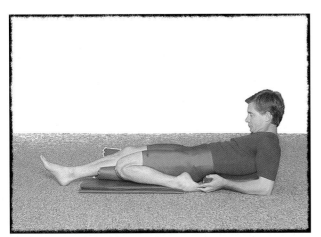

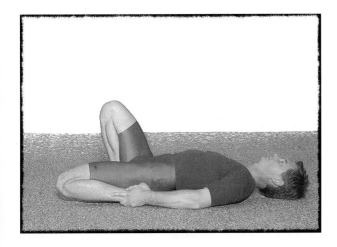

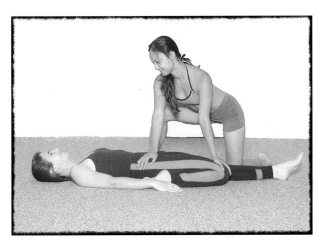

cycle. Do both sides, and remember which is the tighter. Do the tighter side once more.

40. Partner seated/lying single leg quadriceps

Review the instructions for exercise 26, seated/lying single leg *quadriceps*, as your start position and way of getting into this pose is the same. Once you are in your final position, ask your partner to hold the hip and knee of the leg being stretched, as Jennifer and Julie are showing in the last photograph. Once held, curl your trunk forwards—this will increase the stretch considerably, whichever position you are in.

Now two **C–R stretches** may be applied: the first is to try to lift the held knee from the floor (this will engage the hip flexors in addition to the *quadriceps*), and the second is to try to straighten the leg. You may do each **C–R** by itself and restretch, or do both and restretch. Compare the flexibility of each leg and stretch the tighter leg a second time.

In addition to adopting a stronger stretch position (from a reclining to a lying position, for example) your partner can help you roll your hips further backwards, so the lower back is pressed more firmly onto the floor, by leaning more weight on the hip. Do not sacrifice the neutral lower back shape just to be able to lie back on the floor—so doing will make your back sore and will not increase the stretch in the thigh. Getting the stretch in the right place is paramount.

Cues (left page)
front foot in front of knee
partner holds hip of front leg, and supports under bottom of back leg
move forwards into stretch position
C–R: drag back knee forwards
restretch: partner moves you forward

Cues (this page)
hips level; abdominals tight
partner holds hip and knee
C–R: try to straighten leg
restretch: move further into stretch

41. Partner standing suspended hip flexor, with support

Review all directions for exercise 25, standing suspended hip flexor, as this exercise is essentially the same, except your partner is going to hold your hips square for even greater effect. Two support positions are shown, the second being particularly effective if the hip flexors are tight.

Assuming that you are in the start position of exercise 25 (top photograph), your partner holds you by the hip bone and below the buttock as in exercise 39, above, as Olivia and Jennifer are demonstrating. Now slowly try to straighten your back leg as before, maintaining the vertical trunk and neutral lower-back position (using the abdominal brace is best here). The emphasis here is to keep the hips square during the leg-straightening phase. The first **C–R stretch** is to try to pull the whole back leg forward against your partner's resistance. Your partner, perhaps surprisingly, will find it much easier to hold your hips square in this exercise than in exercise 39, because of leverage advantages (the hip flexors are required to try to move the whole leg, rather than the thigh alone, in this exercise). After the contraction, let your back leg bend and lower both hips closer to the floor. The stretch is then achieved by again trying to straighten the leg from this lower position. This is a very strong stretch and the most effective of all the hip flexor movements. It is also an excellent stretch for the upper *quadriceps*.

Now the partner moves their hands to the positions used by Kevin in the bottom photograph. In contrast to the hand-support position just described, in this version the **C–R stretch** is to try to pull the back *knee* forwards. Because you can feel your partner's hand on your knee, the contraction direction is easily understood. The restretch and final position directions are as described above; only the **C–R** support position is different.

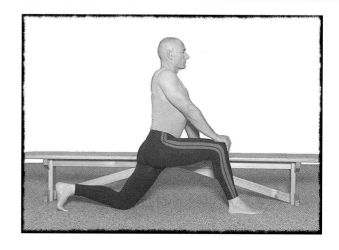

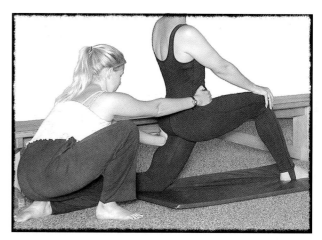

Cues

two support positions:

front hip and under buttock of back leg or under buttock of back leg and knee

C–R: draw back leg knee forwards

restretch: try to straighten leg

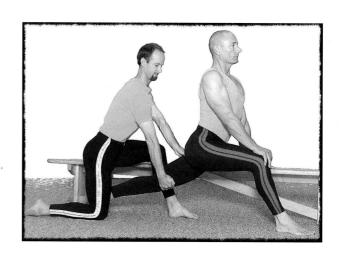

Cues (right)

ensure back muscles stay relaxed

lift only with arms

curl up to finish

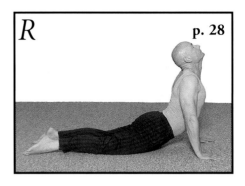

R   p. 28

Try either the floor or suspended version of exercise 2, again. As we have stretched *quadriceps* and the hip flexors, you will be able to bend backwards rather more easily than before.

A support may be used to great effect in a variation of the backward bend. In the photograph, I am hanging from a bar, letting gravity pull me to the floor. My position creates a traction effect on the shoulders and the location of the maximum stretch is higher than either version of the floor backward bend. To tighten the position, use your toes to move the hips closer to being under the support. In time, you will be able to hang with the arms vertical. Because the hips are drawn down from the shoulders, there is a pleasing effect throughout the entire trunk.

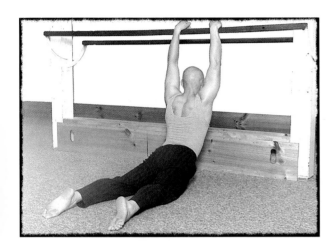

Cues (above)

let yourself hang from support

use feet to bring hips forwards

breathe and relax completely

Exercise 27, Partner backward bend over support

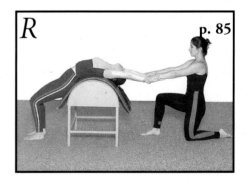

R   p. 85

Continuing the backward bending theme, do exercise 27 again. Here, *let* yourself be stretched; too many students try to force themselves to become flexible—if this were possible, many more men would be flexible than is the case. Breathe and let yourself relax.

Cues (right)

extend arms off body

partner presses hands to floor

C–R: press hands to ceiling

restretch: partner presses hands down

42. Floor feet held back bend

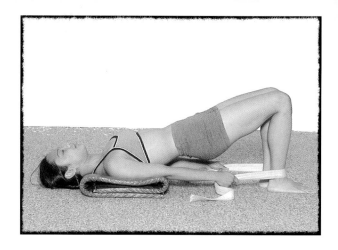

The ease of doing the final backward bend in this lesson depends more on one's proportions than many of our exercises, so give it a try and see if it suits you. This exercise is also a strong *forward* bend for the neck, so if your neck is tight you may care to put a mat under your shoulders to reduce the angle of the neck's final position, as Julie is doing.

Lie on your back with the legs bent, as shown. Reach down one side and grasp an ankle; then reach down and hold the other. I suggest a hook grip—wrap as much of the fingers around the ankle as possible and leave the thumb alongside the index finger. For most people, this unfamiliar grip will provide a stronger hold. Alternatively, a strap may be used.

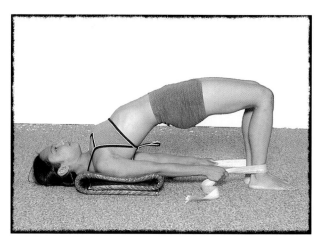

Check your grip and push the hips up to the ceiling using the buttock muscles. This is the second position; hold this for a breath or two to get used to the sensations. Now slowly *try to straighten both legs.* This action will pull you into a bow-like shape: the whole front of the body will be stretched. The most common mistake is to try to arch yourself backwards with the back muscles, but this is unnecessary. Try to keep the back muscles relaxed and use the large muscles of the thighs to do the work.

Use one of the standard recovery movements that stretch the spine forwards (exercise 1, or the last photograph of exercise 2).

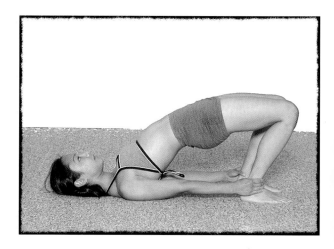

Exercise 36, Partner/solo floor lying bottom leg folded rotation

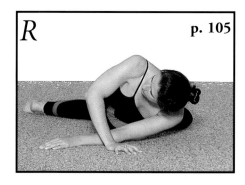

R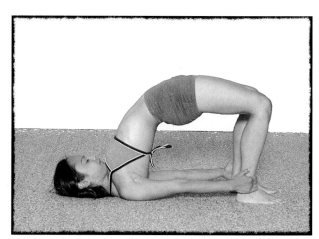

p. 105

Try this exercise again; with what we have done since, you should find that you can go further this time. All the rotation exercises can also be used as recovery poses for strong backward bends.

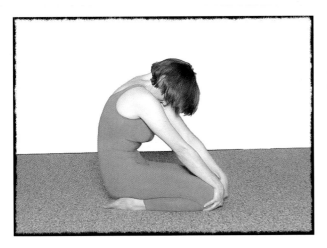

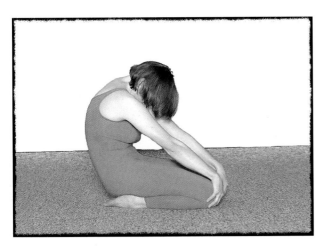

43. Folded legs clasped knees upper back

This is what we term a minor pose, but it can be wonderful for some people (and a strong stretch)—it all depends on where you hold the most tension in your body. This movement stretches all of the muscles that extend the middle and upper back (usually grouped and termed the paravertebrals), the muscles that pull the shoulder blades together (*rhomboideus major* and *minor*), and a number of smaller muscle groups. A stronger version follows.

Kneel as shown (this may be done from the front of a chair or a bench if you wish) and hold your knees with both hands. Now tighten the abdominal muscles and push the hips backwards—a strong stretch for the middle and upper back will result. To make it stronger, pull the shoulders towards the knees by pulling gently with the arms.

You may also try a moderate rotation of the shoulders once in the final position (this is wonderful after hours of typing at the computer), which will move the stretch further down the back on each side.

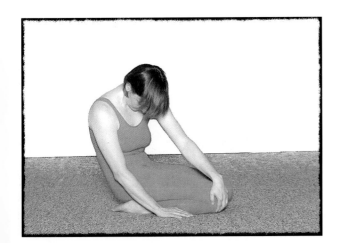

Cues (left page)

hold ankles with hands or strap

push hips to ceiling

try to straighten legs

curl up to finish

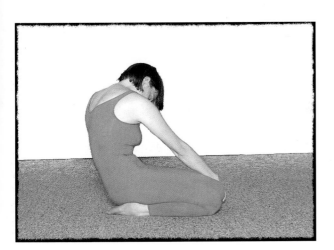

Cues (this page)

chin on chest; let trunk slump

push middle back backwards

pull with arms

rotate at waist to move stretch

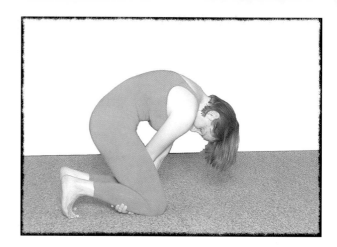

The stronger version can be done only from the floor: hold the legs as shown and, using the bottom and thigh muscles, lift the hips until the stretch is felt in the middle and upper back. Slightly increasing the pull on one arm at a time will induce a small rotation and will move the stretch around the middle and upper back accordingly. Carol is holding her shins from inside the legs, each hand grasping the opposite leg, but the stretch can be done by holding the outside of the legs directly, too (left arm holds left shin and vice versa). Experiment to find the version you prefer.

In this stronger version too, a small rotation may be added to the hip and arm actions to move the stretch further around the back. In the third photograph, Carol has added a rotation and sideways bend to the basic movements. Experiment to find the most pleasing stretch positions. The last photograph shows the details of the holding position.

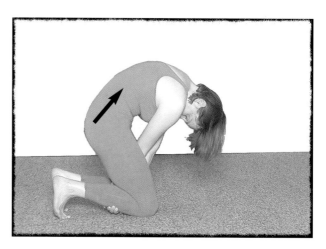

Cues

hold opposite shin through legs

while holding, left hips up and forwards

incline trunk left and right
to move stretch from side to side

push forwards in neutral position

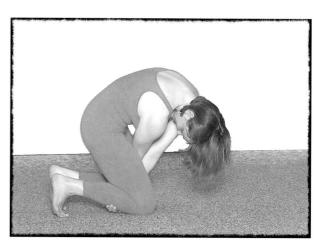

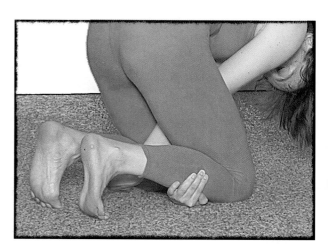

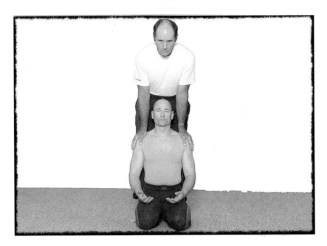

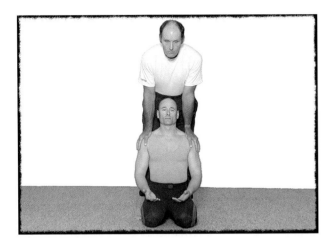

Cues

lean back slightly against partner

palms up on lap

partner leans weight on shoulders

C–R: lift against unmoving resistance

restretch: partner eases shoulders to floor

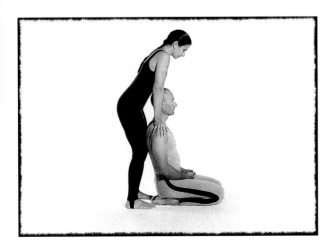

44. Partner shoulder depress

This exercise is one of the most popular in the *Posture & Flexibility* classes because it always makes the students feel good, and they have found it excellent to do with their partners at home, too. It stretches the upper fibres of the large muscle spanning the neck and shoulders (*trapezius*) and *levator scapulae,* as well as many neck muscles. See the illustration overleaf for details. It is also a mild stretch for the *scalenus* group, tightness in which can lead to shoulder, arm and hand pain. Having this stretch done to you immediately makes you feel lighter and more relaxed, as your body's primary reaction to frustration, anger, resentment (and stress more generally) is to tighten these very muscles. The hunched shoulder pattern of tension is characteristic of both aggression and fear. Accordingly, combining exercise 44 with any of the trunk backward-bending movements can be an effective physical approach to altering these states.

Many seating positions are suitable: cross-legged, sitting on the legs, or sitting on a bench or chair. If you and your partner use a chair, make sure that it cannot roll away from you. In all support positions, ask your partner to stand close, with a space between you, as shown in the bottom photograph. Lean back slightly from your upright balanced position, so that the middle of your back is supported (either by your partner's legs or the back of the chair). If you do not lean back slightly, your back will bend forwards when your partner leans on you.

Ask your partner to place their hands on your shoulders, with the fingers out to the sides, lightly cupping the shoulders with the whole hand. Your partner will need to *lean* on you, not push (the sensations of these two actions are completely different from the receiver's perspective, as a moment's experimentation will reveal) and, consequently, your partner's arms need to be straight. After you get used to the sensation, ask your partner to hold your shoulders in the stretch position for the **C–R stretch.** Lift your shoulders *gently* against your partner's resistance—they will have to lean harder during this phase—and then stop; of course as you stop they must reduce their leaning somewhat. Pause, take in a deep breath and, as you breathe out, your partner should lean more weight on you. If your partner watches your chest from above, and concentrates on when you are lifting and when you are relaxing, the exercise is technically simple.

Do not lift with so much effort that your partner cannot hold you in position. For leverage reasons, these relatively small muscles are extremely strong. *Trapezius* and *levator scapulae* enjoy enormous leverage, as their combined contraction forces pivot the shoulder girdle on the *sternoclavicular* joint; together they form a *class II* lever (see the illustration), where the effort and load are almost coincident, and the fulcrum is at the end of the lever. What this means is that the muscles lifting the shoulders are incredibly strong in absolute terms (but the load is not moved very far—compare with either *biceps*) and everyone will be strong enough to lift their partner off the ground in the movement. Accordingly, lift gently, so that your partner can hold the shoulders down. When you stop lifting, do it relatively slowly, so they can adjust their leaning weight. Hold the end position for five breaths in and out or longer, and be aware that, even if you think that you have relaxed your shoulders maximally, they will still drop a little further *if you let them*.

Do the following two exercises again.

Exercise 7, Neck side bend

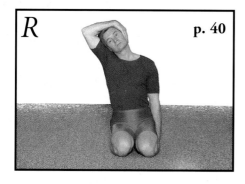

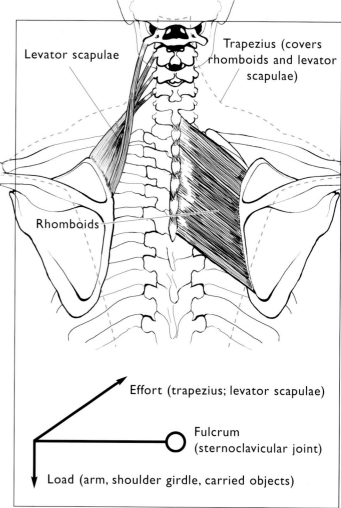

Levator scapulae details and Class II lever

Cues
restrain shoulder and lean away
C–Rs: lift shoulder, and press head to hand
restretch: lean and take head further to side

Exercise 6, Chin to chest

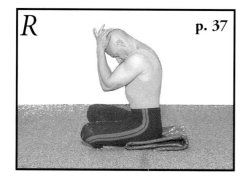

Cues
chin to chest
fingers behind back of head
C–R: press head to fingers
restretch: gently pull head forwards

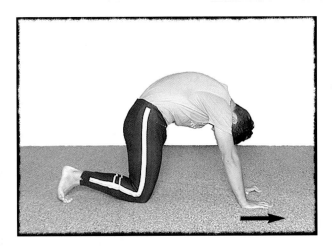

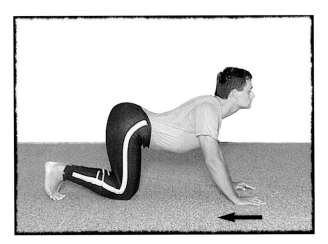

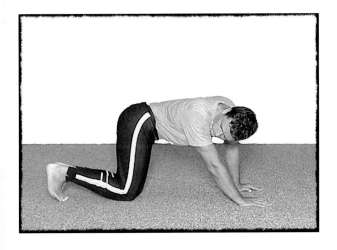

45. Upper back on all fours

This a minor pose which can have a pleasant recovery effect when done after strong forward or backward bending movements. This simple series of movements can be made surprisingly strong with the addition of two **C–R stretches**.

Begin by resting on the floor on your hands and knees; you may wish to have a mat under the knees for comfort. Ensure that your hands are directly under, or slightly in front of, the shoulders, and that the knees are under the hips. Let the head and neck hang down to a comfortable position and contract the abdominal muscles until your trunk is tightly curled; this action stretches the muscles along the back. Hold this position for a couple of breaths in and out. Then relax the body and let it return to the neutral position. Next, arch the back backwards, beginning with the neck. You will feel all the muscles (that act to extend the spine) contract, from neck to sacrum. Hold the arched position for a couple of breaths—breathing will be slightly laboured as with all backward bends. Return to the start position. Once the spine is straight, bend to one side as far as you can and look at one heel. You will feel all the muscles on one side contract; this stretches the opposite side's pairs of muscles. After a breath or two, return to the neutral position and bend to the other side. Bend briefly to the first side to finish.

C–R stretches may be added to the forward and backward components of this movement in the following way. In the curled position, push on your hands as though you were trying to slide the hands away from you (friction keeps them in place). This action increases the stretch in the middle of the spine considerably. When in the back-arching position, try to *pull* the hands back towards you; this action will engage *latissimus dorsi* and other muscles, and their combined action will increase the backward bend appreciably. So that the body feels relaxed after doing these stronger movements, finish the exercise with a gentle curl forwards.

Cues

curl forwards; push hands away

arch backwards; pull hands towards you

return to neutral position

look to heels on both sides

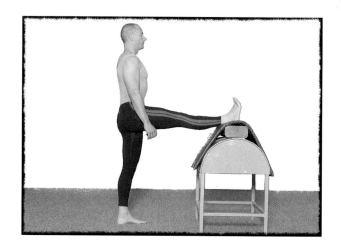

LESSON SEVEN: HAMSTRINGS, HIP FLEXORS AND PARTIAL FRONT SPLITS

This lesson is shorter than the ones preceding, but it is a very strong lesson nonetheless. You may be surprised to be exposed to front splits at this half-way point, but we have had a great many people with only average flexibility tell us that they had their best-ever stretch in the hamstrings in trying this. Because the front-splits exercise is intense and has a number of parts, I feel that devoting some time to it is time well spent.

It will be obvious to anyone who watches dance or gymnastics carefully that the front-splits position is usually achieved by a measure of turnout of the back leg, by considerable hyperextension of the lumbar spine, or by having the hips aligned at less that a 90 degree angle with the line of the legs. The reasons were canvassed in exercise 39, partner hip flexor. Those of you who have tried to sit in front splits will know that there is an intense stretch in the hamstrings of the front leg. What most people do not realise is that the stretch occurs because the *back* leg is insufficiently flexible in extension. Look at the photograph. Many people are loose enough to be able to bend the front leg at 90 degrees at the hip, as I am showing. However, only a tiny percentage of people can allow the back leg to extend the same amount—because of this, as the leg extends, it takes the pelvis with it as well as the hamstring attachment points (the *ischial tuberosity*). Accordingly, the hamstring muscles are stretched way beyond the 90 degrees mentioned above. By working on the back leg, much of the stretch on the hamstrings can be reduced and, for those of you who are loose enough to sit in the position, your alignment will be enhanced considerably.

Cues (right page)

heels on floor

squat rhythmically

pause in bottom position, then

rise until hips just below knees; pause

lift higher; hips just above knees

pause 30 seconds; stand

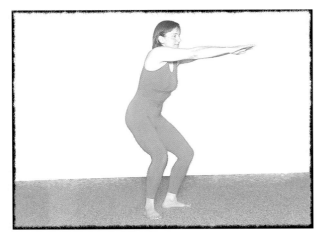

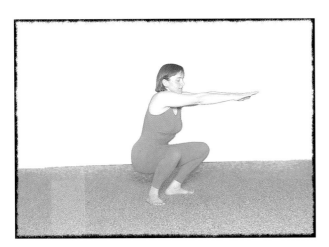

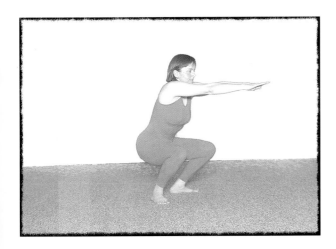

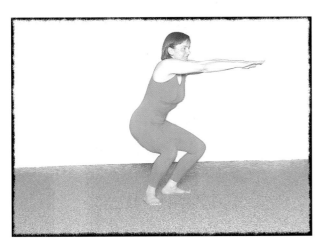

Free squats warm-up, with held positions

We begin the lesson with a more intense version of the free squats introduced in lesson 4. Look at the sequence Carol is demonstrating in the photographs before trying the various held positions. The effect of the stationary points has to be experienced to be believed. Simply holding the three recommended points will elevate body temperature and core muscle temperature by a tangible amount and, as such, is an excellent warm-up. Research in Germany in the late 60s showed that increasing core muscle temperature by one degree Celcius increases flexibility by 15–20 per cent—this makes a huge difference to the sensation of stretching, and can be achieved by this simple sequence.

Do 15 to 20 repetitions of the free squat (recall that it is fine to hold onto something if you cannot keep your heels on the floor). On your last squat, hold the bottom position, letting yourself sink as low as possible. Holding your arms out in front will make balancing easier. Now comes the fun part: lift yourself until your hips are *just below* the level of the knees, and hold this position for 20 seconds. Do not cheat by coming up too high. Wriggling your fingers will help to take your mind off what is happening in your thighs. Next, lift the hips a little more—when the hips are just *above* the knees, the sense of work being done increases dramatically. People who train with weights and do the full squat will know this as the sticking point—the hardest part of the movement. Try to hold this position for 20 to 30 seconds; this will be hard. Next, lift the hips up until the thighs make roughly a 45 degree angle with the floor, and hold this final position for another 20 to 30 seconds (fingers wriggling all the while), and then stand up.

Holding these fixed positions will make you stronger, too, in addition to warming you up. Where I trained in Japan, we would hold these stationary positions for what seemed like an eternity (up to 10 minutes in the second, most difficult position) and similarly hold positions in the wider 'horse riding' stance that we will be trying in a forthcoming lesson. In contrast to weight training movements, these positions involve only body weight, and will not be particularly stressful to the knee joints. Do not be alarmed if your legs start to shake; this is normal. Carol is using a shoulder width stance, but wider foot positions work well, too. All directions remain the same with the wider foot positioning.

Martial arts warm-up with partner

The next warm-up involves the adductor muscles as well as the *quadriceps*, hamstrings and large hip muscles worked by the last sequence. This lesson's version requires a partner; if you do not have one, hold onto a support. I suggest the partner or supported version be used the first time you try this, because considerable stretch will be experienced in the adductors and it is better to be able to lower yourself into the deep stretch position with all possible control.

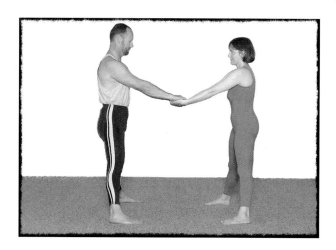

Look at the first photograph, where Greg and Carol are showing the start position. You will need to be standing at arm's length from your partner, with your legs wide apart. Turn one leg out (your partner turns the same leg out, as shown) and you both sink to a squat position on the other leg slowly, keeping the heels on the ground. You may need to adjust the feet the first time you do this to get the right distance apart. The straight leg will experience the stretch, both in the hamstring and the adductors. Refinements in the squat position include distance from your partner (the further away you are, the further you will be stretched towards their hands as you sink) and in the bottom position you can stretch sideways over the straight leg. No balancing will be required: you can hold yourself in position easily using your partner or the support, even if normally you cannot squat down by yourself with your heels on the ground.

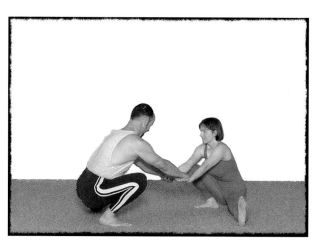

From the bottom position, lift up to just below the halfway point, turn the straight leg *in*, until the foot is pointing straight ahead (at 90 degrees to the line of your feet, in other words). Keeping the hips as low as possible, move sideways; in the centre position both legs will be bent, and then straighten the other leg, and sink down into the squat position again. At all times the foot of the leg you lower yourself towards must be positioned at 90 degrees to the line of your feet; this will avoid strain on the knees, and will help you to avoid rolling inwards on the ankle you squat towards. To avoid over-stretching the adductors, lower yourself slowly into the bottom position using full control on both sides the first few times you try the moves. Use five to eight transitions side-to-side as the complete warm-up.

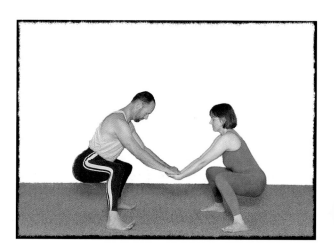

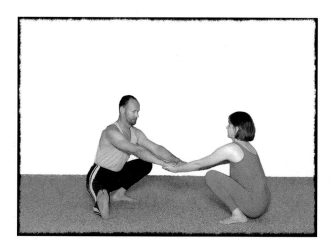

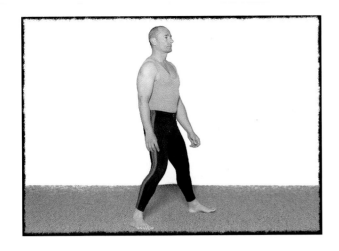

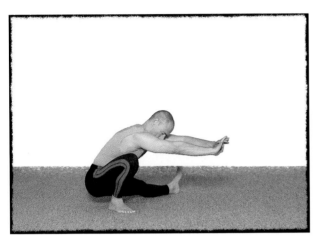

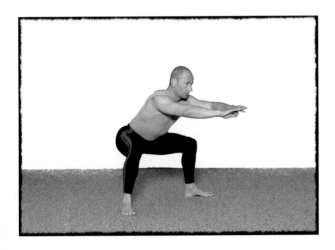

The sequence of photographs on this page shows how the solo version is done. Once you have tried the partner or supported version, you may try the solo version if you wish. If your ankles are relatively tight, you may warm-up for the solo version by doing exercise 18, floor folded leg calf, and exercise 19, wall standing calf. For the solo martial arts movement, exercise 18 is the more important, as folded leg ankle flexibility is essential in the squat position.

Keep the back as straight as possible and do not hold your breath during the movement. Take in a breath before lowering yourself and breathe out as you lift yourself. Keep the hips as low as possible in the transitions from side to side.

Exercise 25, Standing suspended hip flexor

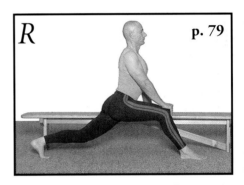

Familiarise yourself with the key form points of exercise 25 (see lesson 4). Increase the intensity of the stretch by trying to straighten the back leg from a deeper position than you did previously. The closer to the floor your hips are, the more difficult it will be to straighten the leg, but remember the effectiveness of the stretch does not depend on getting the leg straight; too many people compromise this by letting the hips rise. The **C–R** contraction will be effective no matter how bent the back leg is.

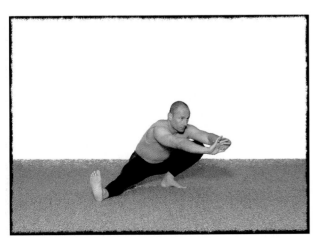

Cues

heels stay on floor
squat under control
lift slowly
keep hips as low as possible

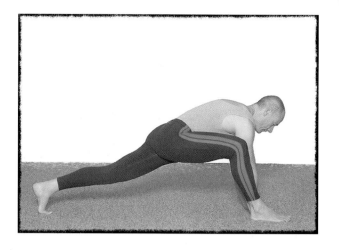

Exercise 21, Buttock and hip flexor, revisited

Review the instructions for this exercise, first taught in lesson 3 (page 66), and move into the final position. Look at the angle made between your thighs, as seen from the side. The looser the hip flexors, the straighter this angle will become (the thighs will get closer to the front-splits position). Having done the **C–R stretch** component for the front leg, and having lowered the hips, straighten the back leg. The stretch for both legs can be tightened from this position.

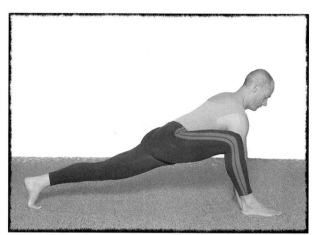

To make the stretch stronger on the *back* leg, look to the front and pull back on your hands as you straighten your back, as I am doing in the second photograph. Hold this position for a few breaths in and out.

To tighten the stretch in the hip of the *front* leg, breathe in, and on a breath out, let your arms bend while keeping your back straight. Hold this position for a few breaths in and out.

To add a lower back stretch to the mix, breathe in and, on a breath out, let your arms bend further, also letting your back bend. If you can, touch your forehead to the floor. You must keep the hips level throughout; the tendency will be for the hip of the back leg to tilt towards the floor; this will avoid the stretch. Hold the final position for a few breaths, relax and stand up. After your breathing returns to normal, change leg position and stretch the other pairs of muscles.

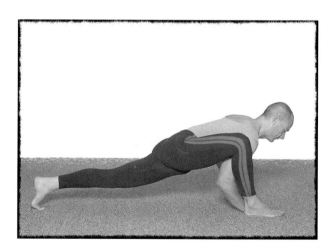

Cues

weight supported on hands

pull back on hands to straighten back

on breath out, keep hips level and
let arms bend to stretch spine forwards

hold final position for a few breaths

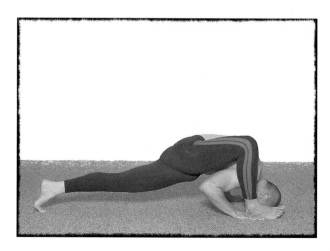

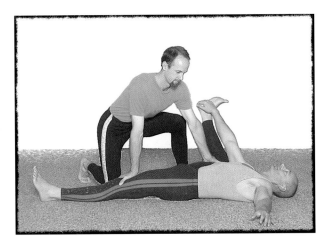

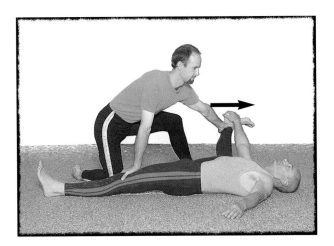

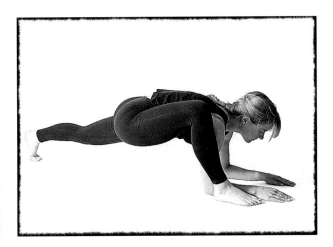

Cues

partner holds straight leg to floor

partner helps you straighten bent leg

C–R: pull heel to bottom

restretch: partner helps straighten leg

46. Partner floor hip and hamstring

Unlike most hamstring stretches, it is almost impossible to cheat in this one. The exercise may be done with one partner but, if you are flexible, you will need a second partner for best effect. Alternatively, you may slide the straight leg under a piece of gym equipment or a similar support and restrain it this way. The reason it is relatively easy to avoid the full effects of most hamstring exercises is that, in the contest between holding the back straight and stretching the hamstrings, the hamstrings usually win. In this exercise, your lower back is held on the floor, both by gravity and by the leg that is restrained. Evidence of this is that many people feel a strong stretch in the front of the leg on the floor—in the hip flexors and *quadriceps*. In fact we are using these muscles to hold the pelvis in position so that the hamstring muscles on the elevated leg will be stretched in the final position, shown overleaf. The important form point is to ensure that the hips stay square to the line of the trunk; the hamstring muscles of the elevated leg will tend to rotate the hip on that side towards the shoulder and the tension in the hamstrings can also lift the hip off the floor.

In addition to the ease of maintaining correct form in this hamstring movement, one of the features of this exercise is that we can stretch the hamstrings in a number of *different* ways in the one exercise. Conventional hamstring exercises move a straight leg (or legs) into the stretch position. In addition to a strict straight-leg stretch position, this exercise can also work the hamstrings from a hip-flexed and knee-flexed start position (as Kevin and I are doing) with the stretch achieved by straightening the bent leg, an entirely different stretch sensation. The closer the thigh of the bent leg is held to the body (or past the body as I am doing), the less you will be able to straighten this leg, but even straightening the leg slightly past 90 degrees will provide a strong stretch if the hamstrings are tight.

We can also move a straight leg into the stretch position. This exercise can also target the different hamstring muscles by varying the angle the leg makes with the centre-line of the body, which is dealt with below.

Petra is demonstrating an alternative support position; she is resting on her forearms, before lowering her head to the floor (final photograph opposite).

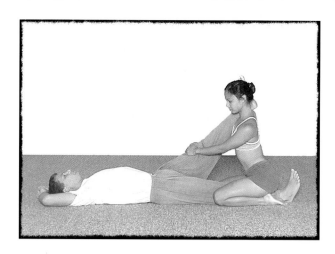

Review the revisited version of exercise 8, partner lying rotation, that is detailed in lesson 3, page 70, where the emphasis is on the hip stretch. This end position can be the starting position of exercise 46, depending on your level of flexibility. Alternative start positions are illustrated: if your hamstrings are fairly tight, have your partner sit on your lower leg, as Julie and Mark are showing in the top frame. If you do not have a partner, you will need to find a way of restraining the leg on the floor, and you may need a strap to loop around the foot of the other leg. The final two frames of the sequence show the recommended partner-support positions if your starting position for the leg to be stretched is better than 90 degrees from the floor.

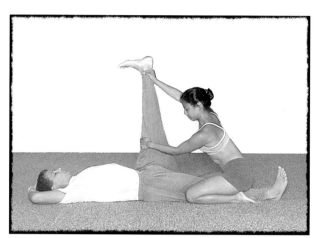

The first part of exercise 46, regardless of whether your leg is bent or straight, is to try to pull the heel to the buttock. This first **C–R contraction** makes the exercise unique—this hooking action will engage the bulk of the three hamstring muscles and, accordingly, will provide a powerful stretch effect. Your partner must make sure that this pulling action is not permitted to move either part of the leg at all. Pull for a count of 10, beginning very gently, and slowly increase the contraction throughout the count. Stop, take in a breath, and on a breath out, restraighten the leg and ask your partner to move the leg further in the stretch direction. A common mistake in this phase is for the partner to try to move the leg too quickly. Hold the end position for at least a ten-breath cycle; a longer stay in the final position will yield additional benefits.

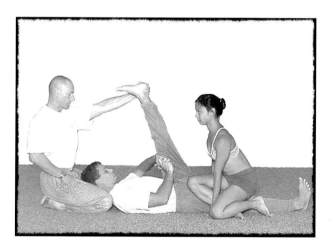

If you are doing the movement from the bent-leg start position, the second **C–R stretch** is done by coming out of the restretch position until you can straighten the leg fully. If you are doing the first contraction from a straight leg position, the second **C–R** will be done from that restretch position. If your partner is sitting on the leg that is on the floor, they can help you keep straight the elevated leg by placing a hand to the hip-side of the kneecap and pulling back slightly as the top hand takes the leg into extension, as Julie is doing in the second photograph. Ask your partner to slowly lean forwards to take the leg as far as possible into extension, while keeping the leg straight. Pause in the new stretch position for five breaths.

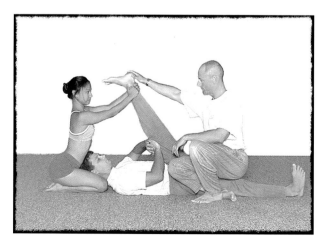

The second **C–R stretch** is provided by pressing the whole leg back to your partner—that is, by holding the leg straight (using *quadriceps*) and pushing back (using hamstrings).

partner sits on leg

partner elevates straight leg

C–Rs: pull heel to bottom and press straight leg back

restretch: partner moves leg in stretch direction

Other powerful hip extensors (*gluteus maximus*) can be engaged to do this, so try to feel the hamstring muscles before trying to push back with them—one reason for doing the hooking movement as the first **C–R stretch**. In many contractions in compound movements, muscles other than the ones we want to stretch can be used to provide the effort, and these will be the ones that will demonstrate the stretch effect. Accordingly, for best results, you will need to isolate the target muscles. Press back to your partner for a count of 10, relax and, on a breath out, ask your partner to take the leg further in the stretch direction until you feel the desired effect. Hold the end position for a ten-breath cycle. Repeat both contractions for the other leg. If you are doing this exercise on your own, a strap and the use of both your arms will provide the necessary support and restretch efforts.

Exercise 22, Lying hip

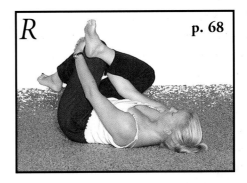

Repeat exercise 22. When in the initial stretch position, feel precisely which muscles are being stretched and try to use only these to generate the contraction effort.

Cues (above)

with foot in position on knee, pull held leg back

C–R: press foot into leg

restretch: move leg further in stretch direction

Cues (two partner version)

one partner sits on leg

second partner supports head and helps you take leg back

C–Rs: pull heel to bottom and press straight leg back

restretch: partner moves leg in stretch direction

Exercise 17, Floor single leg forward bend, revisited; folded leg variation

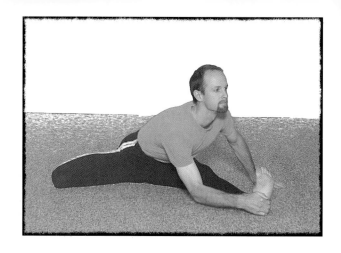

Review the directions for exercise 17, page 70; the version here is one of the standard variations. Look at the first photograph. Kevin is sitting on the floor with one folded leg taken to the side around 90 degrees. Notice that both hips are firmly in contact with the floor. This exercise is done incorrectly in gyms everywhere—and usually by people trying to do it with shoes on. The folded leg's foot *must* be tucked alongside the leg, as shown in the second photograph, to avoid strain on the ligaments on the inside of the knee.

In order to lean forward without tilting to the side, you will need to lean towards the folded leg a little, *before* you lean forward—if you do not, the tension in the *quadriceps* of the folded leg will tend to lift the hip on that side. We want both hips to stay on the floor as we lean forwards.

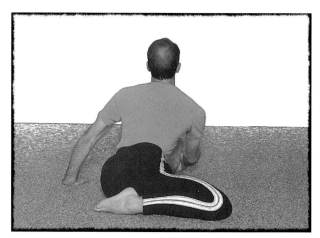

Keep your back straight, and take the body as close to the leg as possible, grasping the foot with both hands, or by using a strap. A **C–R stretch** can be achieved by lifting the chest from the final position and trying to pull the hands away from the foot for a count of 10. On a breath out, slowly pull yourself *along* the leg towards the foot, and hold the position for five to ten breaths.

Exercise 26, Seated/lying single leg quadriceps

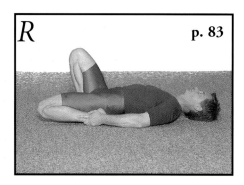

R   p. 83

Repeat this exercise, trying to get a little further in the movement than previously. Remember to keeps the hips horizontal—it is far preferable to use mats for support to keep the form than to have the hips tilted away from the stretch in the *quadriceps*.

Cues (above)

ensure folded leg's hip is on floor
lean forwards with straight back
C–R: lift chest; pull hands from foot
restretch: pull body along leg

Cues (left)

ensure hips level
tighten abdominals
C–R: straighten leg
restretch: tighten position

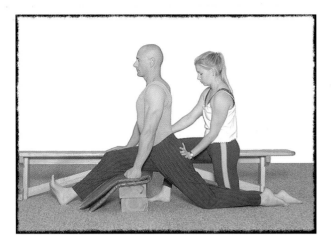

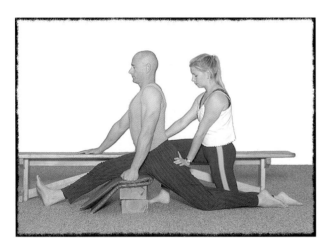

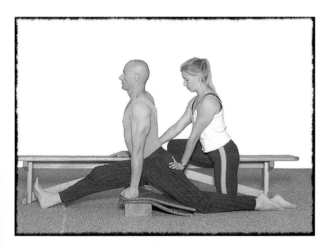

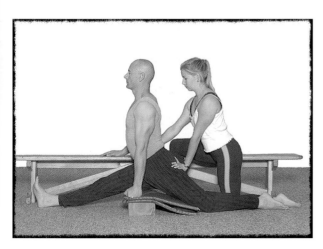

47. Partial partner front splits, off support

47. Partner partial front splits, off support

Although described as a partner exercise, and although most effective if done this way, exercise 47 may be done solo quite well, providing you make an effort to maintain the suggested form. As mentioned previously, good form in front splits is rare but, once we know how the body moves itself to avoid the stretch, we can counteract this tendency. Done as suggested, this exercise will provide as strong a hamstring stretch as you will ever need, safely, and in a way that gives you full control over the end position. Gravity works to assist you and you can hold the end position with little effort; as well, the support effort required from your partner is small. Olivia and I are demonstrating.

In essence, exercise 47 allows the use of the same pair of contractions as exercise 46 above, but gravity provides the supporting force rather than your partner. The hamstring stretch effect is much stronger, because the pelvis is rolled forward by the back leg being taken into strong extension (recall that moving the back leg into extension *hyperextends* the lumbar spine); this effect is used to your advantage here to keep the lower back completely straight. Further, because we will begin the exercise in a modest position that all will be able to achieve, even people with tight hamstrings can enjoy the benefits. All your partner will be required to do is to keep your hips square to the line of the leg.

Imitate the form shown in the first frame: you are on the floor with the front leg bent at the knee (a 90 degree angle is a good place to start) and your back leg is as far behind you as you can place it. Your front leg is resting on a support of suitable height, if you wish. Your partner holds your hips square. Holding you this way, your partner moves your hips forwards—this is identical to what we did in exercise 39 above. Once in the hip flexor stretch position (and you can use the **C–R stretch** of exercise 39 to get into a deeper position if you wish), you can try to straighten the back leg, too, to increase the stretch. Let yourself sink as low to the floor as possible. Then *slowly* try to extend the front foot *without letting the hips rise from the floor*. As you do, you will feel a strong stretch in the hamstrings of the front leg, long before you get the leg straight (this will feel similar to the first contraction of exercise 46 above). Stop in this position.

The first **C–R stretch** is to try to pull the front foot back to you, thus engaging the bulk of the hamstring muscles, for a count of ten. Relax, breathe in, ask your partner to check the squareness of your hips, and then slowly straighten the front leg a little further, again without letting the hips rise. Stay in the new stretch position for at least 10 breaths.

The second **C–R stretch** requires you to press the front foot into the floor, regardless of the knee angle (this engages the hamstrings and the hip extensors) for a count of five to ten. On a breath out, try slowly to further straighten the front leg. Because the contractions engage different muscles (or different proportions of the same muscle's strengths) the stretch effects of the contractions are tangibly different. The most common mistakes in this exercise are to try to straighten the front leg completely or quickly, to let the hips rise from the floor when trying to straighten the front leg, or to let the hips skew around in the direction of the back leg.

Once in the best stretch position (even if the front leg is bent) you can increase the stretch even further by bending forwards from the hips, keeping the back straight. This will provide an intense hamstring stretch. Hold the end position for at least 10 breaths in and out. Rest for a moment and stretch the other leg.

You may need a support substantially higher than the one shown—some of our beginners have needed a support around chair height. Ideally, this support will be able to deform slightly, so that, as your hips sink, the support increases. All phases of the exercise may be done this way, reducing the size of the support as you become more flexible. The value of the support will need to be felt before it is fully appreciated. We feel that the effects are derived from the body's awareness that it cannot be overstretched if the proprioceptors can feel the presence of the support. Additionally, your muscles will not need to exert as much force to support the body's weight (the stretching agent in this movement) because some of that weight is supported.

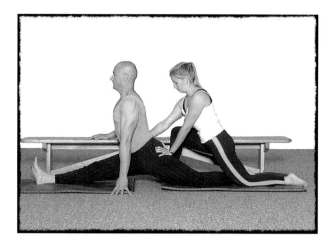

Cues

have suitable support under front leg

partner holds hips square

C–Rs: pull front foot back; press front foot into floor

restretch: slowly try to straighten leg

Cues (right)

chin on chest; trunk slumps

pull head to floor in between knees

pull head towards feet

pull body forwards

add rotations to move stretch

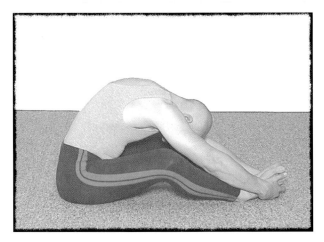

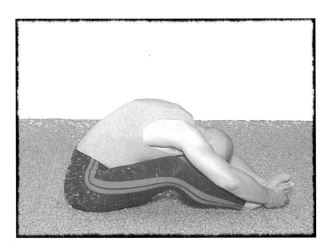

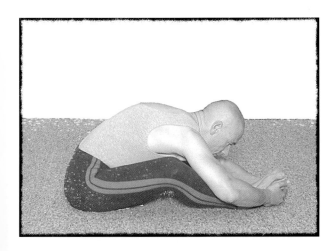

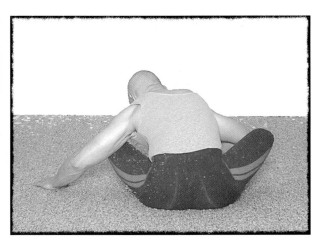

48. Floor forward bend over bent legs

We call this a minor pose, but the effects can be strong and it is a useful recovery movement whenever hip flexors or backward bending is involved. Unlike most forward bends, this exercise is intended to stretch many small, and important, muscles of the back side of the trunk, from the back of the neck to the base of the spine. Read all the directions *before* trying the movement.

Sit on the floor as shown, and hold your feet. If you feel a strong stretch in the buttocks, move the feet a little closer to you or a little further away—the hip position can be a strong *piriformis* stretch for some. Let the chin go towards the chest and let your back slump slowly. Rest in this position for a few breaths; this start position can be quite a strong stretch.

Assuming that your start position resembles the second photograph, use your arms to *very gently* draw your face straight down in the direction of the floor, towards a spot in between your knees. Drawing the face in this direction will bend the upper and middle back; accordingly, that is where you will feel the main effects. Hold this position briefly. Now gently draw the head towards a spot in between your shins: moving the trunk in this direction will stretch the *middle* of the back maximally. Lastly, draw the head towards your feet; this will move the stretch into the lower back, the lumbar spine area. Hold these positions for a breath or two; this stretch is designed not so much to improve your range of movement as to make the back feel good after other exercises. Your proportions strongly affect precisely where you will feel the main stretch effects, so you may need to alter the pull direction to get the stretch in a desired place.

Once in the position that affects your lower back, you may induce a gentle rotation by holding alternate feet as shown. Make sure that you add the rotation *after* moving into the maximum lower-back stretch position to feel the full effects. If one side is tighter, stretch it a second time.

49. Partner all fours rotation

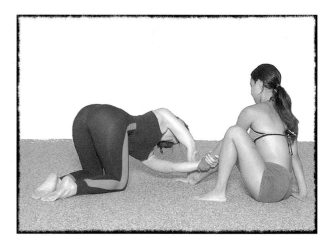

This exercise feels marvellous, and is one of the favourites of the classes. In essence, your partner is providing the support to stretch your whole spine in rotation but, because they are pulling on one of your arms to do so, that shoulder is being drawn off the body in the process. This adds a feeling of overall lengthening and expanding that most rotation exercises lack entirely; the combination will leave you feeling excellent. All levels of flexibility are catered for in this pose—both the stiffest and the most flexible can use the same basic approach. You can do exercise 49 on your own if you have a suitable support, as I show in the final frame.

Look at the first photograph. Position yourself as Jennifer has done, on all fours with your knees under your hips (this is essential; if your knees are too far forwards, there will be insufficient weight on your supporting hand). Your partner has positioned themselves alongside and you reach under your chest to grasp their arm in a trapeze grip, as Julie is doing. Your partner braces your support forearm, and places a foot on your hip. The hand of your support arm needs to point *across* your body to your other shoulder.

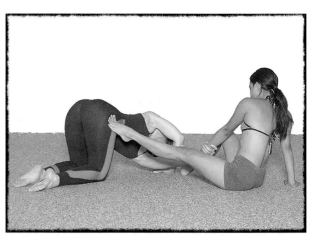

Breathe in. On a slow breath out, ask your partner to slowly pull your arm through; in the process you bend the support arm at the elbow, so your trunk rotates around both your shoulder *and* your elbow. Go as far as you can, until you feel a stretch in the trunk and shoulder.

The **C–R stretch** is to try to pull your arm back from your partner; try to gently use your whole body in this effort. As always, your partner must not let you move at all; it is an isometric contraction. Stop pulling, breathe in and, on a breath out, have your partner draw the arm further towards them. Let yourself *be* stretched; the key to this exercise is to let yourself go. To this end, your partner must make sure that they make their movements slow—if they are quick in any way, your trunk muscles will contract to protect you, and the effect will be lost. Stay in the final position for a 10-breath cycle.

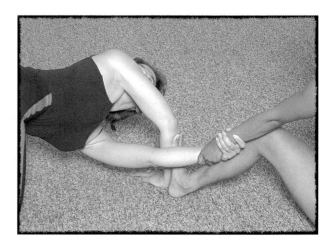

For correct form, the arm that is drawn by your partner and your support arm must be touching each other; if they separate, a twisting moment will be introduced to your shoulders and it will be impossible to be rotated without your being pulled out of alignment. Your partner will need to provide a stable forearm support, too. Stretch both sides.

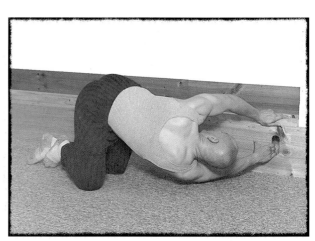

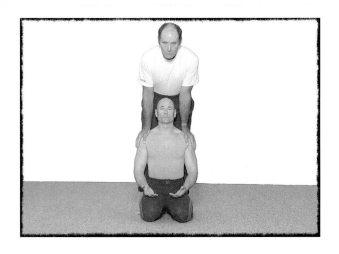

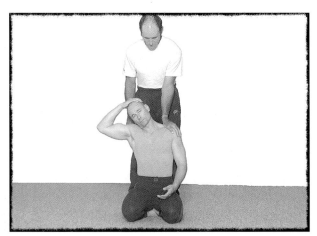

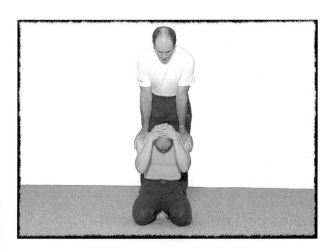

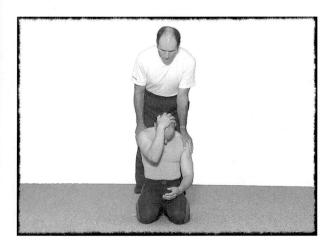

The solo version requires a suitable support. Look at the last photograph on the previous page: while hanging from one arm, I am using the top arm to push the shoulder away—by combining the hanging and pulling forces you can induce a very pleasant rotation in the whole spine. Experiment with different distances away from the support, and try the movement while flexing or extending the spine slightly to change the location of the main effect. A **C–R stretch** can be achieved by twisting the trunk back against the support of the arms. Lean back and hang from the top arm to restretch.

50. Partner shoulder depress with flexion and lateral flexion

This is the strongest of the neck movements and the most precise stretch for *levator scapulae* in particular. The movements can be done very effectively in a chair (in fact more effectively than on the floor) and are the most important of the neck exercises for the office environment.

Refer back to the illustration of this area of the body, on page 122. From the flat, twisted structure of *levator scapulae* you can see that stretching the neck to the side will emphasise the stretch on the shorter fibres and stretching the neck forwards in flexion will emphasise the longer ones. Combining the two movements is will provide the best stretch for this muscle.

Review all the directions for exercise 44, partner shoulder depress; exercise 50 is the same basic form, but with two embellishments. Alan and I are demonstrating the movement. Once in the final position of exercise 44, slowly reach up with one hand and gently pull the head to that side, similar to exercise 7, neck side bend. This lesson's version will be much stronger than exercise 7 because the shoulders are depressed as far as they will go. This action alone stretches many of the neck muscles; when we add a side bend to it, the movement becomes very strong indeed. Do not be overly ambitious the first time you try this.

Once in the stretch position, **two C–R stretches** may be done. The first is to try to lift the shoulder you are stretching away from, working gently against your partner's resistance; the second **C–R** is to try to press the head back against your own resistance. Restretch in between each contraction, or, if you prefer, you can do both contractions and a single restretch. Hold the final position for a few breaths (neck muscles do not require the same stretching time as the larger muscles seem to need).

Once you have had a sufficient stretch in this position, relax and return your head to the start position. The next part requires you to lower the head forward to the chest; the **C–R stretch** requires the head to be dropped forwards slowly towards the chest. As in exercise 6, chin to chest, press your head directly back against the resistance of your own arms for a count of five. Relax and restretch on a breath out; hold the final position for a few breaths.

The final **C–R stretch** is the strongest of all, and combines the effects of all the preceding movements. It is a very strong stretch for *trapezius* and *levator scapulae*. After you have spent sufficient time in the last position, reach one arm up and, *while maintaining the forwards-most position* of the last movement, draw the head to the side cautiously. The major error of form in this part of the exercise is to let the head lift from the forward position. To do so will lose the stretch entirely. It does not matter if you cannot take the head very far to the side—the purpose, as you will recall, is to feel a stretch in the right place.

Once you've stretched as far to the side as you can, restrain the head, and gently press back and to the side at the same time, gently, for a count of five. This direction will be roughly 45 degrees to one side or the other. Notice the head is not turned to the side. Stop pressing and relax, on a breath out, first gently take the head further *forwards*, and then a little further to the side as the second movement. Again, do not sacrifice the forward position of the head just to get it further sideways. Hold the final position for five breaths, and repeat all **C–R stretches** for the other side.

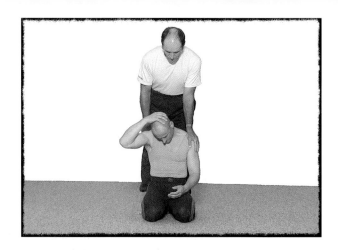

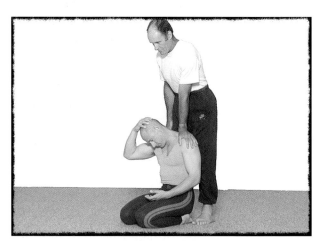

Cues (for all parts)

partner leans on shoulders

C–R: lift shoulders

restretch: partner moves shoulders down

use hand to gently pull head forwards

C–R: press head back against hand

restretch: pull head further forwards

holding head forwards, take to side

C–R: press head back and across against hand

restretch: pull head further forwards, then further to the side

THE UNNUMBERED LESSON: CHECKING YOUR PROGRESS

We have done seven lessons, and we have another eight to do to complete a typical *Beginners* course in *Posture & Flexibility*. To this point, we have adopted a reductionist approach to the task of becoming more flexible, by isolating and stretching specific muscle groups. Now that we have had direct experience of this over a series of classes, it is worth spending a moment or two here to put that somewhat piecemeal approach into the larger context—you. What's required now is *integration* of the small-scale work we have been doing, and this can be achieved by two complementary approaches. The first is to assess what *shape* the body will make when exposed to a whole body task and the second is to assess what the attempts to make these shapes *feel* like. The former can give us invaluable clues as to which parts of the body are looser or tighter than the rest; the latter can provide more subtle information on the state of your muscles and their associated tissues.

Recall from the *Introduction* that I mentioned that the prototypical stretching exercise—sitting on the floor bending forwards over both legs—was an inefficient movement to improve the capacity to bend forwards at the waist with straight legs. To be able to *do* the exercise, in other words, was the outcome, and not the best process by which to achieve it. And I mentioned that whenever you see people doing this exercise, you see it being done badly. People will try to touch their foreheads to their knees and, if they do not have sufficient extensibility in the hamstring muscles, they will bend their spines instead. Bending the spine stretches the muscles that *extend* the spine; accordingly, I argued that doing the whole movement was an inefficient way to stretch the hamstrings. And from there we moved to the kinds of things than can limit the hamstrings' capacity to elongate (the calf muscles, and *piriformis*, perhaps) as well as precise hamstring exercises, some of these by design permitting movement only at the hamstrings.

Pursuing these strategies will make you more flexible in the desired movement; there is no doubt about this—but are we missing something fundamental in the process? I think we are, and this is what I want to consider in this deliberately unnumbered lesson—unnumbered because it can fit anywhere in the sequence (although it will be easier to understand now than if we had tried it earlier) and it will need to be returned to often. Whenever you feel the need for an hour or so of uninterrupted pleasure (which will provide an opportunity to perform a mental and physical inventory), this lesson will provide a check list to assess your progress and a way of alerting yourself to areas large or small that will need further attention for a time. 'Where in the *Beginners* sequence should this lesson be put?' is a little like the conundrum of which came first—the chicken or the egg? If you had not had the experience of the previous lessons, what we are about to do would not mean as much, and most of you would not have the sheer basic flexibility to be able to experience what this lesson has to offer. Now we have both the experience and the flexibility, and are able to refine the basic question of how best to improve a stretching method so it provides the most effective harmonising influence on the body and the mind.

In our work so far, we have concentrated on moving parts of the body through idealised planes of movement—the cardinal points on your stretching compass, we might say. We have stretched the trunk directly to the sides, for example, and we have isolated individual muscles for particular reasons. While analysing movements this way is real in a geometric and anatomical sense, in another sense it is misleading when applied to the task of optimising whole-body function. This is because it is only when we isolate the hamstrings deliberately, for example, do we move only the hamstrings—no movement in daily life or in the most exacting athletic or aesthetic activity ever occurs this way. As long as these simple one-joint movements do not become ends in themselves, this approach can be useful, as you have found. From here, however, we need to find a way to incorporate this vocabulary of movement—focusing on particular joints or muscles—into the sentences and paragraphs that are our dynamically changing structure and its derived functions.

Another problem is determining which muscles need to be more flexible, and by how much? This is why we return our focus to the whole body movements occasionally, to see what shape your body makes when exposed to particular tasks, and, crucially, where you feel the effects (the stress) of such movements. Answers to these questions will alter your developmental trajectory—you will move in the direction needed to supply the stress you require. It will be useful to make notes of tight areas as we go though the positions. To this end, the photographs in this lesson indicate the closest relevant exercise number and page it first appears. Some of these positions, however, do not correspond to specific exercises, so imitate them using the text and photographs and you may find that some of these, at least, provide very pleasing sensations. If they do, add these positions to your routine.

Today's lesson concentrates on subtle movements, too—not the big stretches like front splits, but a myriad smaller movements that pull on muscles, small and large, and the connective tissue that permeates our body, and which, with the muscles, is the means for forces acting on us to be widely distributed. And because we will be stretching while moving from one position to another, we will be stressing the muscles and connective tissue through many ranges of movement that conventional stretching leaves untouched.

Begin by lying face up on the floor, stretching the arms out behind you and pressing your feet and toes away from your body. To get the idea, imagine that you are being pulled gently by both the hands and feet at the same time. Now press one arm and the opposite leg away, and feel how that changes the sensations in the trunk. Now do the opposite pair. Does moving each pair feel the same—if not, where precisely is the difference? Stretch the tighter side once more.

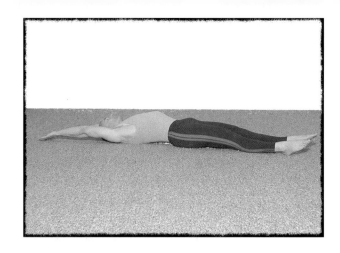

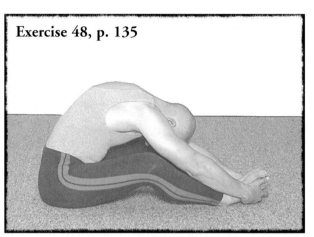

Exercise 48, p. 135

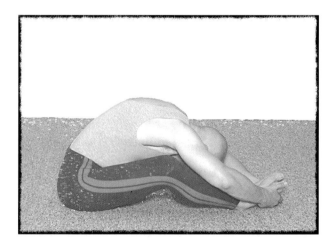

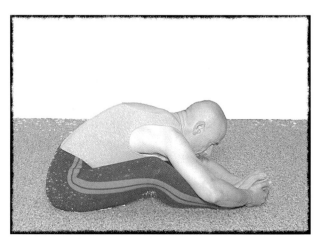

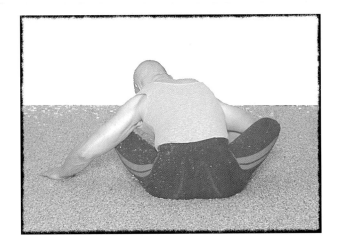

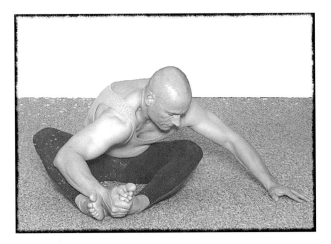

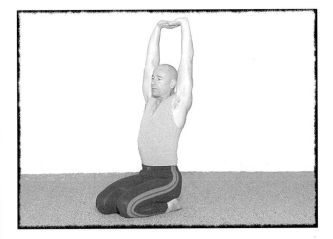

Roll onto one side, and sit up, with your legs outstretched before you, if you are flexible in hamstring movements; if not, have the legs bent 90 degrees or so at the knee, and let them fall to the sides. Put your hands behind your head, take in a deep breath and arch the spine backwards for a few seconds. As you breathe out, let the hands come back to your sides, let the chin go towards the chest, and let the spine slump. Where can you feel the effects of this movement? If you have a partner with you, ask them where you appear to be bending the most—upper or middle back, or is the spine a smooth curve? In your check list, note the tightest area and find an exercise relevant for this area, making sure that you do it once or twice a week in addition to the material in the lessons.

Now let yourself bend forwards at the hips, until you can go no further. Where do you feel this? Let the body go limp on a breath out. Does this change where you can feel the movement? Resume normal breathing. Reach your arms out and hold the feet by placing your fingers underneath. Keeping the chin on the chest, apply the slightest lifting force on the feet, straight up to the ceiling. Your feet will not move if the force is small, but you will increase the stretching effect in the upper back. Try to feel this. Now, while applying this small force to the feet, add a very small pulling effort to the feet; this will move the stretch effect down the spine. Breathe deeply a few times, and feel the breathing action move the ribs near the hips at the back of your waist as you do this. Last in this part of the sequence, stop the lifting effort and instead only pull yourself along towards the feet; if you keep your chin on your chest, this action will place the stretch sensation more in the lower back. Based on where you feel the strongest effects, select an appropriate exercise and add it to your list, too.

Return to the sitting up position, beginning the movement by lifting the head up, and assisting with your hands if you wish. Stretch your arms up and out above you. Relax.

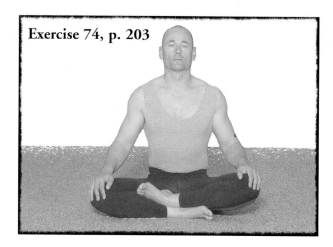

Exercise 74, p. 203

Cross the legs as shown (on top of each other, or one in front of the other), and let yourself bend slowly over one thigh, allowing the whole spine to bend in the final position. You can help yourself move forwards by turning your palms away from you, placing the backs of the fingers under the knees and gently pulling yourself forwards, as I am doing in the last photograph. Where do you feel this? Again lift up, leading the movement with the head and neck. Now move over the other knee, compare sensations, and bend directly forwards; then sit up.

Now swap the positions of your legs; you will be surprised how different this makes the suite of sensations feel. This is probably due to differences in tightness of the external hip rotators of each hip. If movement in one direction is tighter, or both movements are tighter with one leg position, you may care to repeat the movements for that side. Select an appropriate exercise and add it to your list.

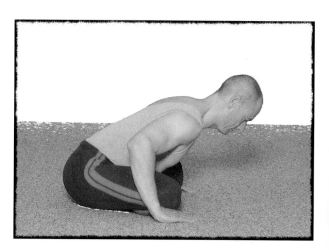

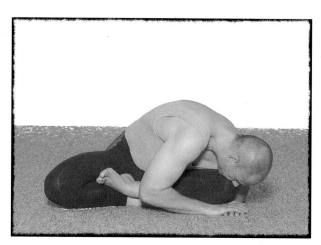

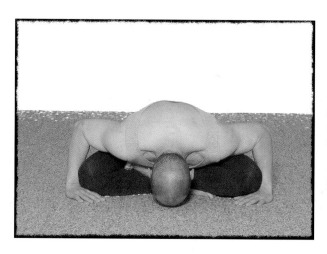

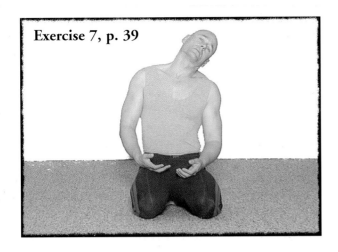

Exercise 7, p. 39

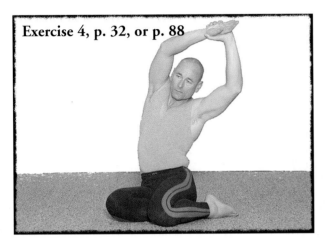

Exercise 4, p. 32, or p. 88

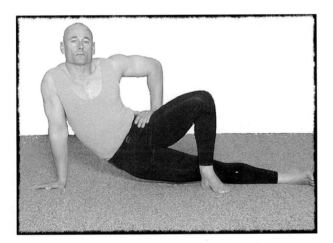

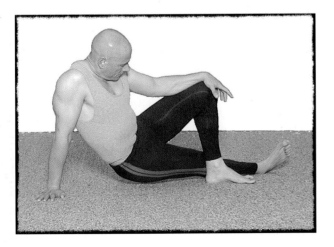

Sit on your folded legs, and feel whether that stretches the insteps or the front thigh muscles, the *quadriceps*, or both. Next, tilt the head to one side (let the shoulder you are stretching rise, if you wish; we are deliberately trying not to be strict here—rather, we want to feel the normal, distributed stretch sensation). Now slowly and smoothly roll the head around on the shoulders, feeling where the tight spots are and making notes as to which directions produce the strongest sensations. Let your bottom slip off your feet to one side and onto the floor as shown; complete this sideways movement of the hips and spine by bending the trunk to the other side. Let the top shoulder roll forwards as you bend to the side. You may support yourself on one arm if you wish; alternatively, you may do the movement a second time with arms outstretched, and by pulling the arm on the stretched side further out as shown. Repeat for the other side, and note any left–right differences. Choose a side bending exercise (seated or standing) if it feels as though this area needs special attention.

Extend one arm and lean on it, then extend the bottom leg until it is straight, as shown. Fold the top leg and place the foot on the floor in front of the other leg's knee. Let your body's weight sink into the floor while leaning on the arm, and feel the rib, chest and back muscles above the hip being stretched in the process. To move the stretch, use the folded leg to roll the top hip, first forwards (this moves the stretch in the back forwards too) and then backwards (which moves the stretch around the lower hip and the back). You can intensify the effects by leaning the whole trunk in the direction of the outstretched foot. Then lie down, roll to the other side and repeat all directions.

Now, lie face up, and do the rotation part of exercise 3, lying rotation. This time, however, once in the rotated position, keep the extended arm on the floor and reach it out past your head as far as you can. Hold this position for a second or two; then, keeping the arm as close to the floor as you can, move it in a large arc down towards your side until the stretch disappears. Reach the arm out to the side again in the normal position for the exercise. While holding the arm to the side and on the floor, bring the knee of the bent leg closer to you (around 45 degrees) and repeat the rotation movement. Once in position, extend the held thigh down towards the straight leg, feeling the effects of this change of angle. Repeat this sequence once or twice more, until you feel you've done enough. Change sides and repeat all directions. This may reveal a tightness across one shoulder or its chest muscle, suggesting the need for additional work. Also, by moving the arms and legs through the arcs described, you may find a few tight places that are not revealed by the standard stretches; make a note if this is the case.

Kneel as shown. Hold your knees and let the back slump, then let the hips roll backwards as far as you can; this will give a lovely stretch across the middle and upper back. You may alter the effects by adding a twist to one side, pulling a little harder on one arm to assist. Repeat for the other side and check any differences.

Next, sit as shown with the legs together, bent at the knees, and reach around behind you to place a straight arm on the floor. Depending on your flexibility, the hand will be about opposite the middle of your hips. Lean on the arm, and with the other reach around and place the elbow on the outside of the opposite knee, as shown. Start with a straight back and, by leaning on the arm behind and gently pulling on the elbow, twist around as far as you can. Note the effects, and vary them by letting the back bend a little or by letting the hips roll backwards. Repeat for the other side, noting any differences.

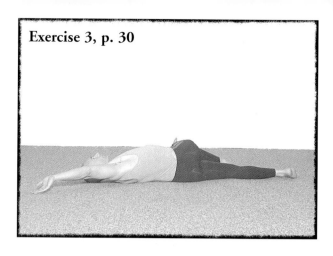

Exercise 3, p. 30

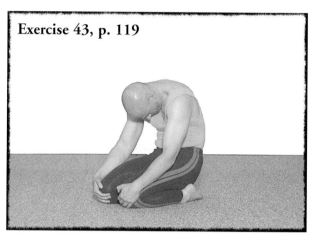

Exercise 43, p. 119

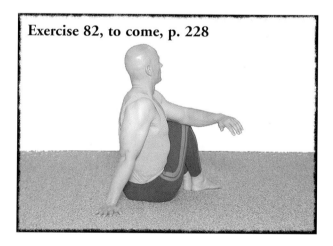

Exercise 82, to come, p. 228

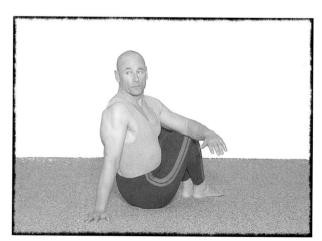

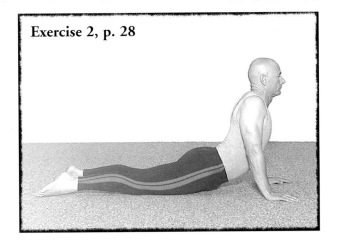

Exercise 2, p. 28

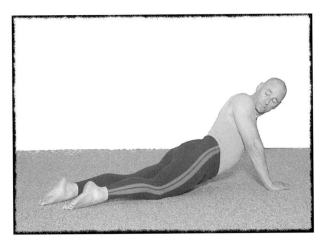

Roll onto your stomach and do exercise 2, the backwards bend from the floor. The key to this exercise today is to let the weight of the body do all the work once you have straightened the arms; so let your weight sink as far down in between your shoulders as you can and let your stomach go towards the floor. Once comfortable, take the shoulders backwards, and feel the effects, then add slow rotations of the whole trunk left and right, trying to look at each foot in turn. The hip that you are turning towards may lift from the floor; let it and feel the effect. Come back to the centre, then take the head backwards as far as you can *without* opening the mouth—we are trying to get an idea of how this movement feels once the entire trunk is stretched backwards. You may add small rotations of the head on the neck once the head is in the extended position. How does this feel?

Next is the deep lunge position, shown in the next photographs. Make sure that the front foot is in front of the knee and that the position you've taken allows you to balance. Support yourself with both hands on the front knee as shown, or with one hand behind the hip of the back leg and let your body's weight pull both hips towards the floor. Feel the stretch; then, if you have enough flexibility lean backwards so the trunk is vertical, at first, and, if possible, past vertical. Again let the head go back as far as you can and feel the effects of this position for a few seconds. Come out of the position, using your arms to let yourself down towards the floor.

Exercise 25, p. 79

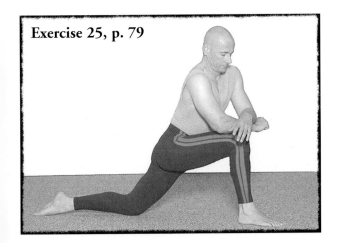

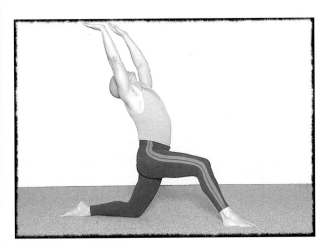

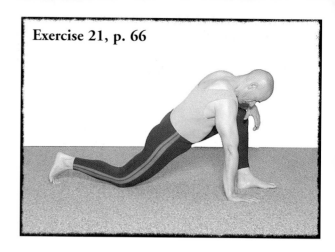

Lean most of your weight on the outside arm, and let gravity pull the hip of the back leg down to the floor, allowing the thigh to move across and down slightly behind you. In the second photograph, you will see that my weight is being supported by the outside arm and the outside of the back leg, which introduces a sideways effect. You will feel this above the back hip, at the side and towards the front of the body. Move the hips to find the best stretch.

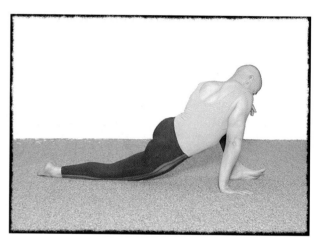

Now come back to the middle position and use your arms to support yourself as you let the trunk go towards the floor to stretch the lower back, hamstring and buttock of the hip of the front leg, in a similar way as we did in exercise 21, buttock and hip flexor. You will need to let gravity work for you here to make this successful; the key is to *relax* into the various positions, and *feel* where the moves stretch you. Repeat all directions for the other side. You may alter the order of this sequence if you prefer, stretching the *quadriceps* and hip flexors of each leg before doing the buttock and hamstring segments.

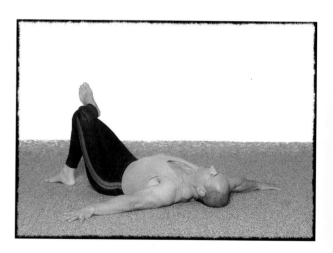

Lie face up again, half bend one leg keeping the foot on the floor and reach the other leg up and outside to hold the leg, as shown. Use the second leg to slowly pull the other towards the floor. Try different arm positions while you do this; I find that taking the arm of the outside leg from the position shown in the last photograph to out past my head, reaching as far as I can, gives the best whole body sensation. Do the other side, again trying to maximise the stretch sensations. Note any particularly tight areas.

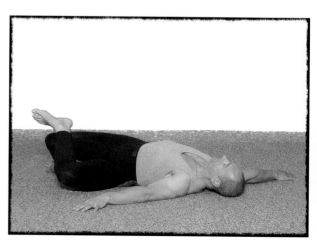

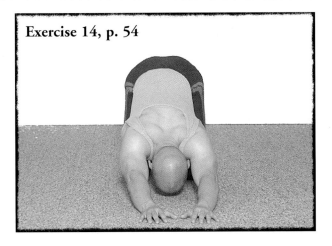

Exercise 14, p. 54

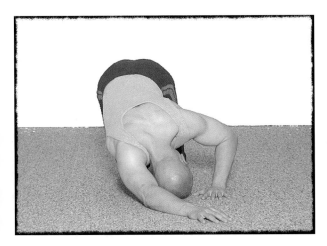

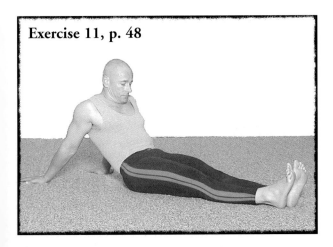

Exercise 11, p. 48

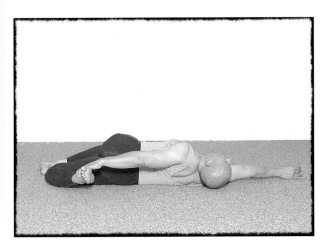

Now move onto your hands and knees, and extend the arms as shown. Let gravity pull the body to the floor, as you try to push your arms as far off the body as possible. Breathe in deeply and, on an exhalation, let the trunk sink as close to the floor as you can. Then, by taking the body's weight mainly on one arm and letting the spine bend gently to the side as you let that shoulder go closer to the floor, you will be able to strongly stretch the muscles of the trunk and the large muscle under the arm, *latissimus dorsi*. The stretch sensation will be much stronger than in the two-arm movement just done, and you can regulate the intensity by taking some weight on the other arm, which will be bent. Repeat for the other side, trying to feel as much as you can.

For the next movement, sit as shown, with both arms extended behind you, letting the trunk slump to a comfortable position. By leaning weight more on one arm, and rolling the hips *away* from that side, you can alter the stretch effect on the arm; this can be further altered by pressing one leg away from you at the same time. Now emphasise the other arm and press each leg away in turn to change the effect.

Next, let yourself down onto the floor, and clasp your arms around your trunk. Lift one shoulder and roll away from that side a little, and do the other side; the legs can be in any comfortable position. I always let myself fall back gently onto the floor; if I let myself relax into it at the same time, the sensation is quite satisfying.

Roll onto one side, extend the bottom arm, and reach the other arm back towards the foot of the top leg, as shown in the last photograph. By pulling on the foot, the leg can be pulled behind you and, by extending the leg to pull further on the arm, the body can be stretched back to the leg. Try pulling on both arm and leg at the same time (imagine you are drawing a bow). Try the other leg to see how that changes the effect—this introduces a diagonal stretch from shoulder to opposite hip. Roll over and sit up. Let the body stretch over bent or straight legs, depending on your flexibility. Roll to the other side and repeat all directions. Finish this sequence by repeating the stretch over the legs.

While sitting cross-legged, grasp one foot in both hands, as shown in the second photograph overleaf. Move the ankle through a full range, including to the inside and outside (*inversion* and *eversion*), then (like wringing clothes by hand) twist the hands on the foot in opposite directions.

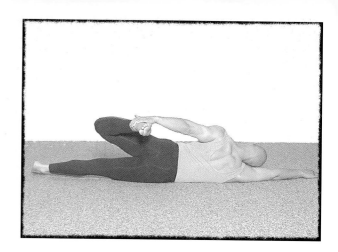

Press the fingertips into the base of the toes and bend the toes backwards; then use the other hand to stretch them forwards, so making extension and flexion movements. Gently pull each toe and give it a twist at the same time. Interlace the fingers between the toes, pressing the fingers through the toes as far as possible, as shown in the top photograph, opposite. In this position, clasp the fingers to the toes, and press the heel of the palm into the ball of the foot, to stretch the toes (second frame). Change legs and do the other foot. Now do similar movements for the wrists, hands and fingers. Rotate the hands and forearms with the hands in both flexion and extension, and feel the effects.

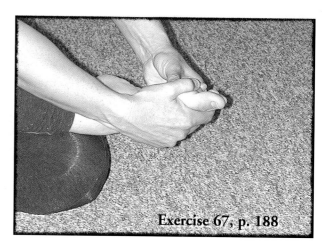

Exercise 67, p. 188

Stand up, bend the knees, and let the body fold onto the thighs with the arms crossed and hanging down near the legs. Let the head hang loose. Slightly straighten one leg at a time, transferring more of the body's weight onto the leg you are straightening. Do this on each side, and feel the stretch. Let your body's weight hang in this position, and let gravity lengthen your trunk.

Now let the arms extend too, and feel that sensation. Make sure you continue to breathe normally throughout. Slightly bend the knees for comfort if you wish. Once in the full hanging position, twist the trunk around so your arms are to one side; feel this for a few seconds and move to the other side. If you can, put your palms under your feet (hold the ankles if you can't) and gently pull on the arms to help gravity. Breathe in and, lifting from the head, arch the back backwards, bend the knees, and stand up. Keeping the knees slightly bent, move the body around as though it were limp, letting the arms move to the sides in the process. Repeat this a few times to each side.

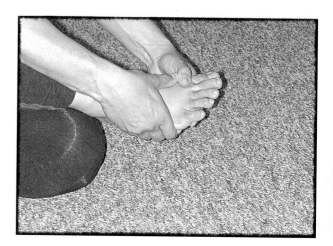

By now, you should feel completely relaxed and have a clearer idea of what areas need special attention. Lie down for a while and run your mind's eye around the body, seeing if you can feel the problem areas. Let yourself relax in any comfortable lying position—you may need to cover yourself. Because the body uses muscle tension to generate heat, one can feel cold after a good stretch. Close your eyes and feel the weight of the relaxed body on the floor. Breathe normally, letting yourself sink that little bit closer to the floor each time. Try not to fall asleep—instead, hover between wakefulness and sleep, and simply feel the suite of sensations coming from the relaxed body. Five to ten minutes will be enough for most people.

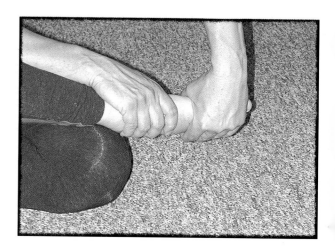

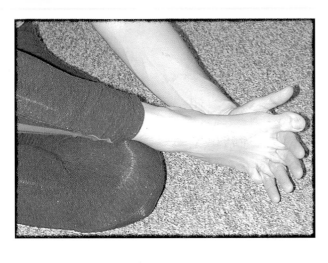

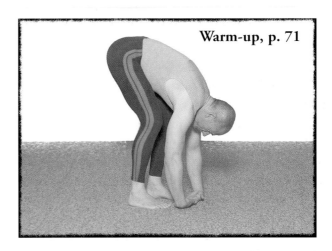

Warm-up, p. 71

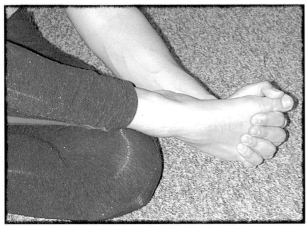

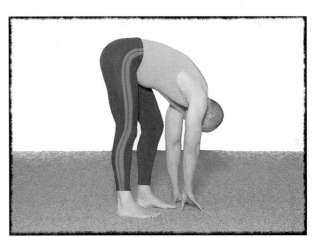

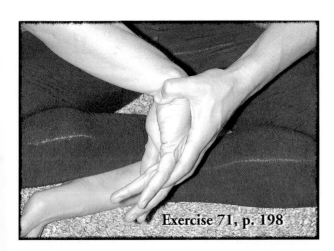

Exercise 71, p. 198

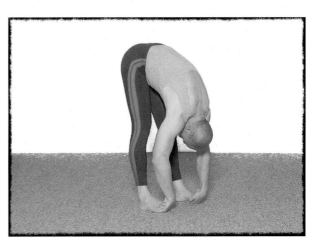

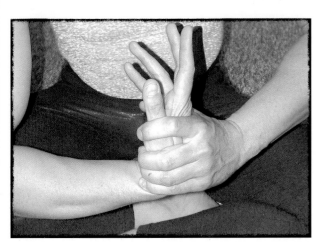

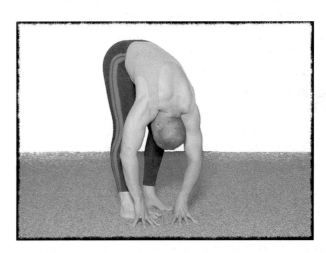

CHAPTER TWO

LESSONS 8–15

By this point, the main elements of the approach will be clear, but it will help to reinforce the principles by considering what we have been doing from a more general perspective. *Form* is the paramount principle. By form, we mean that combination of body alignment and position that causes a stretch to be felt in a particular muscle or group. The requirements of form are based on an anatomical understanding of the relationship between the parts of the body, together with rudimentary geometry, a knowledge of lever systems, and basic physics. We have found this to be sufficient to derive the desired effect in any of the muscles of the body. Where anatomical understanding does not suggest a clear direction (for example, in the *piriformis* stretches), evaluation and organisation of the direct experience of many students and teachers has been an effective substitute—in other words, the empirical approach, unfashionable in some circles.

In all **C–R stretches,** the body is moved into a stretch position, with or without the support of a partner or piece of equipment, and this initial stretch is held until the body becomes used to the position. Then a *contraction* is applied: this term means that the muscle or group that experiences the stretch effect is employed to pull or push back against an unmoving resistance, a partner or another form of support. This point is crucial and a frequent source of error: the extent the support moves is the extent to which any possible stretch effect is reduced. The contractions are gentle— we have found that isometric contractions used to enhance the final stretch effect work better if they are gentle compared with near maximal or maximal efforts. Strong contractions require surrounding muscle groups to contract forcibly for stabilisation. This reaction can reduce the final stretch because the required bracing of the whole body means that it is further aroused neurologically, making the relaxation necessary in the final stretch more elusive.

The final phase of the **C–R approach** is the restretch: after relaxing the contraction you take in a deep breath and, on a breath out (and *only* on a breath out), you move the body further in the stretch direction, until you feel a sufficient stretch in the target muscle. A partner may assist in this phase. The final position is held, usually between three and ten breaths, the time depending on the size of the muscles: most commonly, the larger the target muscle, the longer the final position is held. Breathing is normal and unhurried in the final position and the student is encouraged to concentrate on the sensations coming from the stretch; the stronger we can make the experience of the final position the stronger the effect in terms of the body's map of its capacities.

The other elements of the approach are the use of dynamic warm-up movements that all can do and which often work the body in positions that would be regarded as being between the positions of the more formal stretches, and the progression from easily achievable partial positions to stricter forms later in a class. Many exercises use initial positions that the body finds comfortable, where the elbows or knees are flexed, and the limbs are then further extended, rather than moving into stretch positions with straight arms or legs. This reduces the sense of apprehension that many standard exercises provoke. Later classes usually are more difficult than earlier ones, but occasionally we teach a class that simply feels good to do, partly to integrate the sensations of the new ranges of movement that students display.

In lessons 8 to15, I assume that the paragraphs above have been understood and are thoroughly familiar in a practical way. Accordingly, the directions for subsequent exercises will be briefer and more material will be covered in each lesson.

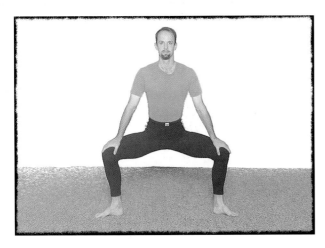

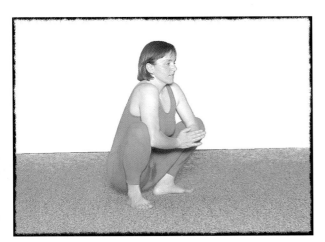

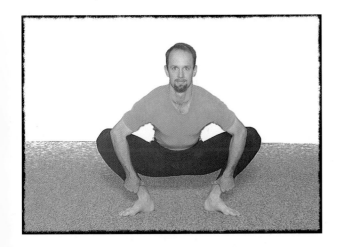

LESSON EIGHT: HAMSTRINGS, LEGS APART, AND BACK BEND

In this lesson we will do three warm-up movements, all of which are excellent stretches in their own right. There are only a few new exercises, but one of them, exercise 55, partner seated legs apart, takes some time to do, and is a cornerstone of flexibility. It is a fundamental movement of yoga, dance, and the martial arts. The final position of this exercise is a compulsory pose in men's gymnastics.

Free squats warm-up, knees pressed apart by elbows

Do 10 repetitions of any version of the free squat, described in lessons 4 and 7, with the feet about shoulder width or slightly closer. Then look at the first photograph: this lesson's free squats are done with a wider foot stance. Do not have the feet so wide that your knees are stressed, and try to use the hip muscles to widen the knee position as you squat. Do 10 to 20 in this fashion, and squat down as low as you can on the final repetition. Kevin is demonstrating the recommended foot placement in the first photograph.

Look at the next photograph; Carol is demonstrating the start position of the hip-widening movement. You will need to shuffle your feet together slightly to be able to lower the hips fully. Squat in the bottom position for a moment, then place the elbows on the inside of the thighs, back from the knees. Put your hands together, and pull them back towards you until the forearms form a straight line: this action will force the knees further apart (bring the elbows closer to you in the starting position for a stronger stretch). Alternatively, use the position Kevin is demonstrating in the last two frames if you are more flexible. Try both of the **C–R stretch** holding positions to find the one that is best for you.

To engage a **C–R stretch**, squeeze the knees against your elbows for a count of five. On a breath out, press the knees further apart and let the hips sink closer to the floor.

After stretching the thighs apart, complete the free squat warm-up by extending your arms to the front. From the full-squat position, lift the hips to the second position (as in lesson 7, the hips are just below parallel—hold for 20 seconds), then the third (hips are just above parallel—hold for 20 seconds), then the last position (hold for one minute). Stand up, and shake legs and arms.

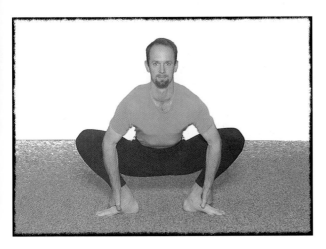

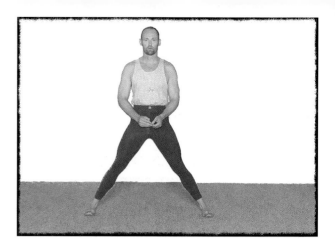

Martial arts warm-up, one foot flat; solo, bars or partner

The more difficult (and in some schools, more traditional) warm-up that we learned in lesson 7 is done here with the feet parallel, and kept on the floor throughout (recall that we turned out each leg in turn the last time we did this). Keeping the feet flat on the floor is a much stronger stretch for the adductors, but it also lets you keep the hips lower in the transitions once you get used to it. This is an excellent leg strengthening exercise too. Do this version unassisted if possible, or hold onto a bar if not. Use the lesson 7 version of this movement if this variation places too much strain on the knees—many people do not like lateral forces on the knees.

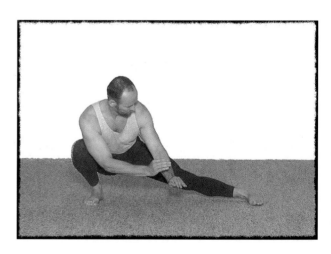

Once the basic stretch part of the warm-up has been achieved, try to keep your weight as low as possible for the strongest effects in the transitions—do not stand up at all during the moves from side to side. Once you become familiar with the movement and find the best foot spacing, move while keeping the hips as close to the ground as possible. Lift from the squat position *smoothly*; when you are good at this, it will be one continuous flowing movement, beautiful to behold and wonderful to do. Each transition should take a minimum of five seconds to complete, and longer transitions are even more effective.

Standing legs apart warm-up

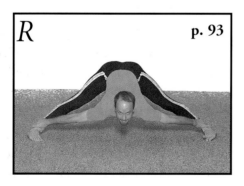

Do this warm-up, described at the beginning of lesson 5. Start the movements with the legs bent at the knees, then try straightening one leg at a time before doing the movements with straight legs. Concentrate on letting yourself relax and allow gravity to stretch you.

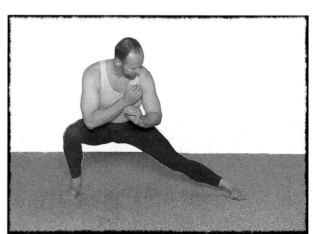

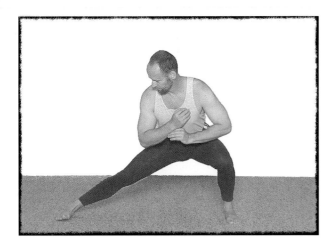

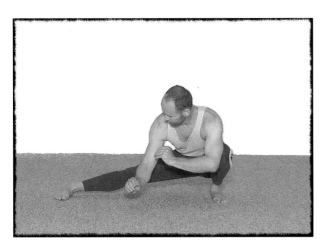

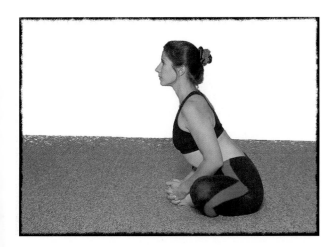

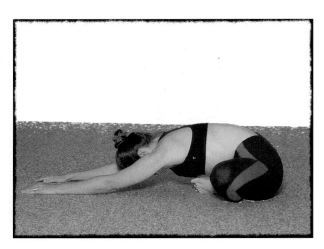

Exercise 30, Wall seated knees apart

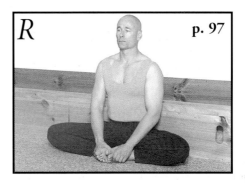

R   p. 97

Review all directions in lesson 5 for this movement, and do the exercise to your capacity. Once you have finished the knees-down-to-the-ground part and, assuming that the legs are on, or very near, the floor, your position will look similar to the photograph above.

Now look at the last two photographs in the left column, where Jennifer is demonstrating the next phase of the exercise. The task is to bend the body forwards at the waist. The most common error in this part of the pose is to bend in the lumbar spine area instead of at the hip joints. Moving properly, the shape of the spine does not change until your ribs come in contact with your feet; at this point your back should be straight and near horizontal. Most of the sensation will be felt in the front of the hip joint itself. Pull yourself forwards only to the extent that you can keep the back straight or even arched backwards.

The elbows can be used to hold the legs down if necessary; I prefer to put the elbows on the floor in front of the shins and use the arms to pull backwards—this action helps you keep the back straight. Lifting the chest at the same time enhances the effect.

This is a fundamental movement in yoga, dance, gymnastics, all martial arts and many other approaches to body work. Many health benefits are ascribed to the final position, including improvement in function of the reproductive organs. In men, the position is said to help regulate the prostate gland.

51. *Standing clasped single bent leg hamstring*

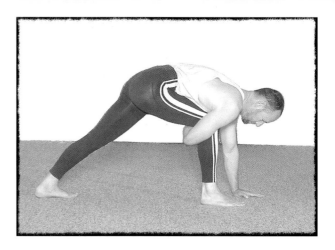

The effect of exercise 51 is similar to, but in some ways stronger than, the first part of exercise 47, partial front splits. In the first part of exercise 47, we tried to straighten a leg bent at around 90 degrees at the knee. In exercise 51, the body is folded alongside the thigh; thus the hip is maximally flexed, and the knee is again around 90 degrees. The fact that the hip is more strongly flexed makes the initial position stronger (in relation to the hamstring) and the use of the hamstring muscles for support adds to this effect.

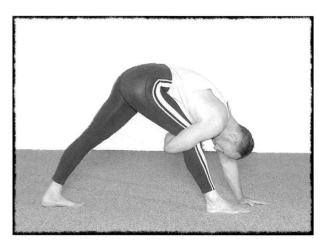

Look at the first photograph. The body (with back held straight) is placed along the thigh, the back foot a full leg length behind the front foot and the feet at hip width for balance. The back foot is turned out to around 45 degrees, to ease the stretch in the hip of the back leg and to assist balance. The stretch is achieved by trying to straighten the front leg. The most common error is that the student sacrifices the body's close position in order to make the leg straighter. The priority here is to keep the body in contact with the leg, while holding the back straight. Greg's final position is not quite as strong a stretch as Carol's, because Greg's ribcage is hard on his thigh, limiting forward movement.

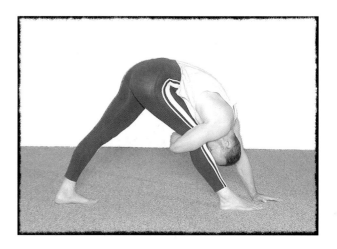

The **C–R stretch** is achieved by lifting the head to initiate a straightening effort and trying to lift the body away from the thigh, keeping the back straight and the body in tight contact with the thigh. This effort should be felt only in the hamstrings. The restretch is to try to straighten the leg slowly from the initial stretch position, but with the body held in place. Most people let the body come off the leg and the stretch is lost. Do the other leg; if one is noticeably tighter, repeat for this side.

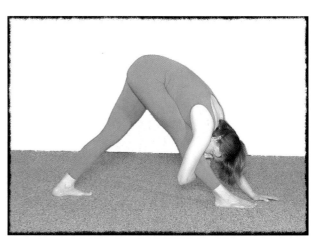

You will notice that the stretch effect is different from bending forwards over a straight leg and is often felt more in the centre and higher parts of the hamstring group. Many people have reported a significant improvement in overall hamstring flexibility after practising this movement a few times. Starting the movement with the body in contact with the thigh seems to reduce the sense of apprehension many people feel in standard hamstring stretches and is one of the reasons this exercise can be so effective.

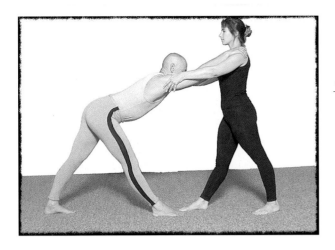

52. Partner/solo standing single leg forward bend

This partner exercise complements the previous one perfectly; together they form an efficient complete hamstring stretch. Jennifer and I are showing the form elements and the support positions.

Stand facing your partner, and take a long pace forwards (we usually suggest one leg's length, but it is amazing how many people have no idea how long this measurement is in their own case). The back foot can be turned out to about 45 degrees. Have the hips close to square across the line of the legs. Lean forwards from the hips, and place your hands on your partner's shoulders for support. Your partner will check to see if the shoulders are level with the floor and that your hips are level, too. Ask your partner to sink down while you hold the back perfectly straight, until the desired stretch is felt. Arching the back (a negative thrust) will emphasise the stretch in the hamstrings of the front leg.

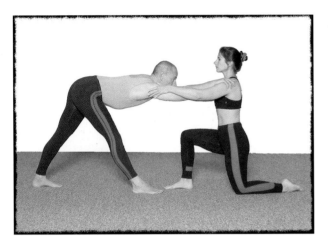

A **C–R stretch** is easily achieved: once in position, either press the heel of the front leg into the floor for a count of eight to ten, or take some of your weight off your partner's shoulders by lifting your body away from their support—either contraction will engage the hamstrings of the front leg. Relax, and restretch; holding the final position is easy, because your partner is supporting you. Check your hip and shoulder alignment once more and change legs when ready.

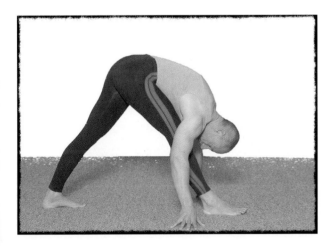

In the third photograph I am showing the shape the body will make once the ribs are in firm contact with the leg and the chin is on the shin. This will be the limit of hamstring stretch in this position for most men. To come out of this position, bend the front leg, lift the head and chest, and stand up.

Jennifer is demonstrating a stronger version of the stretch in the final frame. The differences in our proportions are evident: my face contacts the shin just below my knee and the top of Jennifer's head is in line with her ankle. Always consider your proportions when comparing your shape to that depicted in the photographs.

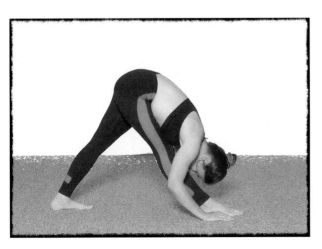

Cues

legs and back straight
use partner for support
C–R: press front foot to floor
restretch: move further in stretch direction

53. Partner wall standing hamstring

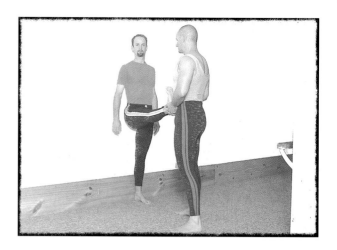

In the discussion of the hamstring muscles (lessons 3 and 7) I mentioned that in forward bending, allowing the leg to be placed to the outside of the centre-line of the body avoided some of the possible stretch. Exercise 53 will make that point in a dramatic fashion—especially if you are flexible. Most hamstring stretches affect the middle and inner parts of this group (*semimembranosus* and *semitendinosus*) more than the outer (*biceps femoris*), because the form of the stretch usually has the leg outside this line.

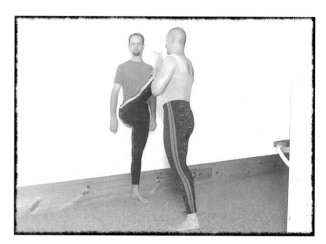

Exercise 53 deliberately brings the leg towards the centre-line of the body (and past it, if you can) because this most strongly affects *biceps femoris*. We have found that flexible people, especially those with good legs-apart flexibility, will find this apparently simple stretch very strong.

Your partner applies enough weight to the elevated foot to keep *both* hips against the wall—otherwise the tension produced by the movement will pull the hip of the leg being stretched away from the wall. The leg is slowly elevated and brought across the centre-line of the body towards the supporting leg. In the third photograph, I have moved Kevin's leg across to illustrate, in the direction indicated by the arrow—this small horizontal movement dramatically increases the stretch effect.

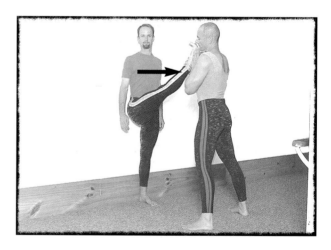

The **C–R stretch** is to press the leg down to the floor and slightly away from the centre-line of the body at the same time (try to use the muscles at the outside and back of the leg). Hold the contraction for at least a 10 count. Restretch following the centre-line or further across to the supporting leg and hold for at least 10 breaths.

54. Partner wall squat knees apart

Unlike our standing warm-ups, holding this position is relatively easy, as your partner is holding you against the wall. Look at the photograph of Greg and Carol: the thighs are roughly parallel to the floor, the back is held against the wall, and your partner is helping the knees apart.

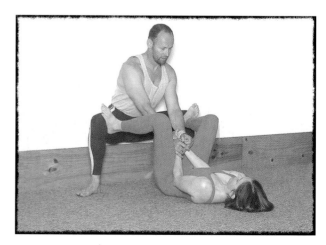

The **C–R stretch** is to squeeze the knees together using the adductors for a 10 count; the restretch is to ask your partner to very slowly increase the pressure on the knees with their legs until a sufficient stretch is felt. Hold the end position for 10 breaths.

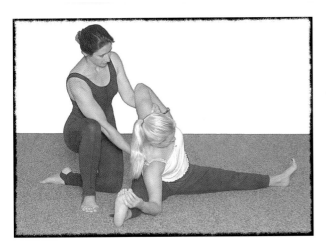

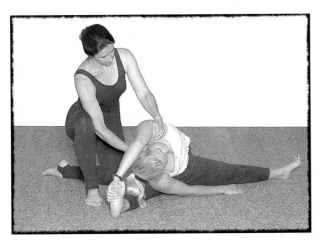

Cues (left page)

lift leg to stretch position

take leg across centre-line

C–R: press leg across and down

restretch: leg further up and across

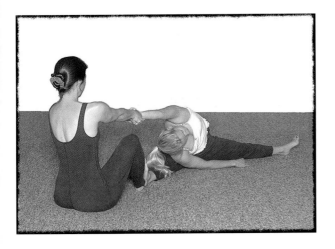

55. Partner seated legs apart

Olivia and Jennifer are demonstrating all the major elements of this fundamental pose. The initial seating position stretches the adductors. The first movement is a strong lateral flexion and rotation of the spine, using the hamstrings to hold the pelvis in position so these stretches can take place; the second movement is a strong single leg hamstring stretch; and the last part is a combined adductor and hamstring stretch. The effect of the final position can vary from mostly hamstring to mostly adductor, depending on how far the legs are apart—the further apart the legs, the more the forward bend movement affects the adductors.

Sit on the floor with legs outstretched and as far apart as you can comfortably get them. Look at the alignment of the first part: Olivia's shoulders are near vertical; she is using a palm-up grip on her foot to enable her elbow to press back into the inside of her leg. This action brings the bottom shoulder forward. By pressing with the elbow the shoulder is held in position; your partner can assist as Jennifer is doing by supporting the bottom shoulder and helping to roll the top shoulder backwards until the shoulders are vertical. If you cannot move the shoulders into this position, a **C–R stretch** will help: try to pull the held shoulder forwards for a count of five; and restretch on a breath out. An alternative support position is shown overleaf.

The stretch is increased by reaching the top arm out in the direction of the held foot; grasp it if you can. If the effect of leaning to the side is felt predominantly in the hamstrings, bend the knee slightly; this part of the exercise is designed as a *quadratus lumborum* and *obliquus* muscle group stretch primarily and, if the hamstring sensation dominates, this will not be the case. If the hamstrings are loose, however, the leg will need to be straight: it is hamstring tension that holds the pelvis in position on the floor so that the trunk movement becomes a sideways bend. An additional **C–R stretch** is to have your partner draw the arm off the body (bottom photograph), in line with the leg you are bending over; the contraction is to try to pull the arm directly back towards you. This contracts *latissimus dorsi*. The partner draws the arm further out in the restretch. This stretches many layers of *fascia* in the trunk in addition to a huge number of muscles, and feels wonderful. (Drawing the arm off the body may be added to exercise 29, floor side bend

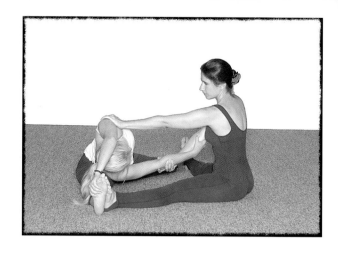

over straight leg, too, adding these additional effects to the basic movement.)

If you can hold the foot with the arm of the top shoulder, there is an alternative support position (from in front of you) shown in the first photograph. This may be an easier position for the partner to hold. The counter-rotation **C–R** contraction can be applied from this position too.

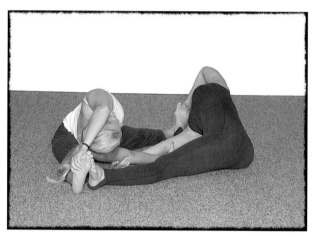

The second photograph shows an excellent dynamic warm-up that can be done from this position. You and your partner sit opposite one another, placing your feet together. You do the same movements together, mirroring each other. Do the side bending movement slowly and on a breath out.

The next pair of photographs shows the assist position for part two of exercise 55, a hamstring stretch over one leg. The partner supports the *roundest* part of your back. The **C–R stretch** is to try to pull your hands away from your feet while lifting the chest and, on the restretch, you can let your back bend slightly to get a little further down towards your foot. Your partner again supports the roundest part of your back, and you hold the final position for a 10-breath cycle.

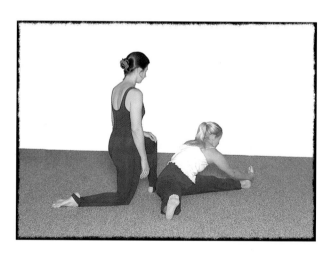

Cues

hold foot or strap; elbow inside leg

reach top arm towards foot

C–R: pull top shoulder forward to partner

restretch: roll top shoulder further back

C–R: press back to partner

restretch: move body closer to leg

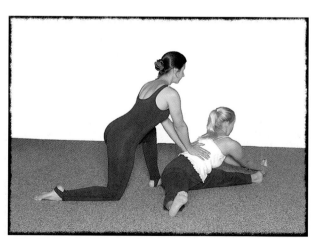

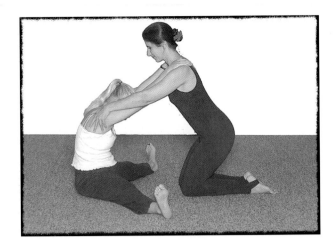

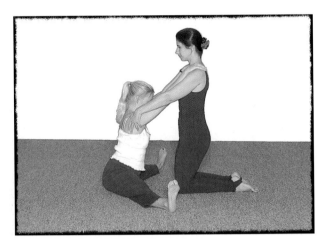

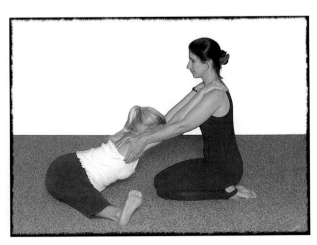

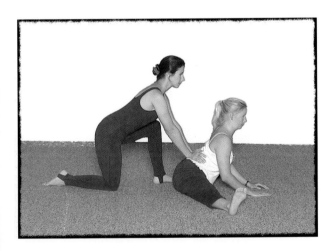

Look carefully at the next two frames. They demonstrate the negative thrust for the pelvis. This movement is essential for the best stretch in part three of the exercise. I recommend that you practise this forward roll of the hips before you attempt the next part. Olivia is sitting in a typical shape: when the hamstrings are tight, many people cannot sit on the floor with their backs and legs straight, because the hamstrings and adductors will not let the bottom bones move sufficiently backwards to allow one to balance. This round back shape is the result. Jennifer is providing the support; Olivia has lifted her chest, arched her back, and rolled her hips forwards. This will initiate the stretch sensation in the hamstrings and adductors—if this shape in the back is held, all movement of the body forwards will further stretch these muscle groups. A **C–R stretch** will be effective here: once in a stretch position, try very carefully to pull back from it, while lifting the chest. This latter direction is crucial; if you pull backwards with a round back, some of the stretch effect will be in the back muscles themselves, and we do not want that in this exercise. I suggest using this support position if you can incline your body forwards from vertical to about 45 degrees from vertical.

The third frame shows Jennifer behind Olivia in the mildest of the support positions, which may be used if your partner's muscles are too tight for the one just described. An alternative support position is shown in the last frame. Jennifer is gently pulling Olivia towards her, lifting her out from her hips, which also allows one to move the hips forwards along the floor to help open the legs.

The lying support positions shown overleaf look dramatic, but, in fact, feel more comfortable than the preceding support version for both people. Use the lying support if you can incline the body 45 degrees from vertical or more. You need to have your hands placed so that your partner can lie on you without stretching you too far. If you have your hands on the floor as shown you can control the stretch position and intensity completely. The **C–R stretch** is performed from this position. Lift your chest, press back onto your partner with the hamstring and adductor muscles (if you feel the effect in your back, you can be certain that the lower back is not held in the slightly arched shape we recommend) and, on the restretch, lower yourself into the stretch by letting the arms bend. You have full control in

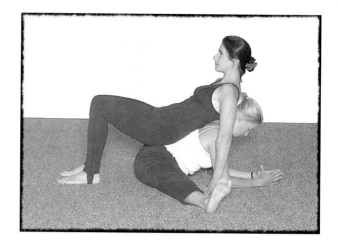

this version, even though it is potentially a stronger stretch position than the preceding version. Do small back-straightening movements once in your final position. You may use rolled mats or other supports between your chest and the floor to lean on, or to to signal to the body that relaxation in this position is possible. Hold the end position for at least 10 breaths; 15 to 20 is even better.

Kevin is demonstrating the bent leg version on the facing page. This is an excellent stretch by itself. Hold your feet if on your own, or a partner can assist as shown—I am sitting on a block to get my hips into the best support position to help Kevin to straighten the lower back (second frame). The bottom two frames show the third part of the exercise.

Exercise 8, Partner lying rotation

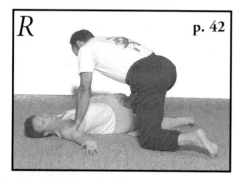

R   **p. 42**

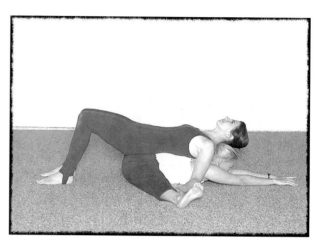

Hold the final position for 10 breaths on each side, and do your tighter side once more.

Exercise 27, Partner backward bend over support

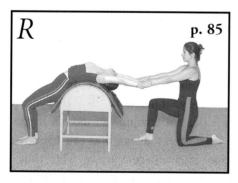

R   **p. 85**

On a breath out, let your partner draw the arms off the body as far as possible. After the **C–R,** take in another breath and let yourself be restretched on a breath out.

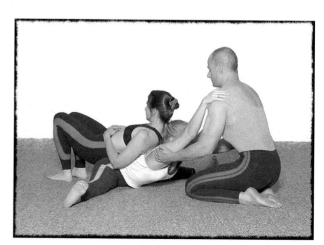

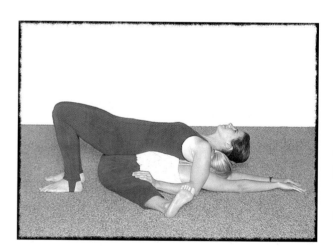

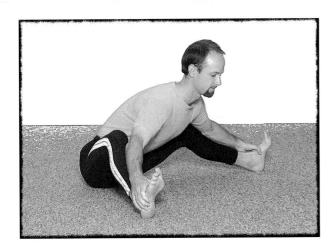

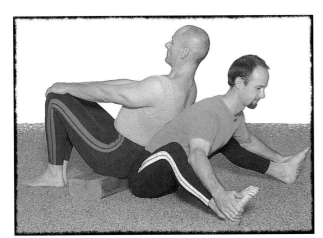

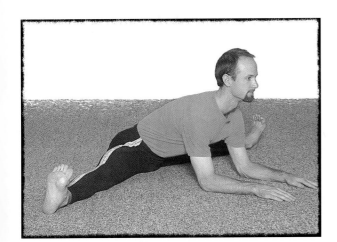

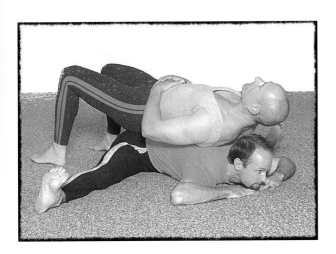

Exercise 1, Floor clasped middle and upper back

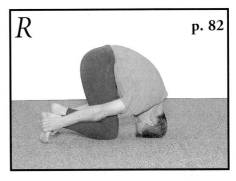

R   p. 82

Do the legs-outside version or the legs-inside version as you prefer. Keep pushing the hips gently forwards each time you breathe out.

Exercise 14, Wall middle and upper back backward bend

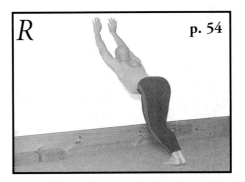

R   p. 54

Concentrate on letting gravity pull your trunk towards the floor. Looking up between your hands will tighten the upper back muscles and can help increase the effect.

Exercise 36, Lying bottom leg folded rotation

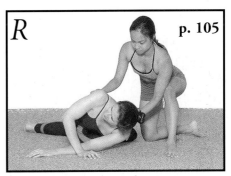

R   p. 105

Repeat this rotation to finish the lesson, if you wish. Let yourself relax into the final position—the only work being done should be by the support arm and shoulder. Relax!

LESSON NINE: UPPER BACK, NECK AND SHOULDERS

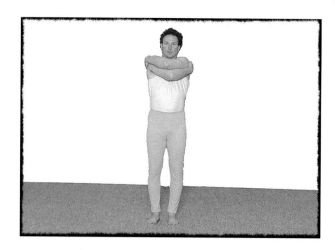

In some ways the exercises presented in this lesson are less taxing than those in some of the preceding lessons, for they stretch mostly small muscle groups. We have found that varying the difficulty of successive classes is much liked by students. As mentioned, small muscles generally require less contraction time and less time spent in the final position for satisfactory results. Of course, if you wish to spend longer in either phase, you are likely to get better results, but it is a good illustration of the principle of diminishing returns: twice as much time will not give you twice the final effect, nor will it help you to become flexible twice as quickly.

Experience suggests that the neck and shoulders are tight areas in most people, and some otherwise comprehensive exercise systems are lacking in these areas. This lesson provides a number of innovative stretches for the neck and shoulders and supplements these with trunk stretches—altogether this lesson should leave you feeling excellent. There is a large number of exercises, but they do not take long to do. People with problems in these areas may care to return to this lesson every week, in between succeeding lessons, for a while, until these areas show improvement.

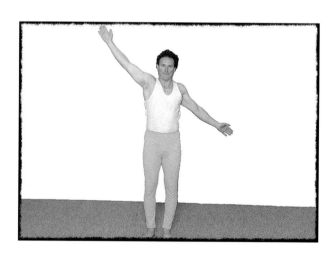

Standing rag-doll warm-up

This simple movement feels good to do and will help you warm-up the shoulders. Do not make too much effort here; the idea is to let the body flop like a rag doll and let gentle momentum provide a gentle pulling force on the arms. Pierre is demonstrating.

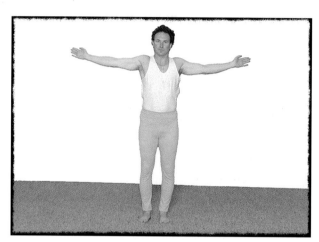

Stand with your weight on both feet and let the knees bend. Do not incline forwards at the waist: keep all the body's weight over the feet. Let the shoulders drop and begin a rotation movement in the trunk by swivelling the hips to one side. As you feel the rotation moving up the trunk, the shoulders will begin to move. As you go from side to side, the arms will be pulled gently out from the body. The turning of the hips moves the arms; do not lift the arms using the shoulders. Turn in each direction five to ten times.

Stand on bent legs and slowly throw the arms out behind you at about shoulder height to stretch the chest and front shoulder muscles. Then do a similar movement with the arms at about 45 degrees, as shown. Finally, throw the arms

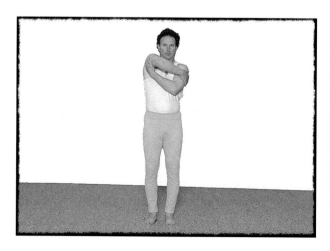

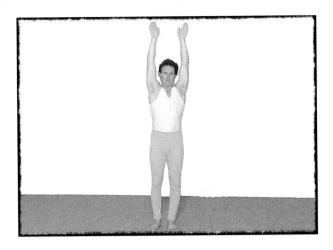

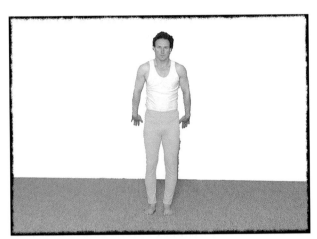

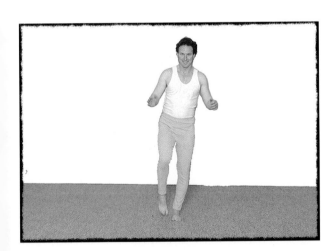

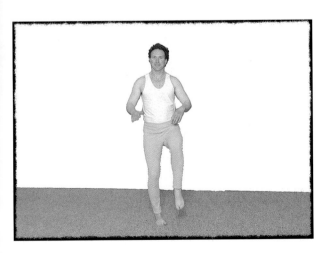

gently backwards and forwards. Stand on one leg and shake the other while shaking the wrists and arms together. Now do the other leg, still shaking the arms. Finish with a few more of the bent-leg whole-body rotations we began with.

Standing alternate leg forward bend warm-up

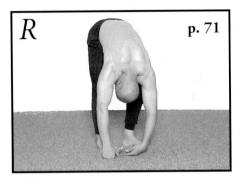

The directions for this movement will be found in lesson 3. You will find the warm-up much easier to do this time. Let yourself relax; you cannot force flexibility.

Exercise 16, Floor face down arm and leg lifts, and abdominal curls

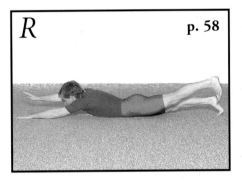

Do 10 to 15 arm and leg lifts, and follow with 10 to 15 slow abdominal curls concentrating on holding a tight top position in each repetition. This sequence is described in lesson 3.

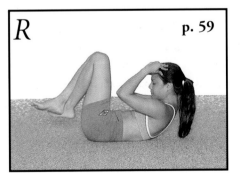

Exercise 38, Lying rotations

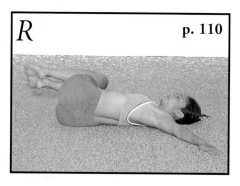

R   p. 110

Do 10 repetitions to each side, using the leg position that is right for you.

Exercise 50, Partner shoulder depress with flexion and lateral flexion

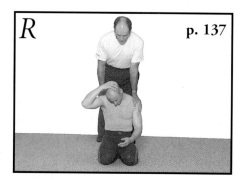

R   p. 137

As your reward, spend a few minutes using this exercise to start the relaxation process in the neck. Make sure that you keep the head as far forward as it can go *before* trying to take it to the side.

Exercise 10, Partner front arm

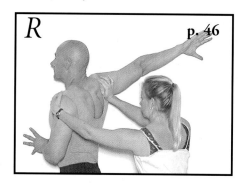

R   p. 46

Review the instructions for this exercise. Make sure you get the arm to body angle correct—if you do not, *biceps* will not be stretched.

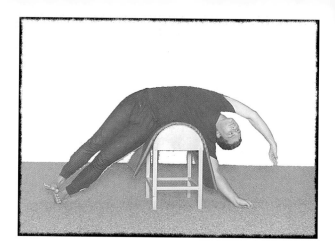

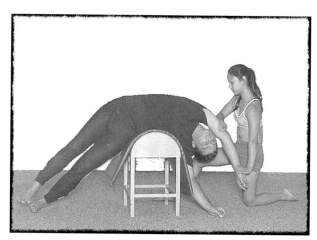

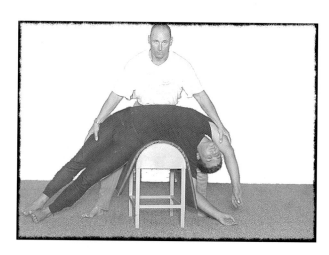

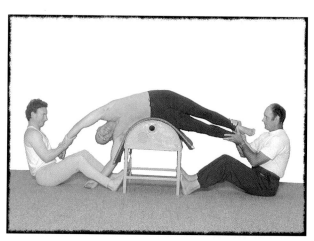

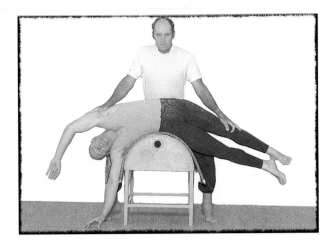

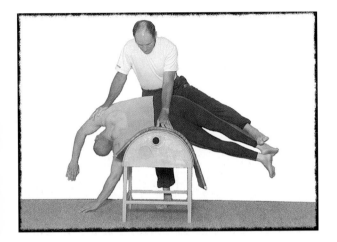

Cues

lie sideways on support

let yourself relax into position

C–R: lift away from support; or pull arm back to body and press leg up

restretch: move further in stretch direction

56. Sideways bend across support

This may be done solo, or with one or even two partners. In its simplest form, you lie across a curved support sideways, with the hips and shoulders vertical to start, and let gravity stretch you. Mark is demonstrating the position in the top frame, opposite page.

One partner may assist, as shown in the next two frames opposite: Julie is drawing Mark's arm off the body to increase the *latissimus dorsi* component of the stretch, and I am applying weight to just under Mark's shoulder and to the uppermost part of his thigh to increase the lateral flexion part of the stretch.

A **C–R stretch** may be achieved by bending sideways *away* from the support (to your partner's hands, in other words); and the partner applies a gentle second stretch. Contract for a count of five and restretch for 10 breaths or so. More stretch effect will be experienced by letting yourself relax, but many people are instinctively apprehensive about this.

A second partner may help, as shown in the last frame opposite: the first partner pulls on the leg first, then presses the thigh in the direction of the floor while the second partner draws the arm out from the body in the direction the arm is pointing. Thus a second **C–R** may be added. As in the first part of exercise 55, partner legs apart, above, the partner draws the arm off the body; you try to pull it back, and the partner applies the restretch. Contract for a count of five and stretch for five breaths. This combination gives a tremendous stretch to the whole trunk.

Breathing will be more difficult than usual because one lung is compressed and the other is stretched open. Trying to breathe deeply in this position is an excellent stretch for the intercostals, the muscles between the ribs.

In the sequence shown on this page, Alan shows how one partner can do the work of two, but in a less intense way. His body is behind me so that the hips and shoulders are held vertical. The second frame shows the leg being gently pressed to the floor.

All the positions shown can be altered to great effect by rolling your hips forwards slightly and restretching and by then rolling backwards and restretching. The entire trunk can be worked in this way. Pay attention to any differences between the sides and restretch the tighter side.

57. Lying legs behind

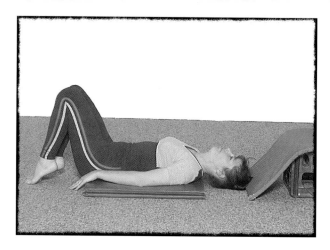

This is a modified version of a yoga asana, the *plough* pose. When performed strictly, the pose requires that the back (from the upper thoracic vertebrae to the lower lumbar vertebrae) be held straight, the body flexed at the hips, and the legs held straight also. Although a beautiful pose to see, this form necessitates a straight neck to be bent sharply forward at the level of the lowest cervical vertebra (C7). Some practitioners believe this to be responsible for some kinds of neck problems, although this has not been my experience. A modified form of the plough pose can be a safe and relaxing upper back stretch.

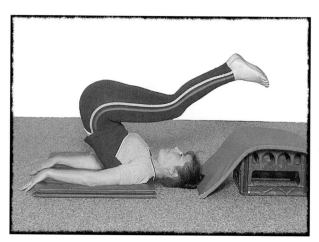

If performed traditionally, part of the effort felt in the muscles at the back of the neck is due to the legs being held straight. Through hamstring tension and leverage factors, considerable weight can be imposed on the back of the neck. For this reason, at least in the initial stages of working with the pose, the legs should be kept well bent at the knees. In addition, because we wish to use this pose to stretch the upper back, make no effort to straighten the back (in contrast to the traditional way of doing the pose). If you suspect that your neck is not sufficiently flexible bending forwards, use a folded blanket or mat under the back and shoulders to reduce the angle the neck will make with the body in the completed position, as shown. Using support in this way will not diminish the pose's effectiveness as an upper back stretching movement.

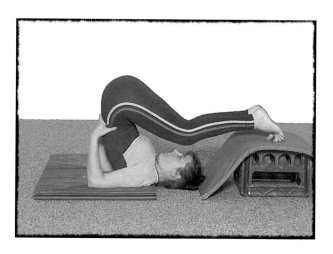

Look at the photographs; Sharon is demonstrating the movements. Before trying the pose, if you suspect that you may not be able to complete the movement comfortably, place a chair or box behind you, where you expect the legs to come to rest. When you try the exercise, your legs will rest on the support, and the difficulty of the pose will be reduced accordingly.

Begin by lying face up on the floor. If you are slender, you may wish to lie on something comfortable, because the *posterior processes* of the spine (the visible bumps of the backbone) will contact the floor as you get into and come out of the pose. On a breath out, lift and bend the legs and, continuing the momentum of this movement, press your hands down to the floor to lift the hips and bring the knees close to the chest. Continue this movement backward. This will lift the body up onto the shoulders and flex the neck

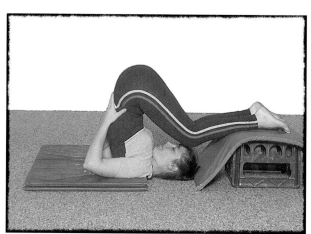

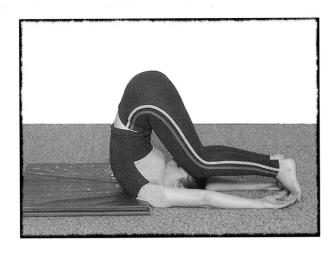

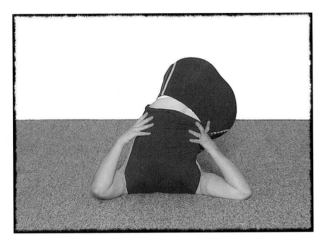

Cues

use shoulder support if necessary

lift legs up and back

ensure legs are supported in end position

let hips tilt to side

stretch neck back then forwards to finish

forward. Be cautious and do not exceed your capacity to bend at the neck. If you have placed a chair behind you (near your head), rest your legs on it. Otherwise, lower the legs slowly to the floor, keeping the knees flexed. Move your hands behind your head so that you can control precisely the degree of stretch in the neck, as shown. Rest in this position for a few breaths.

To increase the stretch, use the feet to walk the legs very slowly further behind you. As you do, let the upper back relax completely. Walking the legs away will increase the stretch in both the neck itself (the muscles at the back) and the upper back. Hold the final position for five breaths or so.

If you wish, you may add a gentle sideways bending component. Bend both arms at the elbows and hold your waist, then gently incline the body to one side until you feel a stretch in the opposite side of the neck. The body's weight will come onto the hand on the side you are leaning towards. Hold for a breath or two, return to the centre, and try the other side.

To return to the starting position, use the muscles of the lower back and the arms and shoulders (by pressing back against the floor) to lift the bent legs off the floor; then let the hips fall away from the previous position. As soon as you feel the upper back on the floor, or as soon as you feel your weight moving over the balanced position, place your hands out to the sides or alongside the body. Use the hands to lower the body slowly to the floor. When the lower back has reached the floor pause for a moment. Rest by letting the legs go down to the floor too.

As mentioned above, whenever we have done a strong stretching movement in one direction it feels good to perform a brief movement in the opposite direction. Accordingly, sit on the floor (or on a chair), straighten the back and open the mouth wide; incline the head backwards as far as it will go, and gently close the mouth and clench the teeth. Hold for a breath or two and return to the neutral position. Lift the shoulders up and down a few times, and turn the head from side to side.

58. Partner bar shoulder flexion with hip traction

This rather oddly named exercise is unique among shoulder exercises. The majority of exercises that use the arms and shoulders to help extend the spine place some compression stress on the shoulder joint. Many people find this the main impediment to improvement. This exercise uses a partner to apply traction (tension) to the shoulders and arms and, accordingly, the extension movement of the upper back imparts far less compression to the shoulders. Sharon is stretching and Jennifer is assisting.

Kneel and hold a suitable support with the hands. The knees are placed under the shoulders, or forward of the shoulders if you want less stretching force. Hold onto the support firmly. Your partner straddles your hips and, after placing their feet next to you, squeezes your waist with their legs. Once the waist is held, your partner leans back to pull your hips backwards. When sufficient traction has been applied, they bend at the waist and apply a downwards force to the roundest (most *convex*) part of the back. Relax into the stretch.

The **C–R stretch** requires that you press your hands down onto the support (your partner must increase their leaning force such that you do not move) for count of a five. On a breath out, ask your partner to restretch you very slowly and gently. Let yourself relax further into the position, and hold for five to ten breaths.

Make sure you do one of the upper-back forward bends to finish (exercise 1, any part of exercise 48 that stretches a tight area, or exercise 56).

Do the following exercises before attempting the two new shoulder exercises presented next.

Exercise 6, Chin to chest

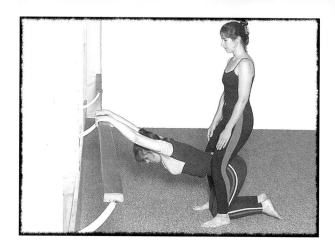

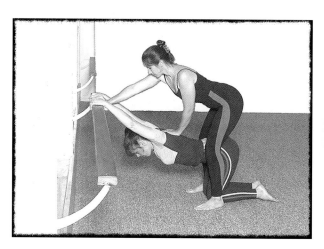

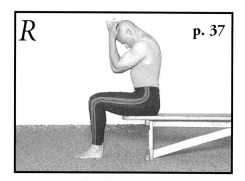

Cues (above)

hold support

partner squeezes waist with legs and leans back to elongate body

partner leans on roundest part of back

C–R: press hands into support

restretch: partner leans gently

Cues (left)

chin to chest

C–R: press head back to hands

restretch: gently pull head forwards

Exercise 15, Floor neck rotation

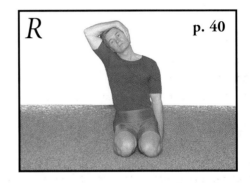

Cues (right)

turn head to side as far as possible

pause

turn head slowly further to side

Exercise 7, Floor neck side bend

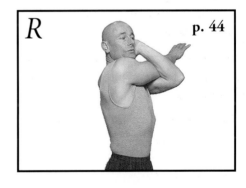

Cues (right)

restrain shoulder; take head to side

C–Rs: lift shoulder; press head to hand

restretch: lean away; take head further

Exercise 9, Arm across body; standing, lying

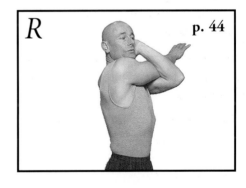

Cues (right)

arm across throat

pull with other arm

C–R: press arm away

restretch: pull arm closer

Exercise 43, Folded legs clasped knees upper back

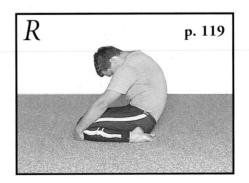

Cues (right)

hold knees

let body slump

push back backwards

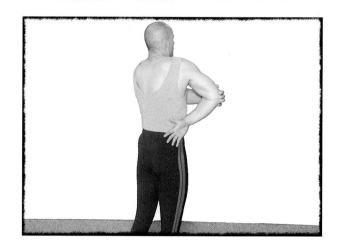

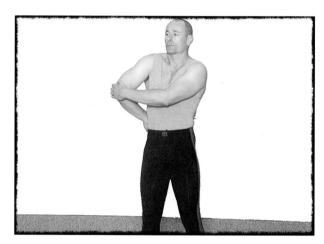

The rotator cuff muscles provide most of the stability of the shoulder joint in its large range of movements. Two muscles pass behind the shoulder joint (the *glenohumeral* joint): *infraspinatus* and *teres minor*. These rotate the upper arm *externally*, and hence are called the external rotators. One muscle is found above the shoulder joint (*supraspinatus*; this acts to *abduct* the arm in the early part of the movement), and one in front (*subscapularis*; this rotates the upper arm *internally*); together they are termed the internal rotators. When all contract, the head of the *humerus* (the bone of the upper arm) is pulled more closely into the cup of the shoulder joint, the *glenoid fossa*. Experimentation has shown that the majority of people have greater strength and flexibility in the internal rotators than the external rotators. The exceptions to this generalisation are rock climbers and gymnasts, in which the opposite pattern is more commonly observed. The following pair of exercises will give you insight to your pattern, and partner and solo versions are shown.

59. Partner/solo shoulder internal rotation

To stretch the external rotators, one must internally rotate the arm, the complementary movement. The external rotators are usually the main limitation to the movement of putting the arm up behind your back (exercise 11, arm up behind back) so you may care to do exercise 11 now to see whether doing exercise 59 yields improvement. The solo version requires you to place the fingers of one hand at the back of the waist as shown. Keep the fingers rigid while you reach around with the other arm to hold the elbow. Slowly pull the elbow forwards; this will rotate the upper arm in the shoulder joint. If you cannot reach the elbow, use a column, or projection from the wall, to move the elbow.

For the **C–R stretch**, press the held elbow directly *back* against the support of the other hand for a count of five. Relax, breathe out, and very slowly pull the elbow further forwards. You will feel the stretch in the shoulder itself, and perhaps behind the shoulder as well. Normal range of movement is to be able to move the arm to at least 45 degrees *in front of* the plane of the shoulders, as might be seen from above.

Cues
hand on side of waist
draw elbow forwards
C–R: press elbow back to hand
restretch: gently pull elbow further forwards

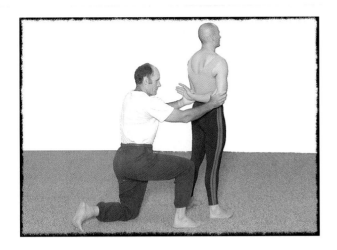

Cues

upper arm next to body

partner holds elbow and wrist;
draws wrist off back

C–R: pull your hand into your back

restretch: partner gently draws hand back

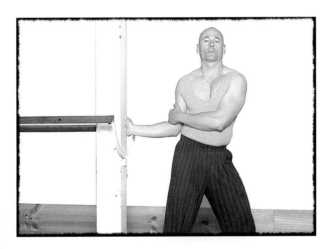

Cues (above)

hold support; hold upper arm to body

rotate other shoulder backwards

C–R: press hand into support

restretch: rotate further backwards

In the partner version (last frame; Alan is assisting) the fibres of the external rotators can be stretched more directly in their line of pull because the upper arm is next to the trunk, making it a better exercise. Put your arm behind your back, with the upper arm as close to the body as possible and the forearm parallel to the floor. Your partner holds the elbow of this arm stable and, holding your wrist as shown, slowly draws the forearm directly behind you, so that the upper arm rotates in the shoulder. Ensure that the upper arm is *vertical*.

In the **C–R stretch**, press your arm *directly* backwards towards your own back in a plane parallel to the floor, against your partner's resistance. The restretch is applied by your partner; ask them to move the arm slowly and gently until the required stretch is felt. Hold for a few breaths. To recover, lightly swing the arm around and, if you wish, try exercise 11 again.

60. *Partner/solo shoulder external rotation*

We now need to move the upper arm in the opposite direction to complete the stretches. Solo, this exercise requires a support that you can hold, and rotate the body away from, to get the movement. Look at the first photograph: the upper arm is held with the other hand, so that the upper arm can stay vertical during the movement— do not let the elbow go away from the body (a common error). Once in position, rotate the whole body around the held arm, so that the upper arm rotates in the joint.

In the **C–R stretch**, press the hand against the support (try to use *shoulder* muscles to do this—many arm muscles can be used in this action too) for a five count; then relax and, on a breath out, rotate the body further in the initial rotation direction until the right stretch is felt. Hold for a few breaths. In the final position, the forearm will be roughly in, or near, the plane of the shoulders, women slightly further.

The partner version is better, for the same reasons that the partner version of exercise 59 is better: greater stability and a more intuitive restretch direction. Your partner stands in front of you (top frame, overleaf), cups the back of your elbow with one hand, and applies the stretch rotation to your hand and wrist. The **C–R stretch** requires you to press the hand back to your partner (again, try to use the muscles of the shoulder joint to provide the force—arm and chest muscles could also be used) for a count of five, then relax and, on a breath out, ask your partner to cautiously take the arm further in the initial direction; hold for a few breaths.

The usefulness of exercises 59 and 60 lies in their ability to give you an idea of the comparative strengths of these muscles, and to provide efficient ways to both strengthen and stretch them. Experience suggests that the combined forces of the external rotators should be at least equal to the internal rotators. You and your partner will be able to assess this roughly by how much contraction force can be provided in the **C–R stretches**. If there is a significant disparity, remedial work in the gym using cables or dumbbells will improve the situation rapidly. The recommended form of the strengthening exercise should be as close as possible to the partner versions of the stretches because, when the arm is in this position relative to the shoulder joint, the line of pull of both sets of muscles is ideal. Accordingly, when doing external rotator cuff exercises, I recommend the upper arm be in line with the trunk and the forearm at 90 degrees to the upper arm. Keep the elbow close in to your side.

Do the following exercises to complete the shoulder stretches. By now you will be acquiring an accurate picture of your own loose and tight parts, and I suggest that you do the exercises only for the tighter parts from now on. Occasionally you can do the exercises for the looser parts, but this is not a priority. The exception to this rule is when particular gym training or athletic movements tighten even your loose areas; use the exercises to return them to normal.

Exercise 11, Partner arms up behind back

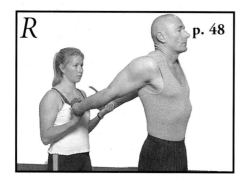

Do this exercise twice and ask your partner to check if the shoulders are level. Lean a bit more of your own weight on the tighter shoulder if they are not.

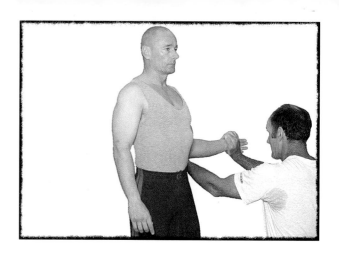

Cues (above)

partner holds elbow and hand
your upper arm next to body
C–R: press hand to partner
restretch: partner gently takes your hand further back

Cues (left)

fingers interlaced or use strap
roll shoulders back to begin
partner lifts arms
C–R: press hands to floor
restretch: partner lifts arms up

Cues

hold elbow; pull shoulder back

C–R: press elbow to side

restretch: pull shoulder further back
and pull elbow across

Cues

pull folded arm behind head

C–R: press elbow to side

restretch: pull elbow across and
press arm back with head

Cues

hands and knees; hips over knees

partner holds arm; supports hip

partner draws arm through

C–R: pull back on arm

restretch: let partner take you further

Exercise 12, Arm up behind shoulder blade

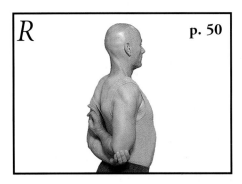

This exercise will be easier to do this time, because we have stretched the external rotator pair.

Exercise 13, Arm behind head

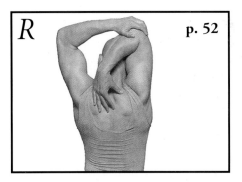

Exercise 49, Partner all fours rotation

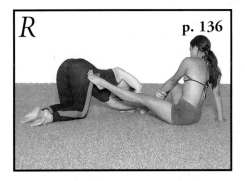

First encountered in lesson 7, this is an excellent whole-trunk stretch to use at the end of a stretch workout. Review the directions, because it is easy to make form errors in this. Slight alterations to the shape of the spine (in a backwards–forwards sense) make significant differences to where you will feel the greatest stretch effect, so play around with this aspect.

partner stands on legs
C–R: lift legs against resistance
restretch: let legs go to floor
incline straight body forwards
C–R: lift chest; press back to partner
restretch: pull yourself forwards

LESSON TEN: LEGS APART AND TRUNK

The main focus of this lesson is getting the legs apart; a goal of all martial artists, hurdlers, dancers, gymnasts, yoga practitioners—and you. No exercise demonstrates your flexibility more clearly in the gym than this one. Quite a few people are loose in the hamstrings without doing any special training, but very few people are naturally flexible in the legs-apart direction.

Free squats warm-up, knees apart version

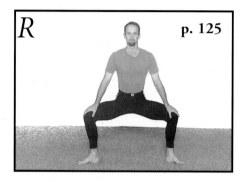

Cues (left)

ensure feet are under knees
use arms for balance
keep heels on the floor

Today, do a knees apart version of the free squat—20 repetitions. Except for the thigh angle, this is the same exercise as done in lessons 4 and 7.

Martial arts warm-up, feet flat

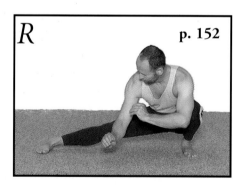

Cues (left)

feet flat on floor and parallel
lower hips to floor
keeps hips low moving side-to-side

Do 10 repetitions once you have managed to get as low as you can. Practising without a partner or a support if you can will develop your balance too. As a warm-up, either version is good. As a rule, do not expect to be as flexible (or more flexible) than the last time you practised. Assess the body's flexibility every time you begin exercising and modify the demands you make on yourself according to how you feel.

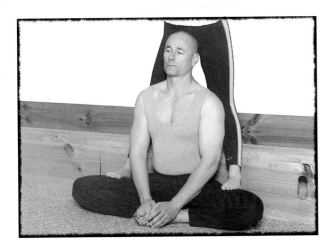

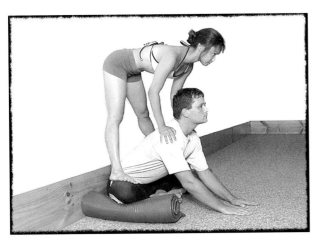

61. Partner wall seated knees apart

A partner can help you in a number of ways in this fundamental exercise; a number of possibilities are illustrated. Please review the directions for exercise 30, wall seated knees apart (lesson 5), before beginning practice. The most gentle partner version is to have your partner press the legs down for you, or support the lower back from behind (not shown).

A stronger version, preferred by most people in our classes, is to have your partner stand on your legs as shown; close to the hip for the least stretch effect (first frame), and out towards the knees for the greatest effect. You may roll mats and place them under your knees to prevent you from stretching too far if you wish and, similar to the supported front splits of lesson 7, just feeling the support under the knees helps the muscles to relax (Julie and Mark, second frame). The weight applied by your partner may be further varied by how much of their own weight they take, by sitting on a bar or support, and by how much pressure they apply to your legs. Recall that in the contraction phase, your legs must not move at all; this means that as you apply the contraction they must increase their support—and when you relax, their effort must decrease, too. Accordingly, make contractions and relaxations relatively *slow*.

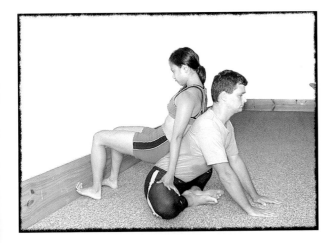

Once the knees are on the floor, or close to it, the second part of the exercise may be attempted. This involves holding your feet and leaning forwards with a straight back, so that the body moves only via the hip joints. To this end, have your partner change their position to apply their bottom to the lower back (so that the backward curve of the lumbar spine is maintained), and support themselves by putting their hands on your knees; this will help to keep them on the floor as you bend forwards.

The **C–R stretch** contraction requires you to straighten your back, lift the chest, and press back gently against your partner using the muscles of the legs. Your arms should feel as though they are being unweighted if you do this properly, but of course you keep the hands on the feet for support. The contraction can be a long 10 count; relax and, as you breathe out, restraighten the back and let yourself go further forwards. In some people the final position causes a compression sensation in the ankles, but this will disappear as soon as you finish the exercise. Once your stomach and

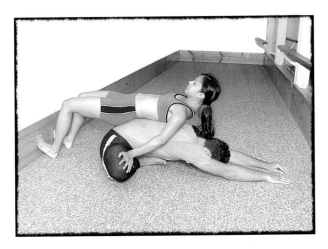

ribs make contact with your feet, you may let the upper and middle back bend forwards, but try to pull yourself over the feet (that is, pull in the plane of the floor, rather than pull yourself down to your feet) to increase the stretch. Hold the final position for 10 breaths in and out.

Any of the assistance techniques for exercise 30 can be used here too, such as widening the distance between the feet and doing the exercise on a low support.

Wall standing legs apart warm-up

The reason this feels different to the free standing legs apart warm-up (first encountered in lesson 5) is that, when the wall is used, your hips cannot move behind the line of the heels (in the standing version, this automatically happens as you bend forwards, to maintain balance over your centre of gravity). Because this cannot happen with your hips against the wall the calf muscles experience a stronger stretch as you bend forwards at the waist. Your partner holds your hips against the wall, by leaning weight against the roundest part of your lower back. The first two photographs show Carol helping Greg to bend further forwards at the hips using this assistance. The next two show bending over each leg in turn, and an additional movement for the arm; you can precede this straight-leg version with a slightly bent leg variation if you wish, as an additional warm-up. Once you have stretched over both legs in turn, come back to the middle position and try a stronger forward bend between both legs.

Exercise 55, Partner seated legs apart

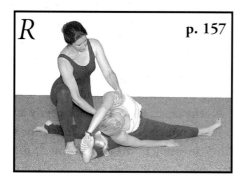

R   p. 157

Use this exercise as a warm-up too. Spend just a few moments doing the first two parts (side bending and bending over each leg in turn). We will return to the third part, bending forwards between both legs, later in the lesson, when we have stretched the adductors properly.

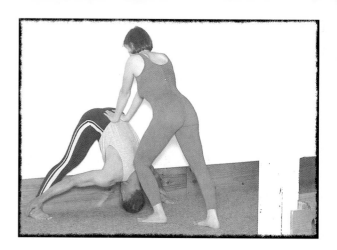

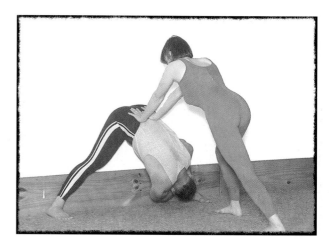

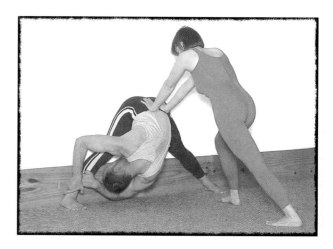

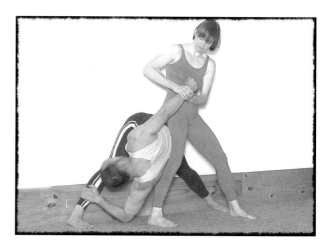

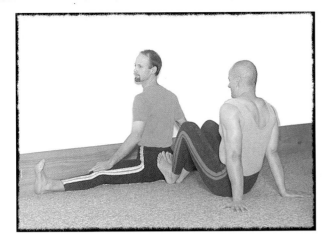

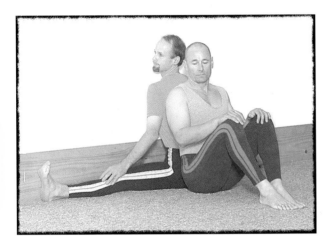

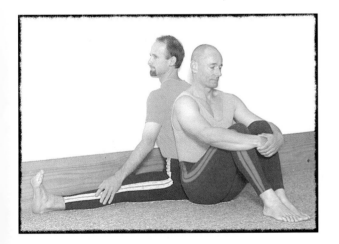

62. Partner wall seated legs apart, facing wall

Achieving side splits requires hyperextension of the lumbar spine in addition to hip abduction, as mentioned above. If we want to concentrate on pure hip abduction, we need to stretch the adductors while keeping the lumbar spine neutral—neither hyperextended nor bent forwards. Exercise 62 does this efficiently. Exercise 34, encountered in lesson 5, describes the solo version; review the instructions if you wish. The advantage of the partner version is that support is provided at exactly the right place and, because your partner is providing the effort to move the hips closer to the wall, you will be able to use a stronger contraction. Take care with your knees, however; as mentioned, some people's knees are sensitive to lateral forces, so you might need to tighten *quadriceps* while applying the contraction, and again while restretching. Two support positions are shown: the first is more difficult for the partner to hold but allows very fine control over how close you move towards the wall, and the second is easy for the partner to hold the final position for any desired length of time.

We have found that stronger contractions in the **C–R stretches** for both the hamstrings and the adductors work well in terms of final stretch positions achieved, in contrast to using gentle contractions which seem to work well for most other groups. 'Stronger' may be a matter of perception: these are large muscles, and even using half one's available strength in a contraction may seem like a lot of effort. Try different effort contractions and see what works best for you. If you are going to try to use more effort, I suggest you begin with a gentle contraction, and then, over the period of applying the force, slowly increase the effort. This way you are much less likely to hurt yourself: your body will tell you if you are trying too hard. Stay in the final stretch position for 10 to 15 breaths.

Cues

feet against wall, pointing up

partner's back against yours

partner helps hips towards wall

C–R: squeeze legs together

restretch: partner gently
helps hips closer to wall

Exercise 27, Backward bend over support

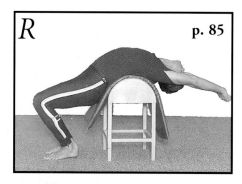

p. 85

To prepare the lower back for the next exercise, do exercise 27 once more (full details are found in lesson 4). Be sure to do the second version that focuses on the middle and lower back, with the middle of the body over the highest part of the support.

Exercise 2, Backward bend from floor

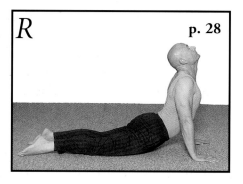

p. 28

Because the maximum legs-apart position occurs together with hyperextension, the lower back will benefit from a good stretch in this position. You can ask your partner to sit on your lower legs, and very gently help you to bend further backwards. Make sure you stretch the lower back out with one of the forward-bending recovery poses.

Cues (left)

middle of body over top of support

extend arms as far as possible

let yourself relax

Cues (left)

back muscles soft

lift only with arms

pull shoulders back; head back

curl up to finish

Cues (right)

use soft support or hands

feet flat on floor

widen legs

C–R: squeeze legs together

restretch: let gravity stretch you

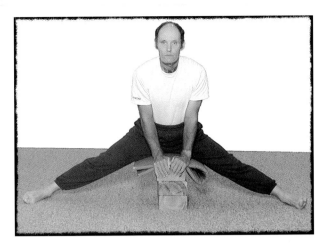

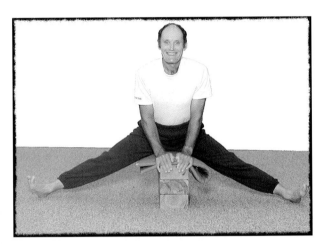

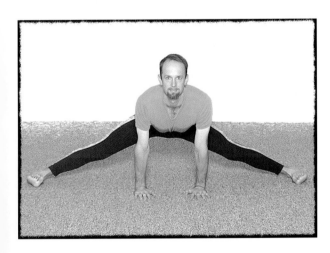

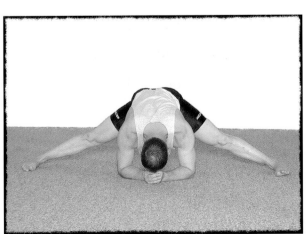

63. Legs apart, off support

This exercise is the most effective movement for achieving the flexibility that will allow you to sit in side splits one day. It is suitable for beginners and advanced alike. Practising the exercise as described will also increase the strength of your legs considerably. The action of exerting your strength in this movement may facilitate the brain's mapping of the leg's proprioceptors—and we have noticed that as the student's capacity to exert the strength of these muscles increases, so does their flexibility. We conclude that for particular leverage and joint protection reasons, the proprioceptors are the major limiters of flexibility in this movement.

Recall the discussion in lesson 5 in relation to position of the pelvis and legs-apart flexibility: the pelvis needs to tilt forwards (*anteversion*) and the thighs to turn out (externally rotated) to achieve the maximum position. If we consider this from another perspective, we can see that a maximum stretch in the adductors will be achieved by taking the legs apart *without* letting either of these facilitations take place, and that is what we did in exercise 62. We can do exercise 63 without turning the legs out (keeping the feet flat on the floor) but we can let the back bend—so, together, exercises 63 and 63 provide three different ways of stretching these muscles.

Look at the first photograph. Alan is using a support that can deform slightly under his weight and he has spread his legs as far as he can with the feet flat on the floor; accordingly, his legs are not turned out. The **C–R stretch** is achieved by trying to bring the legs together, as though through the floor. Begin with a gentle squeeze and, over the space of a 10 to 15 count, slowly increase the contraction force. Do not use more than about half your available strength the first few times you try this movement. You may support yourself by using your hands or, if you are strong enough, do the contractions unsupported. Kevin is demonstrating the legs apart position supported on his arms. Relax, and on a long breath out, slide your feet further apart. Hold the new position for 10 breaths. All the stretch effects will be felt in the muscles on the inside of the thighs.

The next two frames show Kevin and Greg demonstrating two arm support positions that may be used. In both positions the adductors will experience the main effects. The **C–R** is achieved by trying to bring the legs together.

Now, lift yourself from the stretch position and walk around for a moment or two to relax the body. Get back over the support, but this time turn your feet out to the sides as much as you can and rest on your heels with the feet pointing up to the ceiling as I am demonstrating in the first frame. Sink as low as you can, and repeat the **C–R stretch**. This time, you will feel the hamstrings contracting as you squeeze the legs together. Again, use an increasing strength contraction for a 10 to 15 count. Stop, relax and, on a breath out, use gravity to help you get the legs further apart. Hold the end position for 10 breaths. You will notice that you can get closer to the floor and you will be able to feel that your lower back is bending further backwards as you make this attempt. Rest, and repeat this two-part cycle one or two more times until you feel that you cannot improve any more in this session.

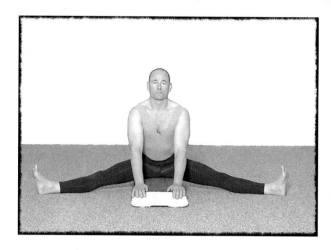

Once you are as close to the floor as you can get, hold the middle and upper back straight and let your trunk go towards the support, moving through the hip joints, as I am showing in the second frame, keeping the hips and feet in a straight line. Any inclination of the body forwards past the angle needed to get into the final position will increase the stretch in both the inner hamstrings and the adductors, so make this lean a slow and gentle move. One further **C–R stretch** can be done in this inclined position by squeezing the legs together. Instead of sinking lower after this contraction, however, let the body go forwards closer to the support, until the body is horizontal. Hold the final position for at least five breaths.

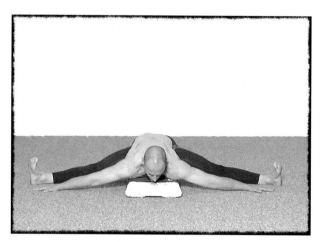

Greg is demonstrating how to position the body so that the inner hamstrings and adductors approximately share the effects (bottom two frames). With the body inclined forwards in this way, strong contractions produce an immediate leg-widening effect. The top photograph on the facing page shows how the legs can be taken wide apart *without* hyperextension, best done by lowering yourself into position, as Greg is doing.

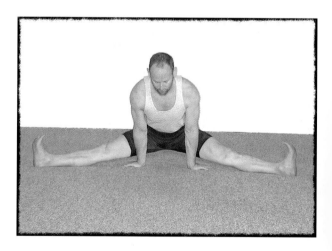

I am demonstrating two assistance positions. In the first, Olivia is holding my legs against the support with her legs, by pressing backwards. This reduces the effect of gravity on my legs, making relaxation easier. The third frame shows a lowering technique where the feet slide apart in the purpose-built boxes; Olivia is assisting by holding my hips directly over my feet, the most difficult position.

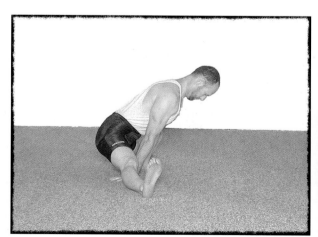

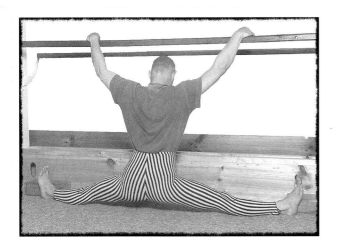

Cues (for legs apart)

use support of correct height

have feet pointing up

have legs 180 degrees (Kit, left, top)

C–R: squeeze legs together

restretch: widen legs and
incline straight body forwards (left, 2nd)

partner holds hips against support (below)

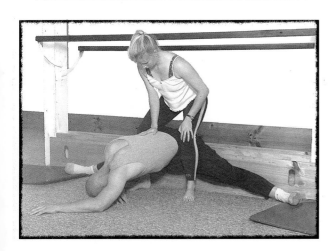

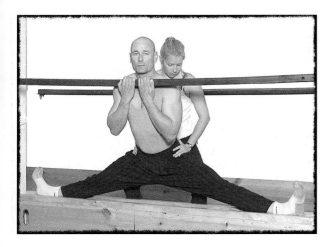

Exercise 3, Lying rotation

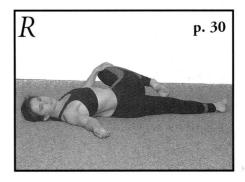

As the last exercise is strenuous, lie down for a moment and redo exercise 3. Take your time and let yourself relax in the final position for at least five breaths per side.

Exercise 4, Standing side bend

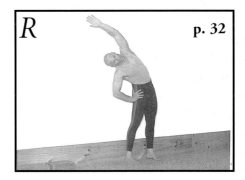

Repeat this exercise, but do not try to improve the range of movement achieved; rather, use it to make the body feel balanced.

Exercise 55, Partner seated legs apart

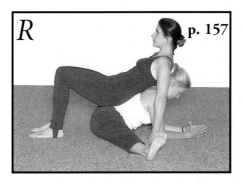

Do this exercise again, and see whether the legs-apart off-support exercise has improved your final position. Most people have a breakthrough in this movement after doing exercise 63.

64. Seated or standing bent leg rotation

This rotation movement can be as strong or as gentle as you wish. If done standing, it is more strenuous (simply because you are having to support your weight on bent legs as well as do the exercise) but, if done seated, is still an excellent rotation. One of its advantages is that body size does not limit its effectiveness (we developed it when Jennifer was seven months' pregnant) and, unlike some rotation exercises, hip flexibility is irrelevant. There is no limit to how far you go, either—as you will have seen by now, some rotation movements are limited by physical constraints. Here, your final position is limited only by your capacity to move the shoulders in relation to fixed hips.

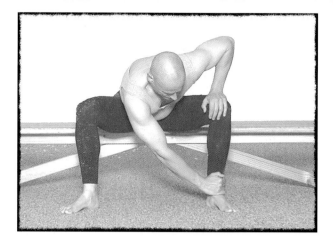

In the first photograph, the body is located in between the knees (standing or sitting version). This body position gives the stretch effect over the largest area of the trunk. Grasp the ankle first, and pull on it so that the elbow bends. The extent of the bend locates where the body will be in relation to the knees. Place the other hand on the knee as shown, and press the shoulder back as far as you can. Pull on the ankle and press on the knee together to feel the stretch you want. The **C–R stretch** is achieved by using the muscles of the waist to try to twist in the opposite direction—but your arms hold you in position. Contract for a count of five, relax, and take a breath in. On a breath out, slowly pull and push on both hands until the desired rotation is felt. Hold the final position for a few breaths in and out.

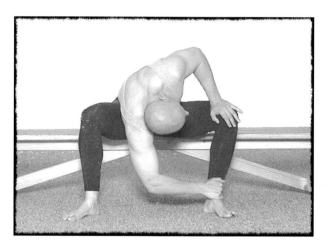

The third photograph shows the exercise being done in a different way—the body is closer to one leg. Try a variety of positions between the knees; each one will focus the stretch in a different place. A number of these different positions can be tried in moments and particular positions may stretch desired tight spots.

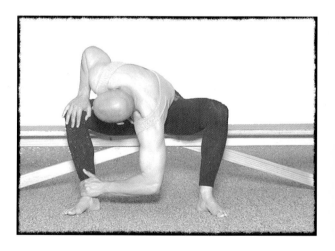

The bottom photo shows my preferred version. Done standing, further alterations to the sensations can be made by the depth of your squat position, as well as by where you position the body between the legs.

65. Partner kneeling arms up and behind

This exercise is a distinct change of pace—it is a minor exercise that nonetheless feels great to do. It is an excellent stretch for the pectoral muscles and, in the final position,

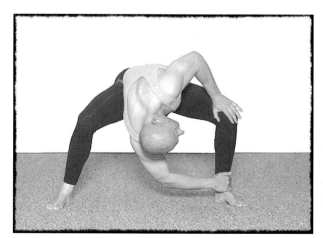

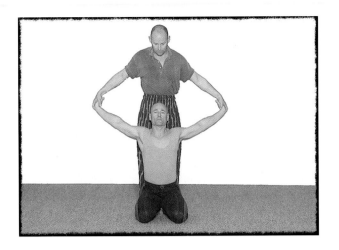

Cues (above)

arms up and back

partner helps find most difficult angle

C–R: draw hands towards knees

restretch: further up and back

the ribs will be lifted, and the front shoulder and *biceps* muscles will be stretched, too. In the flexible person, there will be a gentle extension of the upper and middle spine.

Sit on folded legs as shown. Your partner stands so that their legs are a support for the middle of your back. Lift your arms up so the fingers are approximately level with the top of your head. Your partner holds your wrists from above and takes the arms back while maintaining their height. Let yourself be stretched for a moment or two. The **C–R stretch** requires that you gently pull the arms down and in, towards the knees. This line will pull directly on the middle fibres of the chest muscles, where they attach to the *sternum*; and the restretch will provide a pleasant sensation. Breathing deeply in the final position will work the diaphragm muscle strongly, as it is stretched by the elevation of the ribs.

We will finish with two spine-flexion exercises, the first for the middle and upper back (first taught in lesson 9) and the second for the lower back (presented in lesson 7).

Exercise 57, Lying legs behind

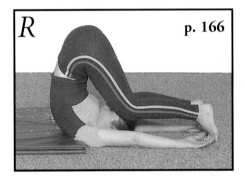

Exercise 48, Floor forward bend over bent legs

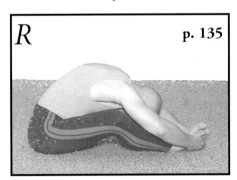

Cues (left)

sit or stand in support position

hold opposite ankle; pull on hand while you push top shoulder back

C–R: twist trunk in opposite direction

restretch: push/pull in stretch direction

LESSON ELEVEN: BALANCING AND STRENGTH

This relatively short but taxing lesson teaches preparation techniques for balancing poses, and two major compound exercises that combine strength and flexibility. Each of these exercises has dynamic and static elements and the transitions from the moving to the held parts provide additional interest. We have found the balancing exercises to be excellent stretches as well—perhaps only because you will be so occupied trying to balance that you won't notice how intense the stretch aspect really is!

Free squats warm-up, knees apart, revisited

Review the directions for the standing version of exercise 64, bent-leg rotation, page 182. Do 20 repetitions of the knees apart version of the free squat (first encountered last lesson). Do not hurry these; the emphasis in this lesson is on making the connection between your mind and your muscles as strong as possible. Feel the way the body transfers weight between its parts during the lowering phase, and how the buttock and hamstring muscles provide the effort for the first part of the lift out of the squat position and how the *quadriceps* take over just below the half-way point. If you do the movements quickly, these subtleties will be lost. Pause in the bottom position for a moment in a few of the repetitions.

In the final repetition, use the elbows inside the knees to gently force the thighs further apart (described in lesson 8). Hold this position for five breaths. Lift yourself up until the thighs are parallel with the floor and, placing one palm on the floor next to one foot as shown, reach the other out as far as you can, rotating at the shoulders until the arms are vertical. Hold this position for a couple of breaths. Bring the top arm back, place it on the floor inside the other foot, and repeat for the other side.

Come out of the second position and move directly into the standing version of exercise 64, which you can follow with an arm supported legs-apart warm-up, with contractions if you desire. Directions for the legs-apart warm-up will be found on page 93.

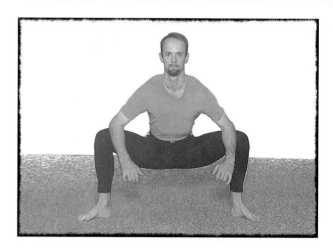

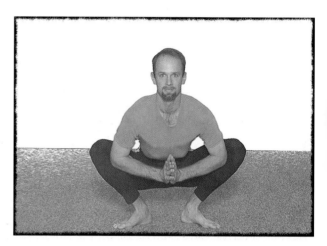

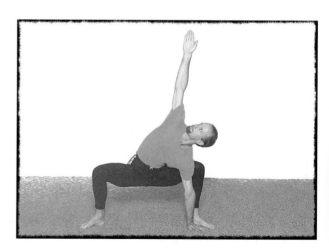

Cues (above)

lower into deep squat position

use elbows to widen knees

C–R: squeeze knees together

restretch: press knees back

using support arm, take top shoulder and arm back; reach up

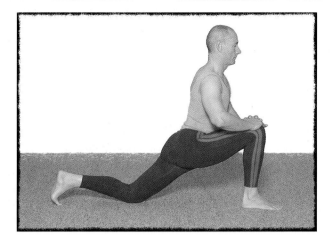

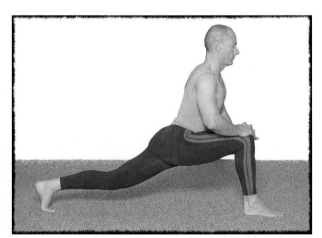

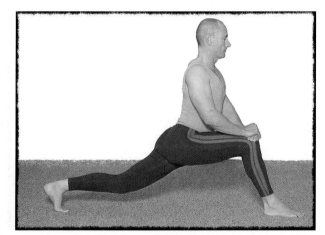

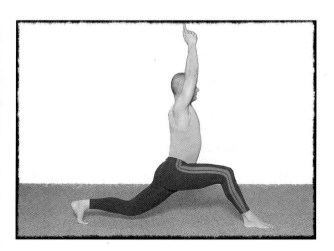

Martial arts warm-up, feet up or flat

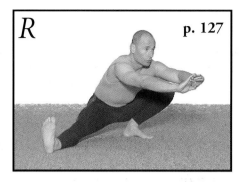

R   p. 127

Choose which version of this exercise you prefer; full descriptions will be found in lessons 7 and 8. You may use a partner or a support if you need to but, as the emphasis of this lesson is on balance, try to do eight repetitions by yourself. Feel how the body needs to fold forwards at both the hips and the ankles, just to be able to balance. Do not let the ankle of the folded leg roll inwards, and check to see whether this foot and the straight leg make a 90 degree angle (both versions). Try to keep your lower back as straight as you can and, in the transition moves, keep the hips as low to the floor as possible.

Standing suspended hip flexor (ex. 25) and buttock and hip flexor (ex. 21) warm-up

Review the directions for exercise 25, lesson 4, and exercise 21, lesson 3. We are going to do a version of exercise 26 without support, so it contains a balancing component in addition to the stretching component, and link the final position to exercise 21. Together, these movements are an excellent warm-up for any activity performed on the legs, and will be the perfect warm-up for this lesson's focus.

Move into the start position of exercise 26, one hand on the front knee, the other behind the hip of the back leg to help you get the hips square. Make sure that your feet are hip-width apart (as might be seen from the front) for balance. The front foot *must* be slightly in front of the knee, to ensure its stability. Use the hand and the hip and waist muscles to rotate the hip of the back leg forwards as much as you can, and press the hand on the knee down hard to activate the abdominal brace. As mentioned when we first practised the hip flexor exercises, you may use the back leg's bottom muscles to tuck your bottom under if that works better than the abdominal brace. Alternatively, you may use both hands on the front knee, if that makes holding the abdominal brace easier. Holding the position, slowly straighten the back leg, keeping both hips as low as possible. Once in this position, maintain the rotation, take your arms out wide and join them over your head, extending the arms towards the ceiling as far as possible. This is the first position.

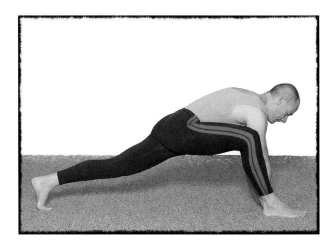

After a few breaths in this position, let the back leg bend again, until the hips lower further and the knee touches the floor. Check the hip rotation once more, keep the hips down, and restraighten the back leg—it does not matter if you do not get it straight; this is a balancing, strengthening and stretching exercise. Lean the trunk back until you are vertical, and hold the final position for at least five breaths.

Breathe out, take the arms out wide, and place them on the floor *inside* the front foot—you will recognise this as the start position of exercise 21. Recall the directions: pull back on the hands to straighten the back as you breathe in, hold the position for a few breaths and, on a breath out, let the arms bend, only as far as you can hold the back straight. Hold this position for five breaths and, on a breath out, let the arms and the back bend as far as possible. Keep the hips level with the floor while you do this. Hold the final position for a few breaths, return to the starting position, and repeat for the other side.

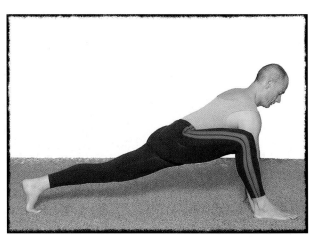

Cues

move into deep lunge position
lift arms up; lean back and reach above
place hands on floor inside leg
C–R: pull back on hands
restretch: let level hips sink deeper
let arms bend (keep back straight)
let back bend while keeping hips level

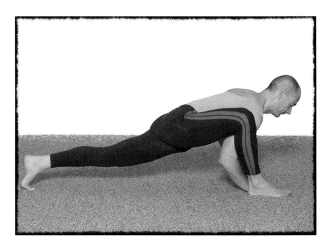

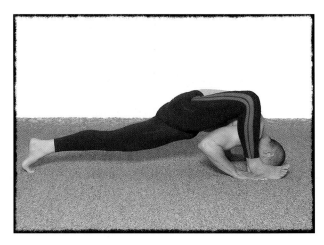

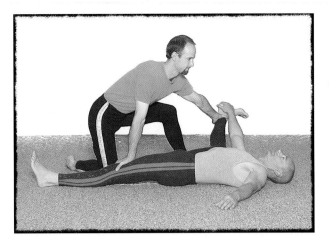

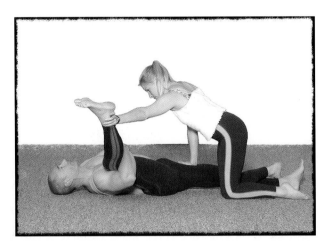

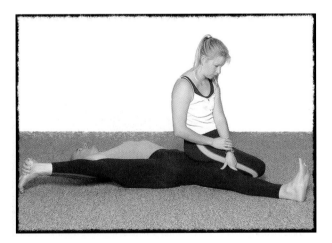

Cues

partner supports leg on floor

hold bent leg next to body

try to straighten leg

C–Rs: pull heel to bottom;
press thigh back to partner

restretch: slowly straighten leg

66. Partner lying 'Y'

This fantastic hamstring and adductor stretch will prepare us for a later exercise. The advantages of the lying version are that the lower back is entirely supported, good form is guaranteed by the floor, and the contractions are easy for the partner to apply. It may be that you will need to work on this version for a while before trying the standing version below.

Exercise 66 is an advanced version of exercise 28, partner lying hamstring, that was presented in lesson 4. Review the instructions for exercise 28 (page 89) before attempting this exercise. The **C–R stretches** are the same, but as we are attempting to put the leg on the floor alongside us, we will need to have the leg quite a bit further outside the body than before.

Lie on the floor as shown. Ask your partner to support the thigh of the bent leg, as close to the back of the knee as possible. If you are very flexible, the *front* of this thigh will be on the floor, with the back of the straight leg held firmly on the floor. The stretch in the hip of the flexed leg is lost if the hip of the straight leg leaves the floor. While your partner holds you in this position, use the *quadriceps* of the flexed leg to try to straighten it. This will be a strong stretch in the hamstring (and the adductors, if the hip is sufficiently flexed) of the leg you are straightening.

Two **C–R stretches** may be done, as in exercise 28; one is to press the thigh back against your partner's resistance, and the other is to try to pull the heel of the flexed leg back to the buttock against resistance (your partner will need to change support position for this). The final stretch is done with your partner's hands in support positions as shown. The key to success in the final stretch is to let the muscles being stretched completely relax. To this end, you and your partner must perform the straightening movement very slowly; one is apprehensive about what will happen because the stretch is intense. Hold the final position for a minimum of five breaths. Change legs and stretch the other side, then walk around for a moment.

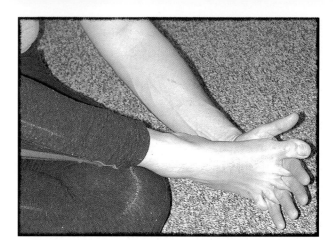

67. Floor feet sequence warm-up

You deserve a rest after the last exercise but, before you sit down, look down at your feet, and try to spread the toes. Can you move them all apart? Let's see if this can be improved. In most people, the feet are their forgotten body part—toes are cramped by shoes, the big toe is pushed towards the other toes by pronating ankles and, in general, the feet have poor flexibility.

This minor sequence will redress some of these problems. Sit on the floor with your legs crossed. Interlace the fingers of the (say) left hand with the toes of the right foot, as shown in the top photograph. Push the fingers in as deeply as you can; you should be able to feel the skin in between the toes being stretched. We have found that stretching this skin—normally moist from wearing shoes—seems to protect the feet from fungal infections. Grip the foot firmly and stretch the instep by pressing the heel of the palm into the ball of the foot (second frame). A **C–R stretch** may be achieved by trying to draw the toes back against the resistance of your hand for a few seconds, and restretching. Do this with both feet.

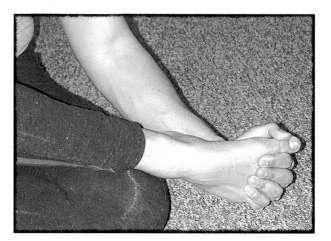

To stretch the toes backwards, sit on the floor as shown in the third photograph, with the ball of the foot firmly on the floor. By sliding the knee forwards slowly while keeping the ball on the floor, you will reach a position where the toes are strongly stretched. To effect a **C–R stretch**, press the toes into the floor gently for a five count, relax, and restretch by sliding the knee a little further forwards. Do both feet.

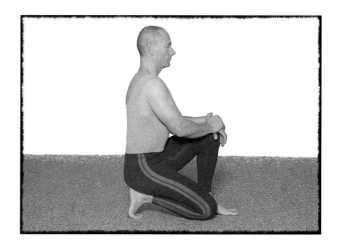

Now stand with the weight on both feet. Try again to spread the toes—any better results this time? Practising the above sequence will activate the toes quickly, and you will be surprised by the control that you will have.

Stand once more; this time, lift all toes off the floor as far as you can. Feel where your feet make contact with the floor. For many people, the floor is felt through the ball of the foot behind the big toe and through the heel. If this is so in your case, look at the shape of your foot—does the ankle roll inwards? You can help correct this by pressing weight on the little-toe side until you feel the foot on the little-toe side contacting the floor too, giving you three points of contact with the floor (ball, little-toe side of ball, and heel). When you have this three-point contact, look at your foot and its arch once again—is the arch further off the floor? The

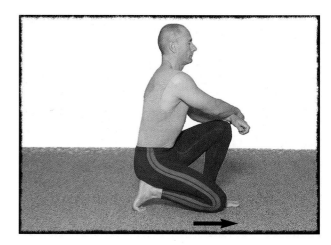

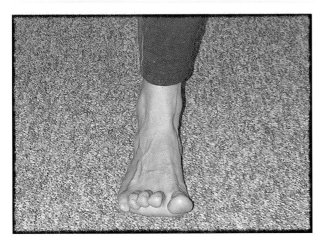

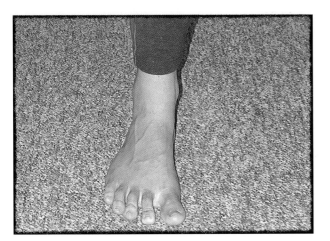

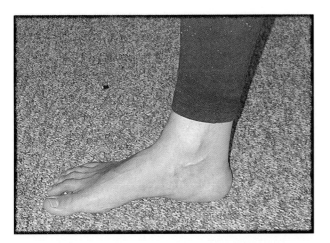

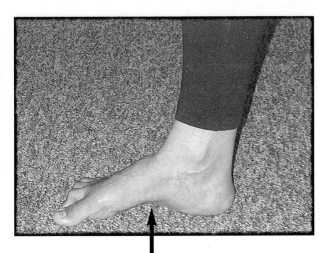

majority who have been told that they have flat feet in fact have pronating or inverting ankles, which is very largely a muscular condition, and can be altered by going through this simple exercise from time to time. You can also practise gripping the floor with your feet, such that the tips of the toes bend backwards as shown in the top two photographs; when you do, you will feel the arch of the foot contract.

The second reason to go through the sequence above is to acquire the feeling and awareness of the foot's natural tripod support, the long (*plantar*) arch between the ball and the heel, and the *metatarsal* arch, between the points of contact behind the big and little toes. Lifting the toes brings this second arch out, and makes us aware of how we might balance—vital in the two new exercises, overleaf.

Exercise 21, Buttock and hip flexor

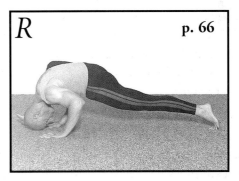

Concentrate on stretching the hip and upper hamstring muscles, one leg at a time. Try to get the body as low to the floor as possible before bending the back.

Exercise 17, Floor single leg forward bend

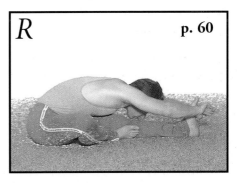

Concentrate on getting the maximum stretch in each hamstring—the two exercises we are about to learn tax these muscles. Hold your best end position for 15 to 20 breaths on each leg, and restretch the tighter of the two for another 10 breaths.

68. Standing horizontal one leg support

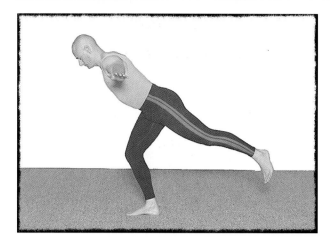

In addition to being an excellent hamstring stretch and an enjoyable balancing pose, exercise 68 is an extremely effective hip and lower-back strengthening movement. It is also effective in revealing subtle left–right differences in the body's balance, strength and flexibility—and just as effective in redressing these. Like many complex poses, its effects will likely be different for everyone.

To maximise the benefits, it will be necessary to get into the pose in the recommended way. Begin by bending one leg and lifting the toes of that foot to make sure that you are standing on *all* parts of your foot. Spread your toes as wide as possible and place them firmly on the floor. Pivot the body far enough forwards until you can straighten the other leg and bring it into the same line as the body. Take your arms out to the sides and keep bending forwards at the hip until the body and leg are parallel with the floor, and as straight as you can make them. This is the first position— have your partner check that your hips are level (the hip on the straight-leg side will want to lift). If the hips are not level, drop the higher one; normally this will make you feel a small stretch high up and under the buttock of the supporting leg.

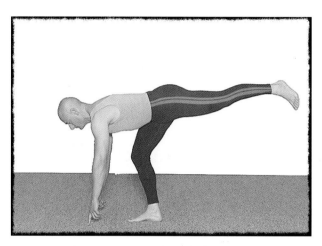

Slowly extend the arms out in front of you, as far as you can. Feel how both hips need to move *back* slightly as this occurs, in order for you to be able to maintain balance. Once the arms are extended as far as possible, imagine that both the foot behind you and both hands are being pulled gently away from each other, so that the body becomes a perfectly straight object. Again check the level of the hips—the support leg *must* still be bent at this point.

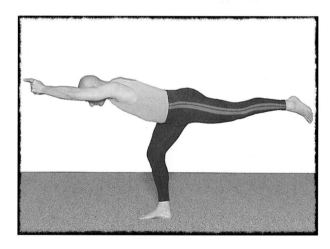

To finish the exercise, very slowly straighten the support leg *without letting the hip lift*. This is far more difficult to do than it sounds—as you attempt it, you will feel a very strong stretch in the hamstring of the supporting leg, so it is essential to try to straighten the leg slowly. The reason this apparently modest hamstring position is such a strong stretch (turn the book to the side, and you will see that the leg is making only a 90 degree bend at the hip) is because the leg behind you has rotated the pelvis into a very strict negative thrust position (the hip flexors and some of *quadriceps* take the pelvis with them as the leg goes behind). Notice, too, how much work the buttock muscles on the

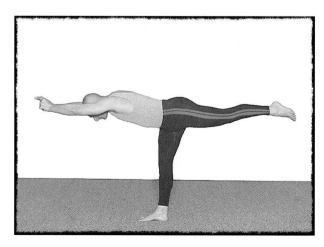

Cues (left)

lean over bent support leg
hips level; reach arms out to side
arms, body and leg aligned
reach arms out to front
check hip level
very slowly straighten support leg

Cues (right)

hold ankles tightly
push hips up to ceiling
C–R: try to straighten legs
restretch: push hips higher

Cues (right)

chin on chest
let back slump
pull face to knees
add rotations if desired

horizontal leg and all the back muscles from shoulder to hip have to do—this is the strengthening aspect and, because of the alignment of the body, you (and your proprioceptors!) become aware of what being in a good line feels like. Hold the final position for at least five breaths in and out.

Do not be tempted to hold a support when trying this exercise. It is far better to lose your balance many times than to do it from a support, in my view. Success will come to you if you try, and the secret is in perfecting the second position (body and leg horizontal on a *bent* support leg). A partner may tell you to lift the leg or the chest, or give you pointers regarding alignment, of course. Do the pose for the other leg and repeat for whichever side was the more difficult—difficulty may be a matter of balance or flexibility.

Exercise 42, Floor feet held back bend

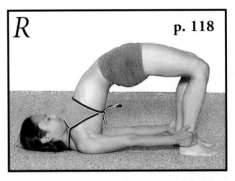

Push harder with the *quadriceps* in your efforts to try to straighten the legs in the final position on this attempt.

Exercise 43, Folded legs clasped knees upper back

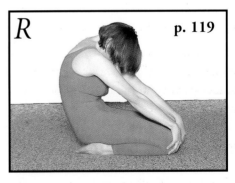

Recall that you may pull on the arms to increase the stretch and induce a rotation by pulling on the left knee with the right hand, and vice versa.

69. Standing 'Y' one leg support

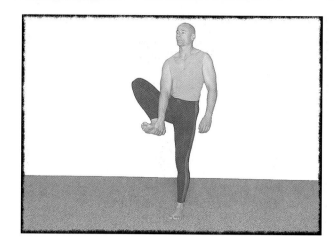

This exercise is a strong stretch for the hamstrings and a good strengthening exercise for many hip and trunk muscles, especially those that stabilise the pelvis. If your hamstring flexibility is limited, loop a strap around your foot—all the strengthening and balancing aspects will be experienced, but with less effect in the hamstrings.

Again, alignment is paramount in this movement. Because your centre of gravity is quite a bit higher than the previous exercise, balancing is more difficult. In addition, moving the outstretched leg from the front of the body to the side involves considerable transfer of weight from the middle of the body to the side. The first position is by far the more difficult exercise in the stretching sense, even though the final position looks more difficult.

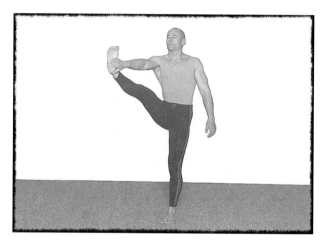

Repeat the toe lifting, spreading and placing sequence described above at the end of exercise 67. Hold one foot from the inside, as shown, making sure the support leg is completely straight and in line with the body. Maintaining this alignment, slowly try to straighten the leg you are holding. Errors include bending forwards at the waist, and bending the support leg. If you cannot straighten the leg as directed, use a strap. Once the leg is straight, breathe deeply and stay as still as possible, elongating your body and lifting the chest to achieve the desired line.

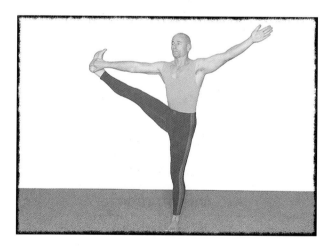

Slowly take the held leg to the side—be aware that this movement will disturb your balance position if you are not careful. As you reach the limit of your hip flexibility, try not to let the hip on this side be pulled away upwards to the leg. Keep the hips as level as you can, as I am demonstrating in the third frame, because this provides the strongest stretch effects. In the final position, breathe in and out for five cycles, let the leg bend, and gracefully replace it on the floor. Do the other leg and repeat the sequence for whichever side was either tighter or harder to balance on.

Cues

spread toes and grip floor

hold bent leg from inside

do not hold onto support

extend leg slowly; use strap if necessary

keep trunk and support leg aligned

slowly take leg to side

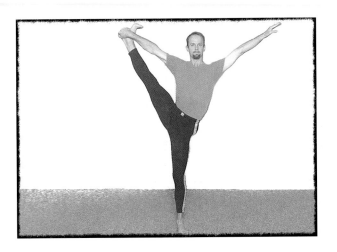

Kevin is showing a more dramatic version of the exercise, where he has deliberately let the hip of the raised leg be lifted to the side. It looks spectacular but is not as effective a stretch as the version above, because the body has accommodated the demands of the position by a tilting of the pelvis and a lateral curve of the spine. It is good to try this version from time to time, if only to experience the alteration in the body's balance that this additional movement requires. Let the body cool down and finish the lesson by doing the following two poses.

Exercise 48, Floor forward bend over bent legs

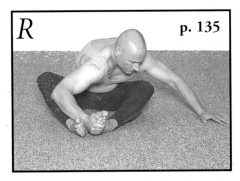

This photograph shows the rotation part of this pose—stretch the whole of spine first. To get the most out of the rotation component, pull yourself forwards as far as possible before going to the side. Finish by bending forwards in the lower back-part of the movement.

Exercise 49, Partner all fours rotation

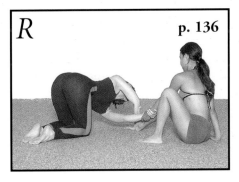

This photograph shows the second position, to demonstrate the positions of the hands; your partner will place a foot on the hips for bracing. Let yourself *be* stretched; this will only happen if you concentrate on breathing as normally as possible and letting the whole body go soft.

Cues (right)

use various pull directions

once stretched forwards, add rotations

stay in positions for a few breaths

let the body relax

Cues (right)

use trapeze grip

partner uses foot on hip for support

ensure knees behind or under hips

C–R: pull arm back

restretch: let partner pull arm through

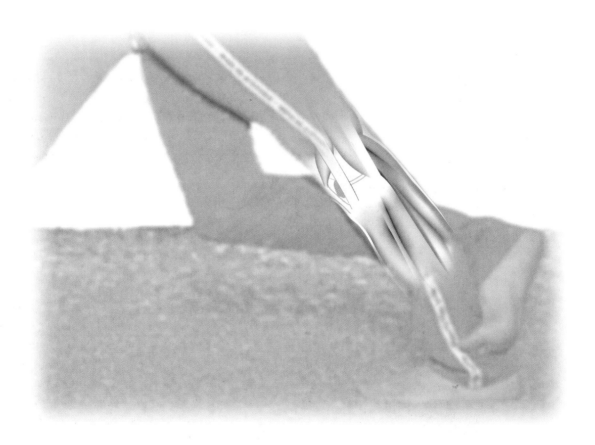

Lesson Twelve: calf, wrists, trunk, and hip (*piriformis*)

This lesson goes over previous work for the calf muscles and introduces one of the strongest of the calf stretches. It teaches stretches for some of the smaller muscle groups of the body: the forearms, wrists and fingers, and introduces some interesting movements for the trunk and neck—especially those hard-to-reach places in between the shoulders. Oriental medicine suggests that the three necks of the body—the ankles, wrists, and the neck—are the first places flexibility is lost as one ages. I have not noticed the accuracy of this teaching over the years (the shoulders and the neck together seem to lose their normal flexibility the most quickly) but the assertion will be a useful organising principle for this lesson. We will finish with powerful movements for the external rotators of the hip, including *piriformis*. In contrast to some others, this lesson is gentle. Control your enthusiasm for the more dramatic stretches and try to emphasise the mind–muscle connection for the next hour or so.

Exercise 19, Wall standing calf

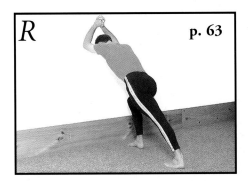

You may need to review the instructions in lesson 3. Do this exercise for each leg, with contractions, and hold the final position for at least 10 full breaths in and out. Remember to keep the stretched leg straight and the heel on the ground.

Martial arts warm-up with partner, or wide squats with partner (shown)

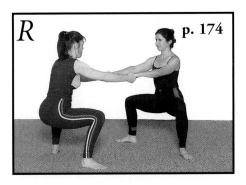

If doing the martial arts warm-up, concentrate on getting the body as far forwards with respect to the squat leg as you can (this targets the ankle in the movement, rather than the hamstrings and adductors on the straight leg), so your start position will be a little further away from your partner than usual. Do 10 to 15 slow transitions.

If doing the wide squat, make sure your feet are in position directly under the knees, with the feet pointing in the direction of the thighs, as Jennifer and Sharon are showing. Squat as deeply as you can, and keep your heels on the floor. If you have tight ankles that would normally limit you from doing this movement on your own, lean back against your partner's support so that the trunk is vertical and you will be able to do it easily. Do 10–15 slow repetitions.

Exercise 18, Floor folded leg calf

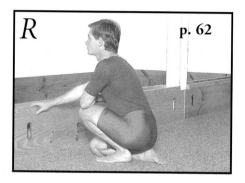

Details will be found in lesson 3. Make sure the arch shape is preserved, and the foot is not turned out to the side. Lean body weight on the knee through the elbow, as Gary is doing. Use contractions, and hold the final position for five to ten breaths.

Exercise 23, Floor instep

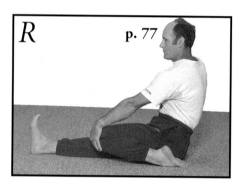

Details will be found in lesson 4. Ensure that you keep weight on the hip while you stretch the instep on the same side. Use contractions, and you will need to let the whole foot go completely limp as you restretch. Most people are resistant to letting this area relax completely, so make a conscious effort to do so.

Exercise 67, Floor feet sequence

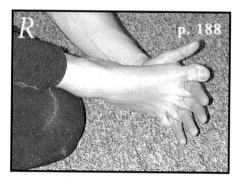

Your feet will be completely warmed up, now. Sit on the floor, and go through the feet-and-toe sequence described in lesson 11. Push the fingers as far in between the toes as you can. You may add an ankle *inversion* movement, by grasping the forefoot in both hands and turning the sole of the foot to face your body (third photograph, facing page), and *eversion* by turning the sole away (bottom photograph, facing page).

A **C–R stretch** can be done by trying to twist the foot the other way, and restretching on a breath out. Hold the final position for a count of five. This can be effective for restoring full movement to those people who have sprained their ankles. When you have finished, stand with your weight on both feet evenly and lift and spread the toes as far as you can. Place the toes on the floor and grip the floor as hard as you can for a five count.

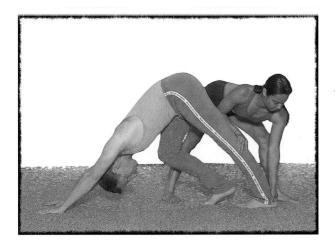

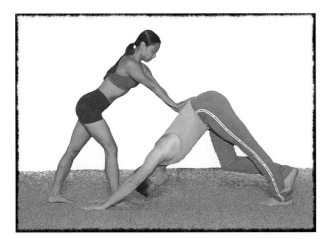

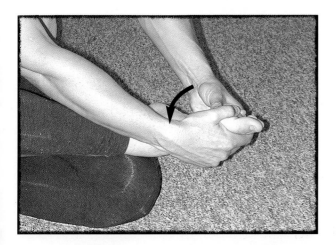

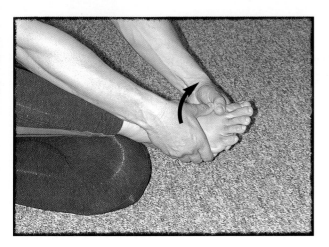

70. Partner floor single leg, both legs calf

This exercise can be done with a variety of intensities and everyone will be able to benefit. Steve is demonstrating and Julie is assisting. We have already encountered a similar exercise in lesson 3, wall standing calf, but the addition of the forward bend at the waist changes the sensations greatly.

Steve is supporting himself with his palms on the floor but, if you are not loose enough in the hamstrings or the ankles, you may lean the hands onto a bench or similar support (shown page 62); however, ensure it cannot slide away from you. Lean on the support and then extend the arms at the same time as you push the hips back, pressing the heel onto the floor. The other leg can be on the floor as shown in the first photograph, or folded out of the way and tucked behind the straight leg, as shown in the second photograph. To increase the stretch, pull your trunk forwards (use the abdominals and hip flexors) which will move the arms closer in line with the body. You will probably need to repeat the instructions, with the foot at different distances from the support, until you find the best position. The first photograph shows an intense position, with the hand support on the floor.

A **C–R stretch** will help; press the ball of the foot into the floor, and restretch by letting the arms bend at the elbows.

There are two ways a partner can assist. The first frame in the sequence shows Julie holding Steve's heel down to the floor. This allows Steve to move his hands and body further forwards, increasing the stretch in the calf. **C–R stretches** can be done in this position.

The second frame shows Julie supporting Steve's lower back, at its roundest point, by leaning in the direction of the heel on the floor. As Julie leans, Steve is able to further straighten his whole spine and, as he does, the hamstring stretch increases; the heel is pressed more firmly on the floor, so it does not slip. The same **C–R stretch** can be done here, too. After the **C–R**, you will need to move the hands slightly further away to increase the stretch in the calf. Hold the final position for five to ten breaths.

The heel of the stretched leg can be placed at the join between floor and wall to stop the foot sliding away; alternatively, the fingertips of the hands can be placed in the same way so the hands do not slip.

71. *Floor wrist and hand sequence*

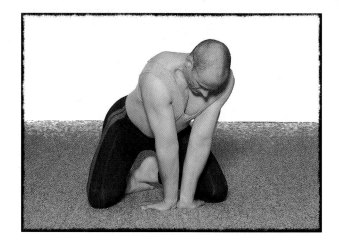

If the feet are the most neglected part of the body—even among those who stretch regularly—then the hands and wrists are probably a close second. Treat this sequence like the foot sequence: do it from time to time, unless there is a more pressing reason or you work out in the gym, as weight training will tighten the wrists and hands unless you do some specific compensating exercise.

We will stretch the wrists in *extension* first (backwards bending) using the floor. Two start positions are shown in the first two photographs—try both and see which one you prefer. If you are sitting as shown in the third frame, make sure that the wrists are in front of the hip joints. Turn the arms so that the fingers point directly backwards, press the heels of the palms to the floor and straighten the arms (you may need to lift your shoulders). Lift the chest to straighten the back, breathe in and, as you breathe out, lean back slowly as far as you can until you feel the stretch in the forearms. If you are flexible, you may feel as though you are having to lean too far back for comfort; if so, place the hands further *forwards* (either position) before you start.

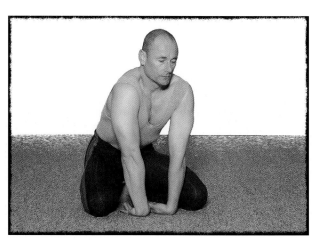

The **C–R stretch** is effected by gently pressing the fingers into the floor once you are in the stretch position. Relax, breathe in and, on a breath out, restretch. Move slowly; this can be intense. Hold for five breaths or more.

Now we will stretch the wrists in *flexion* (forwards). We do this in a similar way, but with the backs of the hands pressed firmly onto the floor. Two positions are shown. The most common fault in this exercise is to let the elbows bend: this will defeat the stretch. As before, you may need to lift the shoulders to straighten the arms. Again, the fingers point directly backwards. The stretch is achieved by leaning backwards; the **C–R** by pressing the backs of the fingers and hands into the floor. Restretch by leaning further backwards. This movement is particularly intense for men who lift weights. Hold for five breaths.

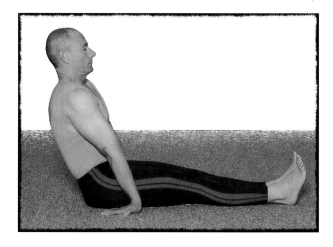

Sit in a comfortable position; we will stretch the hands next. Begin with the little finger. Use the thumb to press the little finger back while holding the base with the index finger of the other hand. A **C–R stretch** is achieved by pressing the finger against the thumb and restretching. Do all the fingers on the same hand, and then stretch the thumb.

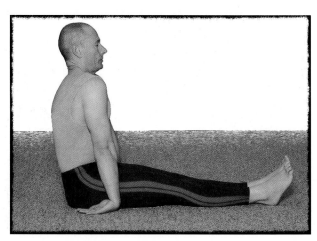

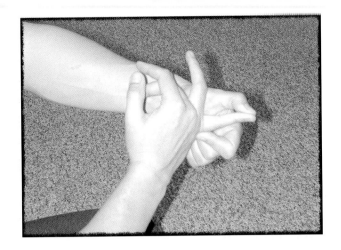

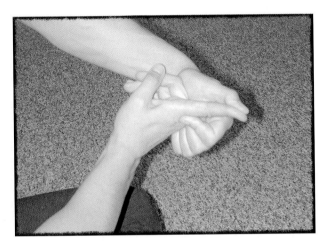

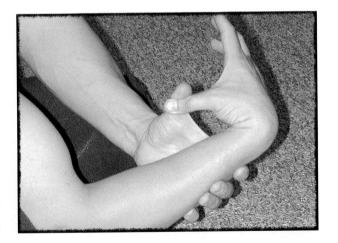

Two stretches are offered: the first affects the wrist more than the thumb. The third frame shows an effective position: flex the wrist of one hand and hold the back of the forearm with the other. Use the thumb of the holding hand to stretch the other thumb towards the inside of the forearm, as shown. A **C–R stretch** is achieved by pressing the thumb back (the effort will straighten the wrist); restretch by moving the thumb further in the initial stretch direction.

Now turn the hand and wrist over, so that the wrist is extended, as shown in the last frame. The stretching hand is in essentially the same position, so the second movement can be done immediately after the first. When the thumb is moved in this direction, the major muscles moving the thumb into the gripping position will be stretched (*opponens pollicis* and *adductor pollicis*); these are the muscles responsible for the pain of writer's cramp, and muscle pain at the base of the thumb. Stretch the other hand.

The two photographs in this column show an additional pair of start positions, where the wrist is both flexed and rotated at the same time. Once the wrist is flexed and rotated as far as possible, the stretch can be intensified greatly by trying to bring both hands *towards* you (third frame) or by gently trying to straighten the arms (bottom frame). Do not lose the flexion and rotation aspects in order to improve the arm position. People with overuse injuries will find these movements helpful.

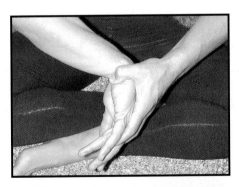

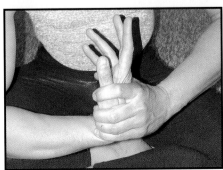

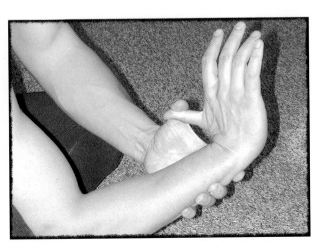

72. Kneeling elbow on floor rotation

The body is able to use its own strength in this exercise to provide a lovely rotation stretch for the entire trunk. A partner may help you increase the stretch in the final position, but it is not necessary if you are careful about positioning your weight and using your strength effectively.

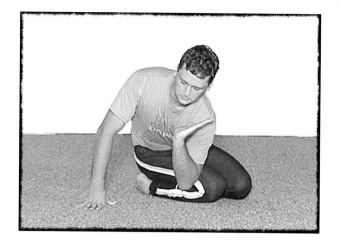

Kneel on your legs as shown. Use mats as supports as necessary, as shown for exercise 23, lesson 4. Take in a breath and, once you have fully breathed out, let the trunk relax completely, bending forward and placing an elbow on the floor as Mark is doing. Use the muscles under the arms to pull the shoulder across the body; to complete the rotation, put your hands together, and lean weight onto the bottom hand to press the other shoulder backwards.

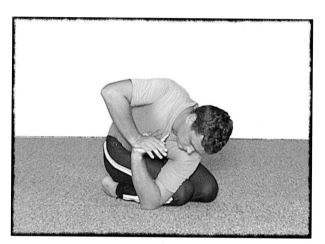

A **C–R stretch** is easily achieved by trying to twist out of the position using the waist muscles for a count of five. Breathe in, and relax; on a strong breath out use the strength of your arms to go further in the initial stretch direction. Hold the final position (breathing will be more difficult than usual, as with all rotation poses) for five to ten breaths, come out of the pose and do the other side.

Interesting variations in sensations and effects can be achieved by changing the shape of the spine—allowing it to bend forwards, or by arching the back backwards. Additionally, a number of body work schools have claimed that beneficial effects on the internal organs can be achieved by trying to breathe deeply when the movements of the ribs are restricted, as in this position. You will find that, because the ribs of the chest cannot move as much as normal, you will be able to feel the ribs at the back near the pelvis move to facilitate breathing (the arrow on the bottom photograph indicates the general area).

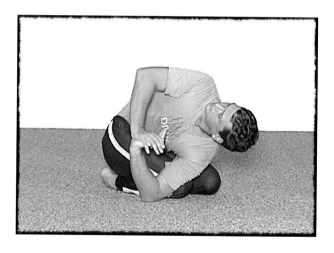

Cues

kneel, and place elbow
outside opposite knee

arch back straight

use top shoulder's arm to improve leverage

C–R: twist back against resistance

restretch: pull further into stretch

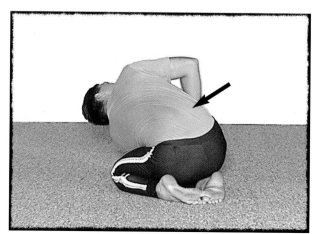

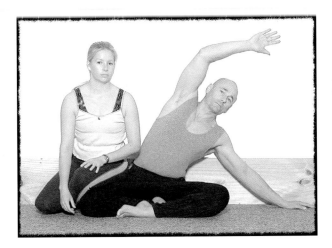

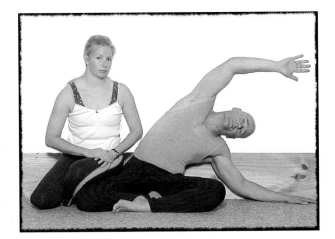

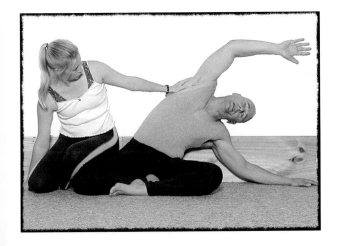

73. Partner floor wall seated side bend

This exercise provides a way to stretch all of the muscles of the side of the trunk, but without hamstring involvement, as the legs are folded. This aspect may enable you to concentrate more fully on the muscles of the lumbar spine (*quadratus lumborum* in particular). Olivia is assisting.

Sit with your back against a wall (this may be done away from the wall as well) and your legs folded. Your partner sits with their thigh across yours, as shown, to hold that hip on the floor. If you cannot sit with your thighs on the floor, roll up a mat and place it under the leg your partner will sit on. Use the wall to guide you and lean directly to the side, supporting yourself with one hand on the floor alongside you until the desired stretch is reached. This may be increased by reaching the top arm across as far as you can, as shown.

A **C–R stretch** can improve the final position dramatically. Your partner places a hand under your shoulder as shown in the bottom photograph; you use the waist and back muscles to press back for a count of five; breathe in, relax, and very slowly lower yourself further to the side. Make sure this restretch movement is slow and controlled. You must move into the restretch by yourself—your partner only assists. You may roll the top shoulder forwards to move the stretch further around the waist into the spine, and an additional **C–R** can be done in these new positions.

If you do the stretch away from the wall, you can feel a strong stretch towards the front of the waist above the hip if you let the top shoulder roll behind the line of the stretch; conversely, if you let the shoulder roll forwards, the stretch will move around from the side of the waist into the lower back, and down into the hip (*gluteus minimus* and *medius*). Experiment to find the most pleasing angles.

Cues

sit cross-legged with hips on floor

lean back against wall to align

lean directly to side; reach top arm out

C–R: press trunk back to partner

restretch: let yourself go further to side

Exercise 27, Backward bend over support

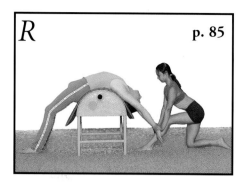

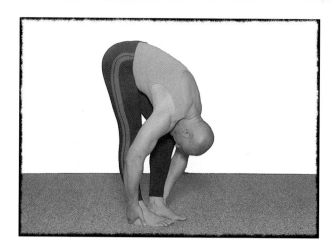

Review the instructions for the pair of stretches we recommend be done over a support, described in lesson 4. You may add subtle rolling-to-the-side movements to stretch new areas (make these extra movements slow and small).

Free squat ankles clasped bottom position

Another variation on the standing forward bending warm-ups, this simple dynamic exercise is an agreeable stretch for the lower back, hips and hamstring muscles, and is perfect to follow the backward bend we just did. Do not force the positions in any way; gravity is working for you here, so let it do what it does best!

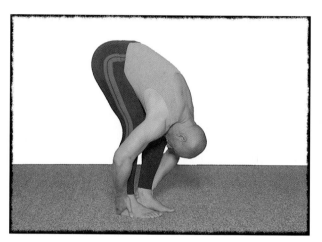

Bend forwards with your knees flexed until your stomach and ribs are pressing on your thighs. Grasp your ankles or your heels, depending on your flexibility. Stay in the bent-over position for a moment; let the body and neck hang comfortably. Keeping the chest against the thighs, slowly try to straighten one leg at a time—unless you are very flexible, you will not be able to, but the action gives a good stretch high up in the hamstring, next to the buttock. Let the leg bend again, and try to straighten the other one; then try both. Gentle **C–R stretches** can be done at all stages.

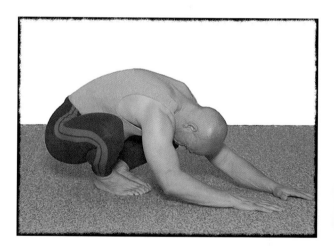

Squat down, and still holding the ankles, let the knees spread apart. Gently pull the body through the knees; this will be an excellent stretch for the lower back and you can make it more intense by using the arms to press backwards on the shins. Follow this by slowly standing up (still with the chest on the thighs) and run through the leg-straightening sequence again. Let go of the ankles and (leading with the head) stand up.

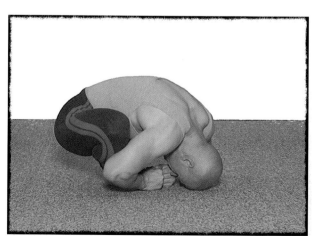

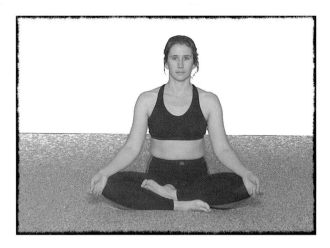

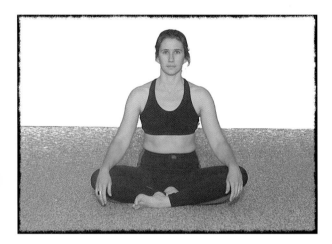

74. Seated legs folded knees apart forward bend

Left–right differences in hip flexibility can be identified and corrected with this next exercise. This is a good exercise for *piriformis*; if this is a problem for you, add it to the list of essential exercises. Jennifer is showing the movements.

Sit on the floor as shown. You do not need the knees hard on the floor for this to be effective, but having the knees spread apart is essential. You may put the ankle of one foot in front of the other or on top of the other—the latter gives the stronger stretch in the hip of whichever foot is uppermost. Lean forwards towards the feet, holding the back straight. You can use a support to pull yourself forwards if you wish, or hold the knees to pull yourself forwards. Return to the start position, rotate the shoulders to face one knee, and lean over that knee, again keeping the back straight. You can place your palms flat on the floor under the knee, and use the arms to pull the trunk forwards, if you like. Return to the start position, and lean over the other knee. Do not be surprised if leaning one way is much harder than the other.

Change leg position, reverse the initial foot placement, and run through the sequence once more. If the same side is tight regardless of which foot is on top (or in front) then a genuine difference has been identified. For most people, changing the foot position changes which side is tight in the movements.

Cues

sit cross-legged, thighs on floor
use arm as brace on opposite knee
lean to both sides
lean to middle; relax over feet

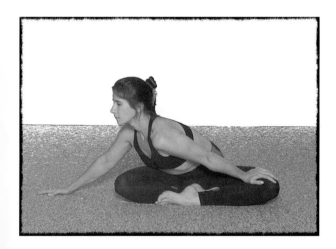

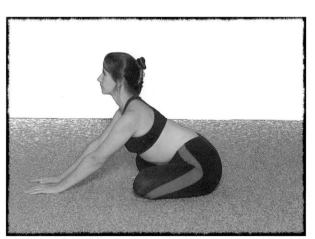

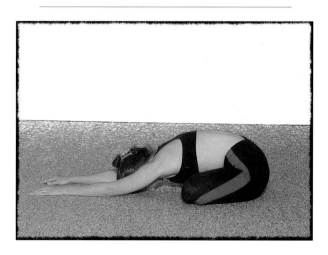

75. Seated clasped bent leg upper back

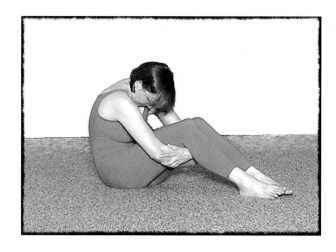

This is an alternative to exercise 43, folded legs clasped knees upper back, first encountered in lesson 6, and should be considered a complementary movement, as the focus of the strongest part of the stretch will differ, depending on your proportions. All of these minor stretches will be excellent for gently pulling tension out of the middle and upper back—particularly for those who spend most of their life in front of the keyboard (I'll just run off and do these now).

Sit on the floor as Carol is demonstrating, and hold the back of the thighs. The first stretch is to simply let the hips roll back as you slump forwards tightening the abdominal muscles. An additional stretch is to incline the trunk to one side while in the stretch position, followed by leaning to the other side, as shown in the second frame.

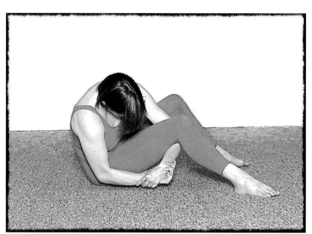

A variation is to open the legs, as shown in the third frame, and hold only one at a time; again slump and let the hips roll back while holding the leg. An additional stretch may be achieved by leaning the trunk to one side once in the stretch position; do both sides.

A final, related stretch is to rotate the shoulders and place both hands outside the leg, and use the back of one arm to increase the rotation, as shown in the final photograph. You can also try letting the chin go to the chest in any of these positions to increase the stretch a little higher in the back.

Exercise 50, Partner shoulder depress; flexion and lateral flexion

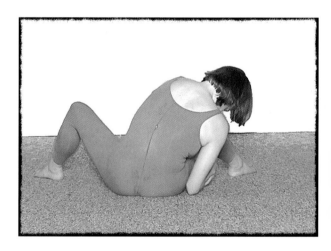

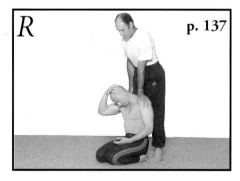

R   p. 137

Follow the gentle, but extremely effective trunk stretches with the partner movements that stretch the muscles between the neck and shoulders. Because the middle and upper back will be looser than normal, expect to be able to

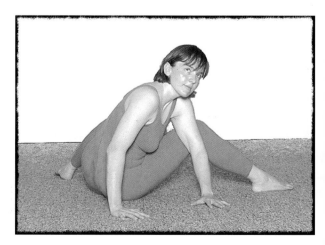

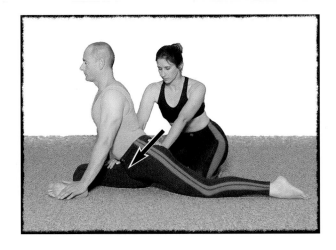

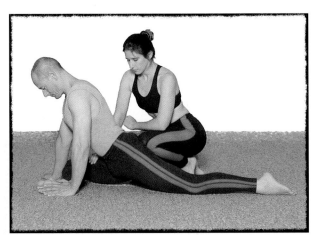

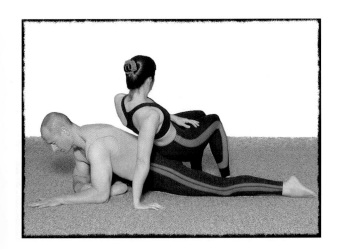

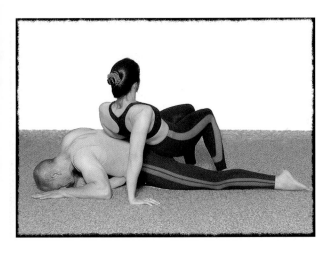

stretch a little further than usual. Review the directions for exercise 44 (lesson 6) and exercise 50 (the last exercise in lesson 7) to make sure that all the subtleties are understood. Be gentle with your neck muscles.

Exercise 25, Standing suspended hip flexor, with support

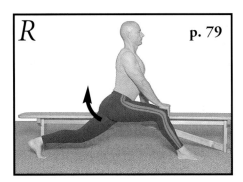

Use exercise 25 as a warm-up for the hip flexors and *quadriceps* only.

76. Partner floor external hip rotator

If done as directed, this is the strongest of the *piriformis* stretches. Look at the photograph: I am sitting on one hip, the knee of the front leg bent at 90 degrees, and the back leg stretched out behind me, as close to parallel with the front thigh as possible. Everyone will be able to sit in this position; the flexibility of the hip of the front leg will constrain how close to the floor you can move the *back* leg's hip. The partner supports you as shown and, for the first movement, tries to roll the back leg's hip *across to the floor*. You will need to assist your partner, using the muscles of the trunk. This movement will place the hip flexor of the back leg under tension, and rotate the pelvis forwards; this action also moves the pelvis in relation to the hip of the front leg, and its position on the floor imparts a strong rotation to the hip. This action provides the initial stretch.

The C–R stretch is to press the outside of the front foot into the floor (try to feel the muscles that do this). The restretch is to ask your partner to move the hip further across towards the floor. You may try two or three brief contractions here; try to move a little further in the stretch direction each time. Hold the final position for at least five breaths. Do the other side. The third and last frames show an alternative support position, and a second movement—when the hip of the back leg is as close to the floor as possible, lean the centre of your body over your foot.

Solo external hip rotator; with support

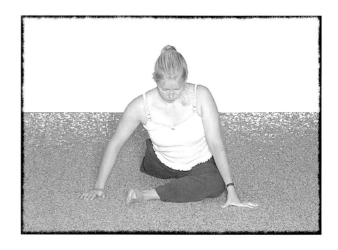

In the photographs on this page, Olivia is demonstrating exercise 76 on her own. To do this, you need enough flexibility in both the external hip rotators and the hip flexors to get into the first position. Use the trunk muscles to twist the hip of the back leg to the floor as far as possible. The **C–R stretch** is the same as the partner version of the exercise; press the front foot into the floor and restretch.

If your hips flexors are so tight that the main effect of the stretch is in the front of the *back* leg, I have added a bench or table-top version of the exercise that, essentially, removes the back leg from the requirements of the movement. Look at the photographs on the facing page.

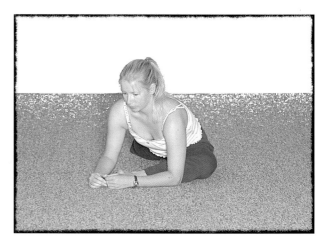

Cues

front knee open at 90 degrees
hips as close to level as possible
use waist to twist back hip to floor
C–R: press front foot into floor
restretch: back hip closer to floor then lean straight body over foot

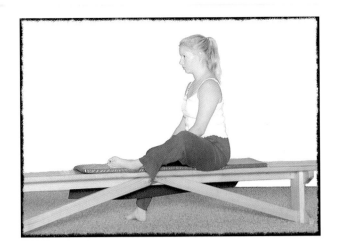

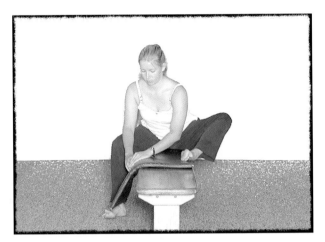

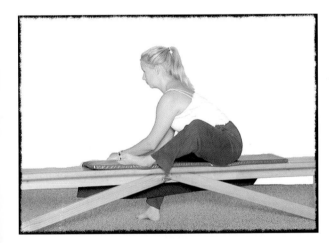

What would have been the back leg in the solo version just described is on the floor for stability and to keep the hips level. Only one hip is on the support. The front leg is folded at the knee at 90 degrees as before, and the foot placed inside the line of the edge of the support (recall that in many *piriformis* exercises the further outside the line of the body the thigh is placed, the stronger the effect in the hip). To get into the initial stretch position, aim the centre of your body at the edge of the support, rather than at the foot. Hold your back straight as you incline the body forwards. Grip the support for balance and to reduce the effect in the hip if too strong; alternatively, if the stretch is not strong enough, the same hand position can be used to pull yourself forwards.

Once you feel the stretch in the hip of the front leg, hold the position for a while to get used to it. The **C–R stretch** requires that the front foot be pressed directly down into the support for a count of five-to-eight. Stop pressing, breathe in and straighten the back and, on a breath out, move the trunk further forwards until the desired stretch is felt. Hold the final position for five to ten breaths; the **C–R** may be repeated from the new position.

Cues

only one hip on support
front knee open at 90 degrees
foot across from edge of support
other foot on floor for stability
lean forwards to edge of support
C–R: press foot into support
restretch: incline straight trunk further in stretch direction

Lesson Thirteen: HAMSTRINGS, QUADRICEPS, HIP FLEXORS, FRONT SPLITS

This lesson concentrates on the muscles that control the legs' movements in the forwards–backwards plane. These exercises should form the basis of the stretching routine of anyone who desires a greater range of movement for the legs in this plane, as well as anyone whose sport emphasises movements in this plane. Gentle and advanced exercises will be found; try them all and make a selection based on how well you can do them and how they feel.

Standing alternate leg forward bend warm-up

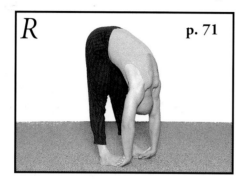

Review the instructions for this sequence in lesson 3. Make all movements gentle: start with bent legs and position yourself for maximum comfort. Once you have explored the bent-leg positions, straighten the legs slightly and do them again. The photograph shows the final position in the sequence.

Free squats, with pauses

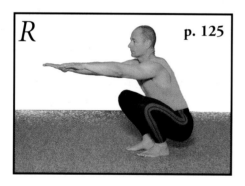

Review the directions for this sequence, first encountered in lesson 7. Hold each of the four pause positions for 10 normal paced breaths—or as normal as you can make them while doing this strenuous movement. Do not lift yourself too high for the first-pause position: your hips should be just below your knees.

Exercise 19, Wall standing calf

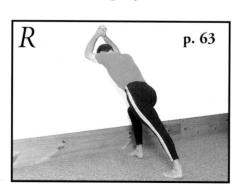

First tried in lesson 3, review the details and practise this exercise again. Do not let the ankle of the straight leg roll inwards and make sure that the leg is pressed straight before you take the hips closer to the wall.

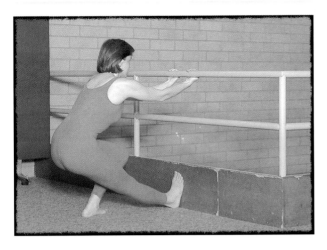

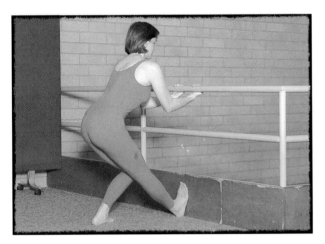

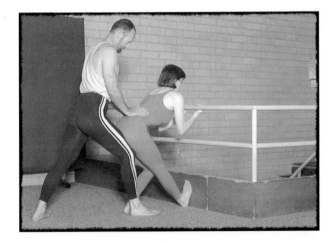

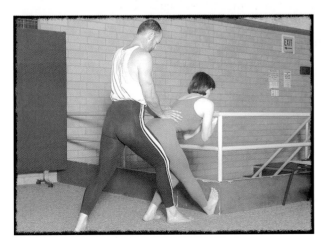

77. Partner bar standing calf

A much stronger calf exercise that provides the maximum stretch for the *sciatic* nerve is shown. This movement is really two stretches in one: the first part stretches the ankle (*dorsiflexion*); the second flexes the trunk forwards over this stretched leg—you will find this position intense.

Hold onto a support, lower yourself until you can jam your heel into the join between floor and wall (make sure the heel is hard against the wall and the leg straight), and lift yourself using the arms and the other leg until the desired stretch is felt. Carol has lifted her hips until this point is reached.

A **C–R stretch** works here, too: press the ball of the foot into the wall for a count of eight to ten, then relax, breathe in and, as you breathe out, lift yourself higher in the initial stretch direction. Hold this position for 10 breaths.

The second part requires you to bend forwards at the waist with a straight back *while maintaining the full calf stretch* just achieved. Greg is providing Carol with support in two ways: his right leg is holding her hip in the calf-stretch position, while his hands are pressing on her lower back to help her keep her back straight as she leans forward. Do not be in too much of a hurry to move into the final position; this is a very strong stretch. You may care to try a second **C–R** for the calf muscle once in the final position.

Exercise 40, Partner seated/lying single leg quadriceps or Exercise 26, Seated/lying single leg quadriceps

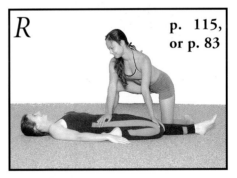

R   p. 115, or p. 83

To help prepare the legs for this lesson, repeat exercise 40, lesson 6, if you have a partner, or exercise 26, lesson 4, if you do not. Make sure your alignment is good: the thigh being stretched needs to be in line with the body and the spine in a neutral shape—no hyperextension.

78. Floor forward bend over straight leg, hurdler's variation

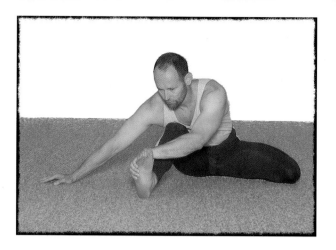

To this point, the single-leg hamstring stretches you have done had the other leg either bent at the knee and next to the stretched leg (exercise 17, lesson 3) or folded and placed alongside (exercise 17 variation, lesson 7). Exercise 78 is a useful hamstring stretch, and it will help to loosen the hips in sideways movements too. You can see this exercise being done badly anywhere stretching is done. If the foot of the folded leg is turned out to the side, there will be potentially dangerous uneven strain on the ligaments on the *inside* of the knee. Look at the second photograph on page 132: the foot is alongside the hip, the calf muscle has been pushed out of the way, and the folded leg taken to the side at about 90 degrees. If you cannot sit this way, you will need to master exercises 23, floor instep, and 26, seated *quadriceps*.

To lean over the extended leg, you will need to incline your body's weight towards the folded leg to an extent, until both bottom bones are on the floor. Tension in *quadriceps* is trying to lift the folded leg's hip, and you will need to counteract this force. If you cannot sit with both bottom bones on the floor, you are not ready to use this variation.

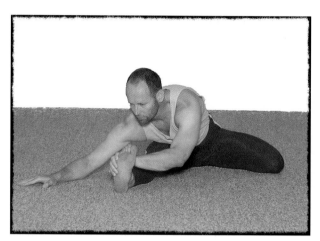

Greg is showing how to use a bent leg to get into position. Lean forwards with a straight back until the desired stretch is felt; a partner can assist by supporting the lower or middle back (whichever wants to bend first) as usual. A **C–R stretch** can be done by trying to pull away from the held foot, using the hamstring muscles of the extended leg, or by trying to pull the heel of the extended leg through the floor. Make sure that your chest is lifted in these contractions. Hold the final position for 10 to 20 breaths.

Standing suspended hip flexor (ex. 25) and buttock and hip flexor (ex. 21) warm-up

Cues

folded leg 90 degrees
foot next to body
body on bent leg; try to straighten
C–Rs: pull heel into floor, or press whole leg into floor, or pull hands away from foot
restretch: straighten leg further

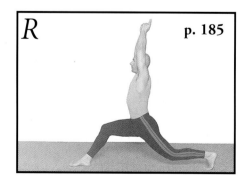

Directions for this warm-up are found in lesson 11.

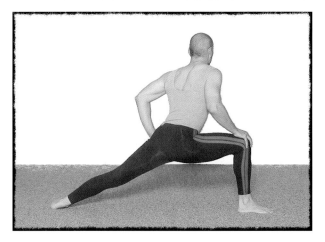

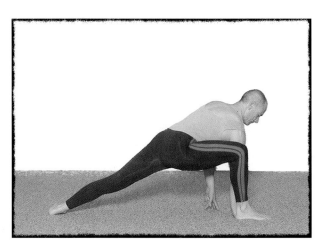

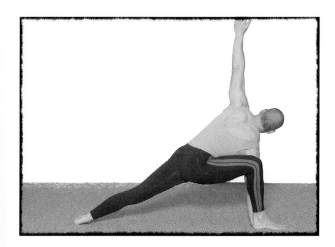

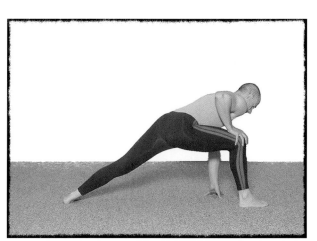

79. Standing forward bend over bent and straight leg

This is a standard pose from hatha yoga, but done with support. It is an excellent alignment exercise, it has a strengthening component, and the final position is an efficient hamstring stretch.

In the first position, the legs should be far enough apart such that, when you bend one leg and sink into the start position, the bent leg's foot should be in front of the knee and pointing in the direction of the thigh. This requires about one-and-a-half leg lengths. The back leg's foot is turned at about 45 degrees in the direction of the front foot. Sink down until the thigh of the bent leg is parallel with the floor, if you can, and while watching the bent leg's knee, roll the other hip backwards slowly. When you have reached the limit of your adduction on the straight leg, you will see the knee move *forwards*; stop at this point and hold for a few breaths.

Running your hand down the thigh allows you to get into position without risk: if you feel that you are going too far, you can stop yourself. Put your palm flat on the floor (or on a block if that helps) and lean your weight on it. Lower the hips as far as you can. Extend the other arm out to the side level with the shoulder, and move the arm and body together around the shoulder of the supported arm until the top arm and both shoulders are vertical. Hold this position for five breaths.

When you come out of the pose, reverse the instructions and bring both hands together on the floor. Using the hand you brought back from the overhead position for support, bring the first hand up onto the knee and use this arm to help you stand up. Repeat for the other side. If you find significant differences between sides, do the tighter side once more.

The second version of this pose is similar in approach (the body's weight is supported as much as you need by the bottom arm) but, because the leg you are bending over is straight, the hamstring stretch is the limiting factor—if you use good form. Many people feel that they are doing the pose well because their bottom hand is flat on the floor, but when you analyse their form, their spines are bent strongly to the side in addition to the desired rotation.

Take a stride of approximately one leg length, with the feet in the same relation as for the pose just described. Now rotate your hips so that they are near square to the line of the legs (that is, the hip of the front leg pulled *back*), check to see if your back is straight and, running your hands down your leg for support, go as far as you can before the lower back starts to bend. You can place the back of one hand on the lower back as a way of checking this or you can watch yourself in a mirror. The bottom hand must be able to support the body's weight for the next part, so hold your ankle, lean on your fingertips, or place the flat hand on the floor. Do not let your back bend. Alternatively, you may lean on a block placed inside the foot. Holding your shin, but with the back straight, is far preferable to bending the back and placing the hand on the floor.

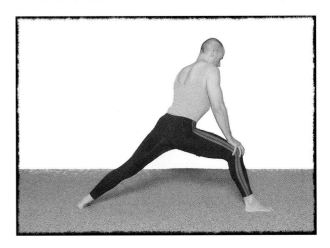

Now very gently pull back on the bottom hand: this will slightly arch your back and increase the hamstring stretch. Maintaining the neutral shape of your spine, reach the other arm out to the side, parallel with the floor. Using the bottom hand as a pivot, extend the other arm as far off the body as you can, and rotate arm and body until the shoulders are vertical. If you have kept the back straight, the spine will be only rotated, and there will be a stretch in the hamstrings of the leg you are bending over. To finish off the pose, push the hip of the front leg forwards (that is, the way you are now facing) until there is a stretch in the front of the hip too. Hold the position for five to ten breaths.

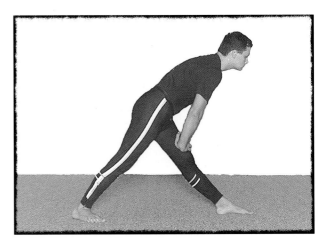

To come out of the pose, reverse the order you used to get into it. Once both hands are near each other on the floor, bend the just-stretched leg, arch the back and, lifting from the head, stand up gracefully. Bending the leg removes the strain completely from the standing action. After a rest, do the other side.

In addition to being an effective hamstring stretch, this pose has excellent strengthening effects. Holding the trunk straight against gravity and the stretching forces of the hamstring muscles requires considerable strength. Do not be surprised to feel the waist muscles the day after you do this exercise well.

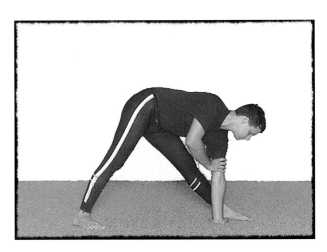

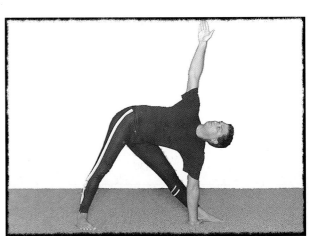

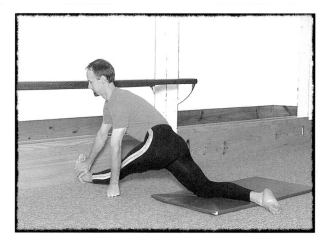

80. Wall and floor kneeling/straight leg outer hamstring

The end position of this pose resembles exercise 47, partial front splits, which we practised in lesson 7. The difference is that exercise 80 uses a board or wall to *dorsiflex* the calf muscle as a preparation, and we deliberately lean the centre of the body to the *outside* of the leg. This action emphasises the stretch in the outer hamstring (*biceps femoris*), which, as I mentioned previously, is often the tightest of the three.

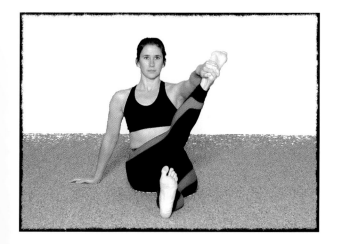

Kneel on one leg with the other extended as far as you can in front, and with that foot pressed on a board, as Kevin is doing. You want the back thigh as far behind you as possible, because its hip flexors will tilt the pelvis forwards (hence straightening your lower back) when under stretch, making good form easier to keep. Try to keep the hips as square as possible, however, and level. Keeping the back straight, lean forwards as far as you can, maintaining the centre of your chest *outside* the line of the leg you are bending over.

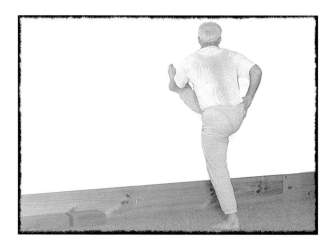

A number of **C–R stretches** are possible. For the first, try to pull the heel to the bottom by bending the knee. The second is achieved by trying to press the heel into the floor. If the calf muscles are protesting particularly, you can use a third: press the ball of the foot strongly into the board. The restretch is the same for all contractions: hold the back straight and bend further forwards across and over the leg. A partner stretch can be done too, by asking a partner to support the roundest part of the back. And if you have a partner, a fourth **C–R** is possible. Once your partner is supporting your back, lift your chest and gently press your body back to your partner's hands. The restretch is the same as before. You may try all four contractions.

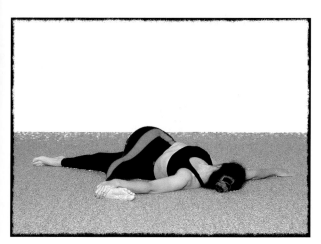

Eldon is demonstrating a wall version: gravity and friction will hold the foot in position and make leaning forward easier. Make sure that you lean *across* the leg as you lean forwards for maximum effect. The contractions are the same: down and across, not just down. Try to feel the stretch in the outer hamstring—to this end, don't put your foot too far up the wall (even if that makes you look more flexible!); use a more modest position and emphasise the leaning across aspect. Jennifer is demonstrating a sitting version (a strap may be used here) and a lying version. Both emphasise the outer hamstring area of the thigh, and you may feel the stretch in the lateral aspect of the calf muscle, too.

Exercise 66, Partner lying 'Y', face-down variation

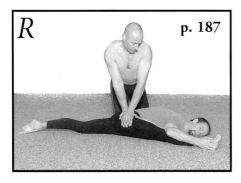

R   p. 187

Cues (left)

held leg can be put against wall

bent-leg position can be used

partner presses hip to floor

C–R: press leg into floor

restretch: partner eases hip to floor

Review the instructions for this exercise (lesson 11) and remember to let the hamstring muscles relax; you will not be able to force them to become flexible. Gravity will help you in this version. Read the **Cues** before attempting this.

Exercise 39, Partner hip flexor or exercise 25, Standing suspended hip flexor

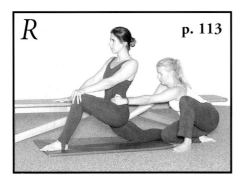

R   p. 113

Cues (left)

use support for balance

partner holds front hip and supports under bottom of back leg

C–R: drag back knee forwards

restretch: go deeper in stretch direction

Keep the hips as square as you can in both exercises.

Exercise 47, Partner partial front splits, off support

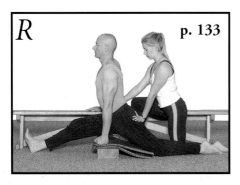

R   p. 133

Cues (left)

use support under front leg

partner holds front hip and supports under bottom of back leg

C–Rs: press or pull front leg and drag back leg forwards

restretch: sink deeper into splits

By this time you will be as warmed up as you are going to be today, so tackle this major exercise once again. Remember, the object of the movement is not to get down to the floor (although that will happen one day), rather it is to feel the stretches in the right places. Review all directions for this exercise, found in lesson 7.

Cues (right)

knees together; feet apart

hold outside of legs

top of head on floor

C–R: shrug shoulders strongly

restretch: push hips forward

Exercise 1, Middle and upper back

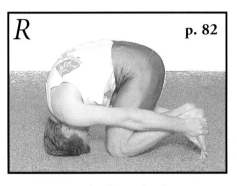

We are going to go back to the beginning with this exercise. Review the instructions; but this time when you do it, hold the feet from the outside of your legs, as shown, and described in the instructions for the more advanced version of the exercise found in lesson 4. Use whichever of the versions feels best for you.

Cues (right)

hands and knees

trapeze grip

let partner draw arm through

C–R: pull arm back

restretch: let arm be pulled further through

Exercise 49, Partner all fours rotation

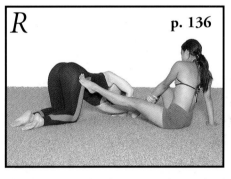

Finish the lesson with these stretches, which always leave the body feeling so relaxed.

Exercise 57, Lying legs behind

Cues (right)

use mats and support under feet if necessary

let body relax completely in position

lets hips go to side if desired

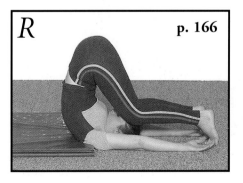

Do not force this movement in any way: relax in it.

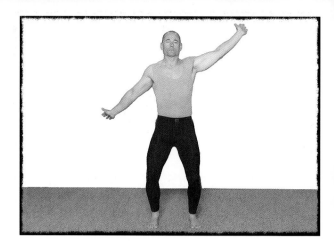

LESSON FOURTEEN: NECK, WRISTS, ANKLES, WHOLE BODY

This lesson has a little of everything: an initial focus on the neck, wrists and ankles, and a number of pleasant whole-body movements in the second half. All but one exercise will be familiar to you, and the photographs will remind you of the main form points. If you are unsure of the details of an exercise, refer back to the lesson in which they first appeared.

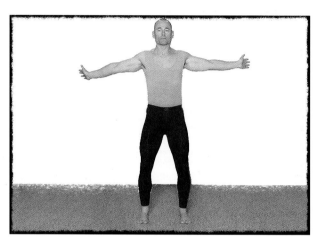

As a general rule, any stretch presented in an idealised form (by this I mean one whose directions use expressions like 'stretch directly to the side', or similar) has many effective stretch positions between it and an adjacent movement (bending the trunk forwards, for example). At this stage in your practice, you will achieve the most effective stretching sensations by doing the idealised movements first, and then finding as many intermediate positions in between as you wish. Once you have developed the capacity to interpolate between the formal positions taught so far, your own body has become your teacher—this is the outcome we have been looking for, without stating it. I cannot overemphasise the importance of maximising the suite of sensations coming to you from your body as you do this work: these sensations are the language of the body, which many of us cannot hear. As I am fond of saying in the class situation, the body has its own imperatives and its own tempos—of change, of rest, of variety. If you want genuine integration of mind and body, you will need to make a real effort to understand these imperatives. So, today's lesson concentrates on a variety of stretches that work small parts of the body, or large parts like the trunk, but in a general way. Your task is to concentrate as hard as you can on what the body is saying to you.

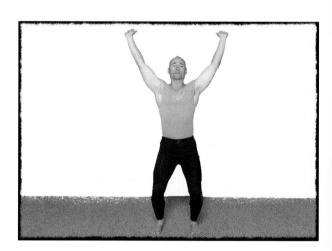

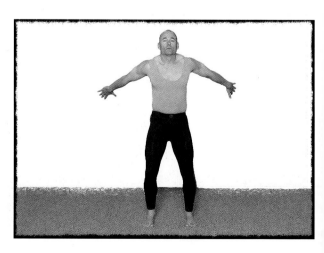

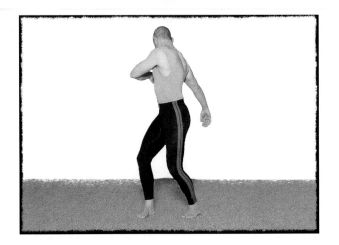

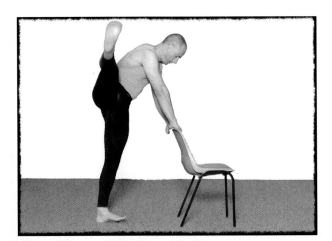

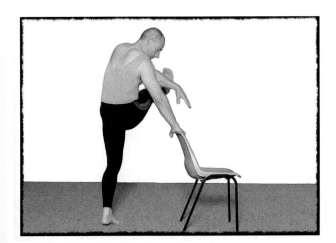

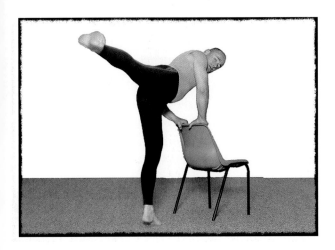

Standing rag-doll warm-up

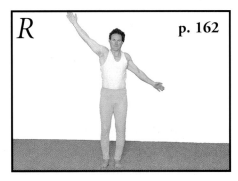

R   p. 162

This sequence, described in lesson 9, wakes up the whole body and reconnects you to all parts. It is the very opposite of some of the strenuous movements we have employed in earlier lessons and it simply feels good to do.

If your balance is good, you may do front-to-back, and side-to-side movements with the legs, as well. This part of the sequence can be done holding a support. Again, do not force the movements and remember that if too much momentum is built up the movements can become dangerous. The core idea is to do just enough work such that the momentum of the leg carries it to a gentle stretch position, increasing with each repetition as far as you can. Notice that I let the trunk bend into the leg movements; do not try for what would be otherwise strict form,

Finally, again with bent knees, initiate the trunk movement with a quick twitch of the hips; this will move your shoulders, and the loose arms will be gently moved out and around. The head should follow the shoulder movement. You will need to experience this to be sure that you have understood: the tiny hip movement initiates the shoulder movement, and this moves completely relaxed arms, whose elbows are kept loose too. It is momentum that straightens the arms, not the arm muscles. The entire body will be moving like a rag doll—completely floppy.

The last moves in the sequence are to shake a leg and both arms vigorously, change legs and repeat. This sequence will leave you feeling energised. If the leg movements are included, this simple sequence can gently stretch all the major muscles of the body in a few minutes, and I recommend this before any athletic activity. The movements affect the stretch receptors that are time- as well as position-sensitive, and so can reset their position to prepare for more strenuous activities. As I mentioned in the *Introduction*, my preference is for slow stretching after the body is completely warmed up, or as a cool-down.

Exercise 44, Partner shoulder depress

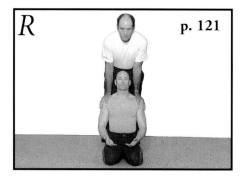

This partner exercise is the best preparation for any sequence of neck or shoulder exercises. Remember that these muscles enjoy excellent leverage, so lift up gently rather than with too much effort. Concentrate on allowing the shoulders to be eased down gently after the contractions.

Exercise 7, Floor neck side bend

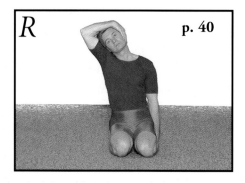

Notice how Gary is holding his shin to hold the shoulder down. You can increase this effect by leaning to the side before you reach up to hold the head. If you do this correctly, you will feel a mild stretch in the arm. Stretching the neck to the side will increase the effect in the arm and add a stretch effect to the neck.

Exercise 6, Chin to chest

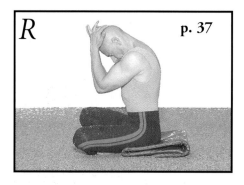

Remember, this and the preceding exercise can be done effectively from a chair or other support, making these very useful for the office situation. Do not pull the head forward with any great effort; it is often better to let the weight of the arms do the restretch movement, while you concentrate on breathing in a relaxed way.

Exercise 57, Lying legs behind

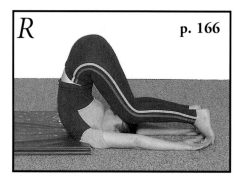

Review all instructions for exercise 57, first practised in lesson 9. Once in the final position, with the neck and the body feeling relaxed, you can add three refinements.

The first is to reach behind you with both hands and grasp the feet. Take in a breath and, on a long slow breath out, gently pull the feet towards you so that the knees are drawn to the front of the shoulders. This tightens the

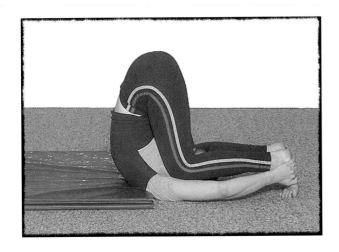

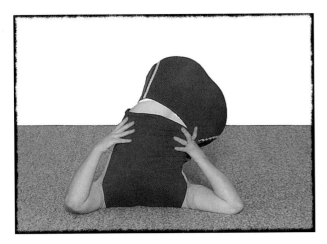

pose considerably, so make sure you do it carefully. Hold the position for a few breaths in and out. This position will increase the stretch in the back of the neck (you can see from the photograph that Sharon's spine has moved closer to vertical, increasing the effect in the neck).

Let the legs go to a relaxed position once more. The next move is to let the hips tilt to one side; to allow the knees to pass over the face you will need to straighten the legs slightly. Let the hips go as far to one side as you can, while keeping both shoulders on the floor. Hold the position for a couple of breaths and slowly move to the other side.

In the final version, slightly straighten the legs once more and use small foot movements to walk them around behind you, as far to the side as you can while keeping both shoulders on the floor. The spine is given a gentle rotation and lateral flexion, and these movements are transferred to the neck in the process.

Make sure that you do the neck extension and flexion movements described at the end of exercise 6 to relax all the muscles of the neck.

Exercise 50, Partner shoulder depress with flexion and lateral flexion

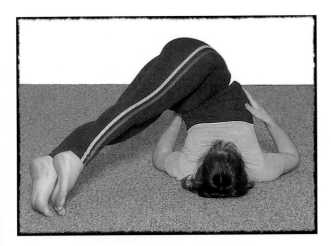

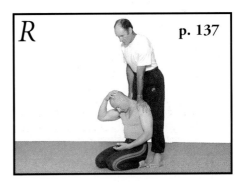

This will feel great to do after the last exercise, and you may find that you are looser in the final positions than normal due to the effects of the preceding exercise.

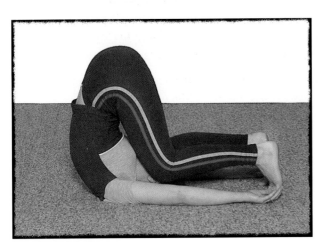

Exercise 15, Floor neck rotation

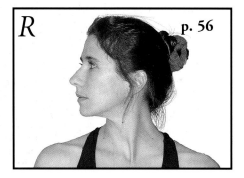

Review the directions (at the end of lesson 2) for this exercise to finish the neck sequence. Make the second rotation after pausing for a couple of seconds and relax as many muscles as you can before making the attempt.

Exercise 71, Floor wrist and hand sequence

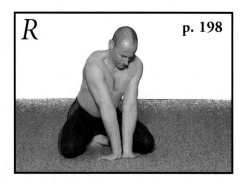

Review the instructions for exercise 71, lesson 12, before practice. Make sure you keep the heels of the palms pressed tightly to the floor while leaning backwards.

Exercise 23, Floor instep

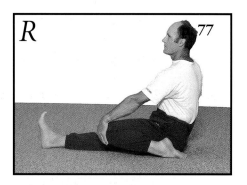

To prepare the foot, review instructions for exercise 23 (lesson 4), and stretch the instep and the toes backwards as far as you can. If the arch of the foot cramps while practising, immediately do exercise 19, below. This will relieve the cramp immediately, so try exercise 23 once more.

Exercise 19, Wall standing calf, partner or solo

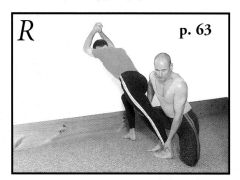

The instructions for exercise 19 are in lesson 3. Make sure your foot is positioned as described and the back leg is pressed straight.

Exercise 67, Floor feet sequence

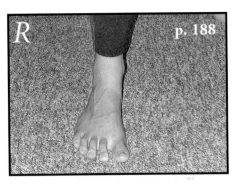

Cues

lift and spread toes

feel three points of contact with floor

spread toes; place on floor

grip floor with toes

Once you have run through the floor feet sequence, spreading and stretching the toes as far as you can, see whether your standing toe spread has improved. Remember to lift the toes off the floor as far as you can to feel the balance points before you spread them. Once you have spread them, keep the toes apart and place them on the floor. Grip the floor as hard as you can, so that the tips of the toes are bent backwards. Once you have done this, stand there for a moment, and experience the sensation of being 'grounded', in the most practical sense. Let your shoulders drop, and feel the weight of the body pressing into the floor through both feet.

Many foot, ankle, knee, hip and lower-back problems have their genesis in poor alignment of the foot in respect of the lower leg. If the ankle is aligned as shown in the photograph, the foot is an excellent shock-absorbing mechanism. Because the control of the position of the ankle is largely muscular, and hence can be altered, it is worth concentrating on these simple exercises occasionally.

Exercise 34, Wall seated straight legs apart, facing wall

Cues

push hips towards wall

hands behind hips to hold position

C–R: squeeze legs together

restretch: press hips closer to wall

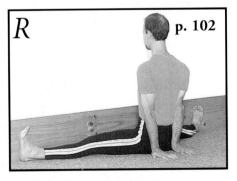

Directions for this exercise will be found in lesson 5.

Exercise 55, Seated legs apart, solo version

Review the directions for exercise 55, presented in lesson 8, page 157. I am showing an intermediate level solo version of this exercise, which comprises three main movements. All form points need to be observed, so you may use a wall for alignment in part one of the exercise (shown in the top photograph), if you wish. By placing the leg you are bending over against a wall, you can get into position by rolling back against the wall, and you can use it to help straighten the back, too. Do not have your legs so far apart that you cannot hold the feet, if you are flexible—it may surprise you to learn that this intermediate legs-apart width is the hardest position from which to incline the trunk forwards, because all hamstrings and all adductors limit the movement. Imagine if you could sit with the legs 180 degrees apart: if you were to bend forwards from this position, all that happens is that you would roll forwards from the back of your legs to the insides, with no further stretch.

Try to keep your back as straight as possible in parts two (bending over one leg) and three (bending forwards between both legs). This sequence stretches a huge number of muscles in the body. Because you are doing the exercise on your own, the strengthening component is greater—assuming that you are trying to hold your back straight in parts two and three!

C–R stretches can be done for all movements. In part one, try to pull your body away from your leg while holding your foot. This will affect the muscles between the hip you are stretching away from, and the ribs. In part two, arch the back by lifting the chest and try to pull the hands away from your foot. If your form is good, you will feel this only in the hamstrings. Part three requires you to arch the back and pull back on both feet; this will affect adductors and hamstrings. Restretch in the usual way; hold for 10 breaths.

Opposite, Petra is demonstrating an advanced alternative to the part one position, achieved while sitting on the floor with one leg folded. Hold the foot of a bent leg and slowly straighten the leg, keeping it as close to the body as possible.

If your back muscles have tightened while trying to hold yourself straight, use any of the recovery poses from backwards bending. Exercise 1, middle and upper back, either version, or exercise 48, floor forward bend over bent legs, emphasising the lower back, are both excellent.

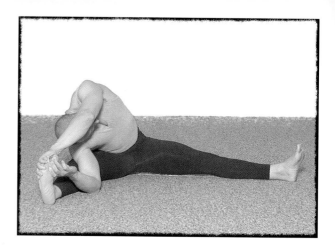

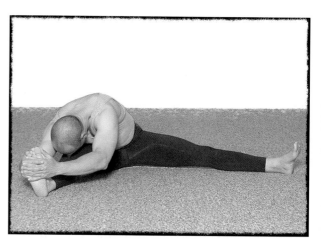

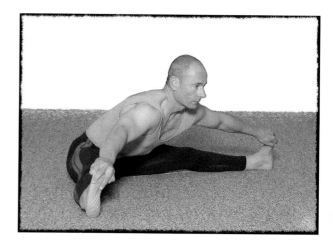

Cues

roll top shoulder back; **C–R**

turn to face leg; pull body to leg; **C–R**

restretch: pull body closer to leg

hold both feet; straighten back; **C–R**

pull body towards floor

Cues (right)

lean back over support

extend arms; partner assists

C–R: press hands to ceiling

restretch: partner presses hands down

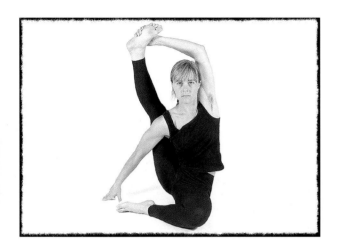

Cues (right)

lie across support; relax

partner presses trunk and legs down

C–R: lift away from support

restretch: partner helps you stretch further

Exercise 27, Partner backward bend over support

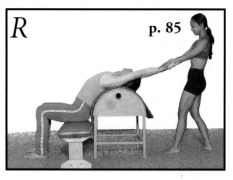

Remember you can let yourself bend backwards over any stable support, even a chair. To make a flat surface more comfortable, roll a mat or a firm cushion to produce a curved surface. If you do not have a partner to assist you, the movement is still worth doing; just stay in the position longer than you otherwise would, and introduce some small sideways rolling movements to stretch the muscles at the sides of the waist. Even on your own, small **C–R stretches** can be done to enhance the stretching effect: simply lift the head and shoulders slightly by tightening the abdominal muscles, and restretch by relaxing and reaching out your arms at the same time.

Exercise 56, Sideways bend across support

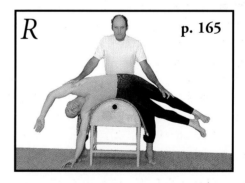

Review the directions for this exercise, first presented in lesson 9. This may be done effectively by yourself, or with one or two partners. Once you have experienced the movement directly sideways, roll the body a small distance forwards and restretch, then backwards and restretch. You will find some pleasant areas to stretch in these intermediate positions.

Free squat bottom position, ankles clasped, straighten legs sequence

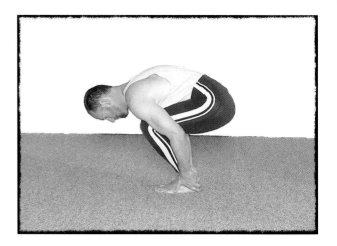

Today, we will use this warm-up as a cool-down: all the muscles we have worked will be given a gentle stretch and, because the form is not strict, you can attend to all the sensations of the movements. Begin in the bottom position of the free squat. If you cannot keep your heels on the floor, you can place your heels on a board, or balance on the balls of your feet. Clasp the ankles and slowly straighten both legs while keeping your chest firmly on the thighs, and your head hanging down and relaxed. Once you feel the stretch in the hamstrings, pause in that position for a few breaths, and squat back down. Repeat the leg-straightening action five to ten times, trying to straighten the legs a little further each time.

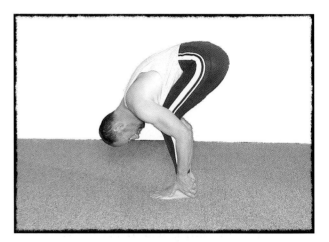

A **C–R stretch** can be done in this exercise, too, to great effect. Once in the best position you can achieve, lift the head to the neutral position and apply a slight back straightening effort. The only place you should feel this is up under the buttocks, in the hamstring muscles. The chest remains tightly pressed against the thighs. To restretch, relax the back, keep the chest on the thighs, and slowly try to straighten the legs further. One leg may be straightened at a time in a separate sequence, if you like.

Exercise 8, Partner lying rotation

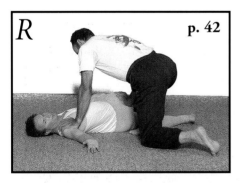

R p. 42

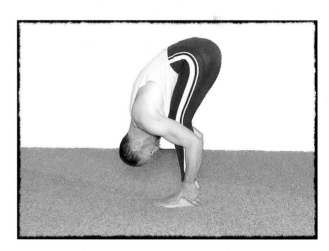

If you have a partner, do this exercise; if not, do exercise 3 from lesson 1 to finish, or any of the other rotation exercises you like. Rotation movements are a lovely way to settle the body into a comfortable state after any vigorous exercise.

Cues

squat and hold ankles
use slow leg-straightening efforts
relax and pull body onto legs
C–R: apply slight back-straightening effort
restretch: try to straighten legs

LESSON FIFTEEN: A FINAL CLASS OF MAJOR POSES

In this, the last lesson, we will concentrate on the more difficult versions of most of the poses we have learned and introduce a few new exercises and variations on ones you know. To do all the exercises will take you approximately an hour and a quarter, and will stretch most of the major muscles of the body. Doing a series of difficult poses is challenging, and the feeling when you finish is fantastic. Spend a moment or two relaxing at the end of the class as a reward—simply lie face up, arms and legs by your sides, close your eyes, and enjoy.

Exercise 70, Partner floor single leg calf

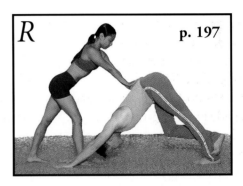

This exercise can be done solo (exercise 20 in lesson 3) or with a partner, the version suggested here.

Exercise 25, Standing suspended hip flexor

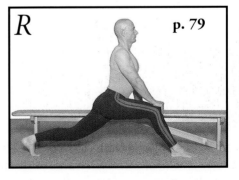

Do a partner version of this exercise (exercise 39, lesson 6), or the partner version of the suspended movement (exercise 41, same lesson) if you prefer. Try to keep the hips as low as possible to the floor when trying to straighten the back leg. Use a **C–R stretch** to improve the final position—you can use a little more force in the contractions now that you are used to doing them.

Cues (right)

hands on suitable support

heel flat on floor; leg straight

partner supports lower back

C–R: press ball of foot into floor

restretch: arch back straighter

Cues (right)

trunk vertical; hand on knee

apply brace; let hips sink to floor

rotate back hip forwards

C–R: drag back leg forward

restretch: sink, restraighten leg

81. Partner wall reverse legs apart forward bend

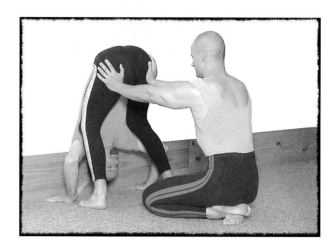

Unlike some two-leg forward bends that can strain the back, gravity and a wall's support of the lower back make this an excellent hamstring exercise; and depending on how far you have the legs apart, an excellent adductor stretch too.

How far away from the wall you place your feet depends on the answers to two questions: how loose are your hamstrings, and how much stretch do you want in the calf muscles? The looser the hamstrings, the more acute the angle the body can make with the legs and the closer you will be to the wall as a result. If you are loose in the hamstrings, however, and want to increase the calf muscle effect, deliberately stand further away than necessary—the extra lean into the wall will flex the ankles strongly, making the whole stretch in the back of the legs stronger.

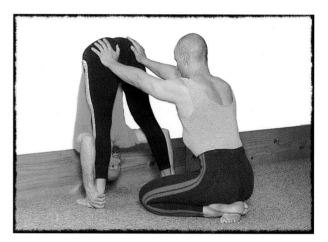

To get into the first position, stand next to the wall at roughly the right distance, bend the knees, and turn to the side while bending forwards. Lean into the wall, and bring the body back to the centre. The first part of the stretch is to lean the lower back against the wall with bent legs and ask your partner to support your legs on, or just under, the bottom. Small back-straightening movements comprise the **C–R**.

From here, you may try to straighten one or both legs, depending on your flexibility, and use small back-straightening efforts as in the **C–R** as before. Additionally, you can try moving the body more to one leg than the other, to emphasise the stretch in one leg at a time.

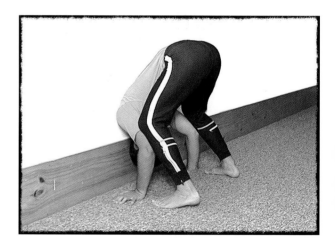

Further, you can try the exercise with various foot spacings, being aware that the wider the foot position, the less the hamstring effect and the greater the adductor effect. Finally, try the stretch again from the centre position, so both hamstrings are stretched together. Once you are held in position, try to relax into the final position, and hold it for 20 to 30 breaths—this will be a couple of minutes or so. If you know that you intend to hold a stretch for a long time, do not be to eager to begin it with an intense position: the stretch will become more intense simply because you are holding it for longer than usual. After a while (usually a minute or so for the hamstrings), the intensity will diminish. Mark is demonstrating a solo version of the stretch, also effective because gravity is helping him hold the final positions.

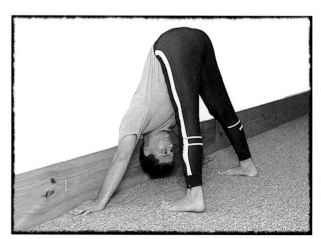

Cues (left page)

bent legs; back against wall

partner presses hips to wall

apply single- or two-leg straightening

C–R: arch back and press into wall

restretch: partner presses hips to wall

Cues (right)

lower body between feet and hands

let body relax

lean back; open mouth,take head back

close teeth; breathe deeply

curl up to finish

Cues (right)

both bottom bones on floor

lean forwards; clasp knee

lift chest; pull knee to armpit

C–R: press knee away

restretch: pull leg closer to body

Exercise 2, Backward bend from floor

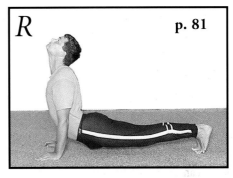

Do either the standard or suspended version (described in lesson 4), or both if you have the time. Make sure you bend the spine strongly forwards after bending backwards, or do one of the rotation movements to stretch the lower back muscles.

Exercise 5, Seated hip

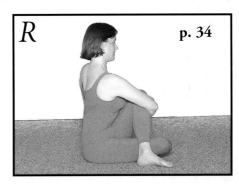

Any of the *piriformis* exercises may be substituted for exercise 5. In increasing order of difficulty, they are exercise 22 (lesson 3) and any version of exercise 76 (lesson 12). By now you should know which is the most effective for you—but don't forget, doing other stretches over time can change the effect of any other stretch. If you have the time, try a few of them.

82. Wall lunge rotation

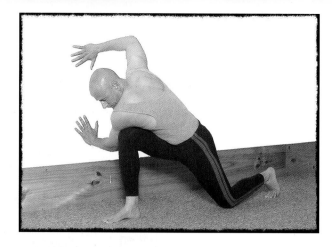

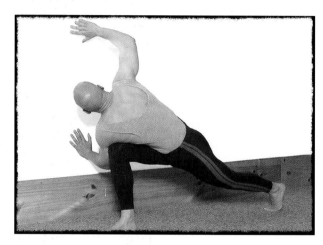

An excellent hip and rotation exercise in its own right, exercise 82 can be applied at various intensities: by how far you let the hips sink, and by how far you straighten the back leg. Look at the first photograph: you need to be one forearm's length away from the wall, with the bent front leg closest to the wall. Lean on the wall with the closest arm while cupping the knee with that hand, and kneeling on the back leg with the ball of the foot on the floor. On a strong breath out, rotate the other shoulder forwards and across until you can put the front leg's knee in behind the shoulder, as shown. At this point, the back will be bent forwards as well as rotated, and the forearm placed on the wall so that it is both level with the floor and perpendicular to the wall. Ideally, there should be no space between your body and the thigh.

As you breathe in, arch the back straight: this will tighten the rotation component considerably. Reach the forearm of the top shoulder up, so that it, too, is perpendicular to the wall, and use the arm to push the top shoulder away from the wall. You can also use the muscles under the arm of the bottom shoulder to help pull the leg further across the body. Hold this position for a breath or two.

To increase the stretch, slowly straighten the back leg, trying to keep the hips as low to the floor as possible. You will feel the effect more strongly now in the front leg's hip; this is an excellent *piriformis* stretch. To tighten further, let the back leg bend a little, sink to the floor as low as you can and restraighten the back, then restraighten the back leg.

A **C–R stretch** can be done from here: while using the arms to hold you in position, use the waist muscles to try to twist yourself out of the position for a count of five. The hands on the wall and the lower arm trapped behind the knee will provide resistance against the contraction. Stop, breathe in, relax and let the hips sink, and restraighten the back and the back leg. Hold the final position for five to ten breaths; breathing will be difficult due to the constraints on rib movement, but this will help you breathe into the lower quadrant of the lungs (between the top hip and the middle of the back), which most people do not use. Pay attention to left–right differences, and do your tighter side once again.

Cues

deep lunge position
forearm's length from wall
position hands; straighten back
straighten back leg to tighten
C–R: twist away from support
restretch: arch back, let hips sink to floor, straighten back leg

Exercise 42, Floor feet held back bend

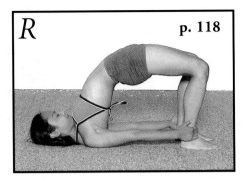

A full description of this exercise will be found in lesson 6. The final position is determined both by your flexibility and by the strength in *quadriceps*. Keep the lower back muscles as relaxed as you can, and make sure you bend the spine forwards afterwards.

Exercise 58, Partner bar shoulder flexion with hip traction

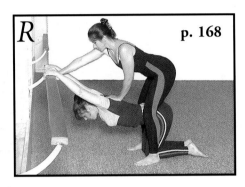

Lesson 9 has the details of this exercise. Recall that the essence of successful performance in this exercise is to let yourself be drawn away from the support, and to let yourself relax under your partner's weight—so, partners, press very gently! Recover with exercise 1, middle and upper back or exercise 43, folded legs clasped knees upper back, emphasising the upper back aspects.

Exercise 6, Chin to chest

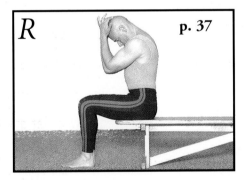

Some neck tension is likely after the last exercise, so sit (or stand) and briefly stretch the neck forwards, as described in lesson 1.

83. Partner floor back bend, off support

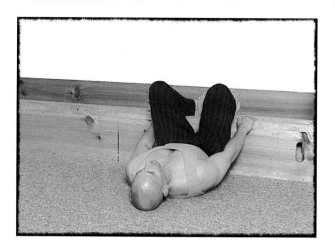

The standard full back bends done off the floor, sometimes called the bridge or the crab, are fundamental to dance, gymnastics and yoga. For most people, however, because of tight hip flexors and *quadriceps*, and tight shoulders, the main effect of floor back bends is to strongly bend the lumbar spine backwards. This can result in an unpleasant compression sensation or can strongly tighten the lumbar spine muscles. It is mainly for these reasons that we concentrate on stretching the muscles mentioned until they are relatively loose, and to practise more passive back bends off supports, as in exercise 27. Once these muscles are loose enough, the full exercise can be done easily and, instead of feeling it in the lumbar spine, you will feel a strong stretch in the front of the body. In a real sense, this next exercise in its various forms is a major pose: all of the muscles mentioned in the ageing process discussed in exercise 14, lesson 2, are strongly stretched and, if a partner helps you, the effect can be transferred to any particularly tight places in the spine. My reservations about doing standard back bends come from observing thousands of students attempt the full exercise, and noting that, if the thoracic spine resists bending backwards (by far the majority of students), the lumbar spine must bend commensurately further. In most students' attempts, if unassisted, there is little backward bend in the thoracic spine. Assisted, the spine can be encouraged to bend at its tightest points and the effect is entirely different. This pose can be enormously exhilarating and can have a calming effect on excited people, and, paradoxically perhaps, a stimulating effect on dispirited students or those whose energy levels are low.

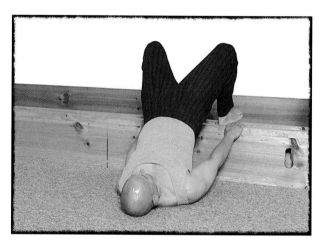

To enable a student to master the full back bend, we have found assistance useful in addition to a support for the feet. Olivia is helping me. The higher the feet are off the ground, the less the spine is required to bend backwards. Supports of up to a forearm's length are useful; above this height, getting into the position is difficult. Look at the first photograph. The feet are placed on the support, the bottom is brought close, and the palms placed on the floor behind, at about shoulder width for the first attempt. Your partner stands next to your hands, so that any tendency for the hands to slip away behind you is arrested against the feet. The partner bends forwards from the hips with a straight back, and places their hands under the shoulders. You breathe in.

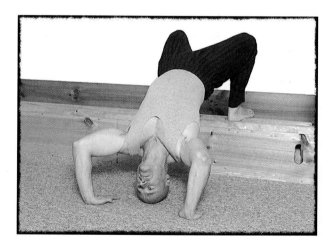

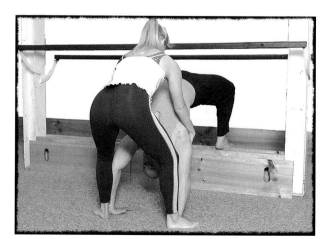

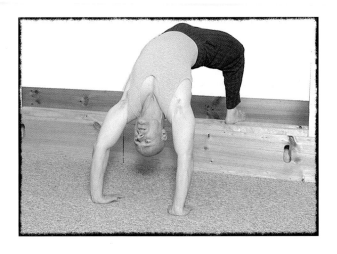

Cues

hips next to support

hands under shoulders

lift yourself onto head; pause and adjust

press arms out and lift up

push hips up to ceiling

use recovery pose

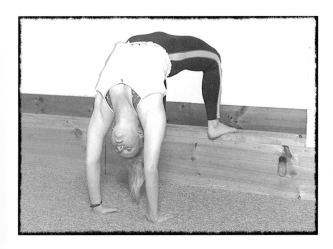

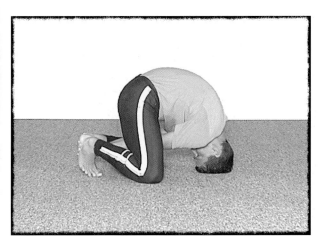

On a breath out, press your hands away behind you to lift yourself from the floor; at the same time your partner helps by applying a *small* lifting effort under the shoulders, until you are resting on the top of your head. Pause in this position if you wish, adjust your hand and foot positions, and then try to lift yourself all the way up. Partners, do not assist too much: if you are not strong enough to do all, or most, of the lifting work you must try anyway—and this effort will make you strong enough in time. Lift yourself as high as you can, and try hard to straighten your arms. Try to breathe normally (breathing is difficult in this position)—under no circumstances hold the breath.

Now your partner can help you move the major bending effect from the lower back. Ask your partner to draw your shoulders back very gently and *slowly*, away from your feet, as Olivia is doing in the last frame, opposite. A note to partners: usually, the effort of only a couple of fingers is needed to achieve this movement. As the partner moves you, the stretch will move into the middle and upper back, and the shoulders. Make your best possible effort to straighten the arms fully (or keep them straight) during this process. As an additional effect, you can try very gently to apply a small straightening effort to the legs; this too will move the stretch higher in the back. In the final position, the shoulders will be directly over, or close to over, the hands. Hold the position for at least five breaths (10 is better) and, to come out of the stretch, slowly bend the arms, remembering to bring the neck and head forwards so you don't bump it on the floor!

Curl up in one of the recovery positions, or roll around on the floor for a moment to relax the back muscles. The best recovery poses are exercises 1 (Mark, last frame) and 48.

Try the exercise a second time after a rest. Generally the second attempt feels much easier, especially the lifting part. If the final position was relatively easy, you may try a lower support, or no support at all. If you choose to do the pose from the floor, place your feet at the join between floor and wall for your first attempt: the tighter you are, the more the hands and feet want to slip away from you. Do not bring the bottom too close to the feet in the starting position for your first try. As you progress, you can bring the bottom closer; eventually you can start with the feet under the bottom. This position and its variations will be explored in chapter three.

84. Wall squatting rotation

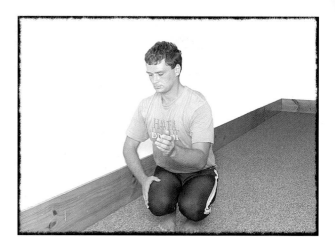

This exercise is similar to exercise 82, wall lunge rotation, but is a stronger rotation for the whole of the spine (especially the lumbar region), and is also a good stretch for *piriformis*, because the outside leg is brought a long way across the body with the hip flexed. Gravity and friction work for you here, so the final position is easily held. Small back-straightening movements will change the focus of the stretch, so spend some time and experiment.

Mark is leaning on his right elbow, holding his knee, and is spaced about one forearm's length away from the wall. To get into the first stretch position from here, breathe out and, while the breath is held out, twist the trunk to bring the far arm and shoulder into position. Lean your weight on the point of the elbow closest to the wall; the forearm of the bottom shoulder will be level with the floor. Your feet are flat on the floor but, if your ankles are not loose enough to permit this, the exercise can be done on the balls of the feet.

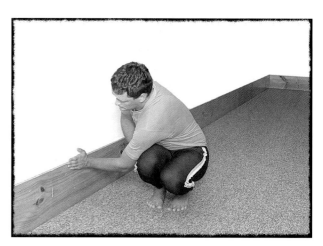

As you breathe in, reach your other arm up and place the hand on the wall, so that the forearm is perpendicular to it. Use both the muscles of the back under the bottom arm, and the muscles of the chest and arm of the upper arm, to rotate yourself into a tighter stretch position. Try to breathe normally.

A **C–R stretch** can be done in the final position: straighten the back by arching it backwards, make sure that you are held in position, and use the waist muscles to try to twist yourself out of the position for a five count. Relax and, on a breath out, use the muscles described above to tighten the position further. Stay in the final position for 10 breaths.

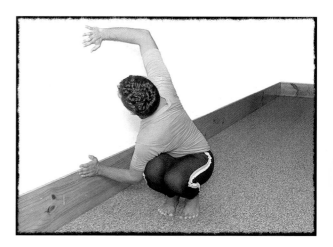

Notice the stretch in the hip—this is due to the leg being brought strongly across the body while the body is being rotated in the opposite direction. For some people, this will be one of the strongest stretches for the hip region; for others it will be one of the strongest lumbar-rotation exercises. The movement is a good strengthening exercise for the trunk.

Cues

squat on flat feet or balls of feet

forearm's length from wall

hands into position; arch back

C–R: try to twist out of position

restretch: arch back,
and pull trunk into tighter position

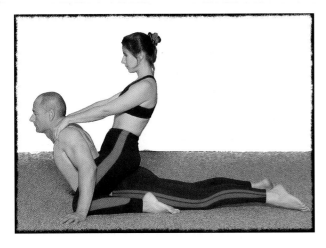

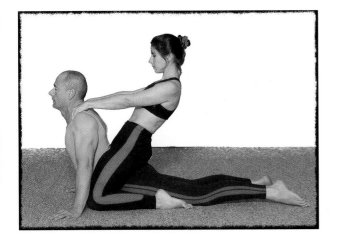

Cues

partner sits on back of legs

support provided by leaning back

let yourself relax

C–R: gently pull shoulders forwards

restretch: partner takes you gently back

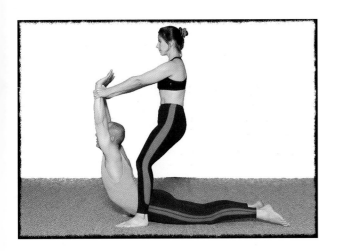

85. Partner floor backward bend

The partner version of one of the first exercises we learned is qualitatively different from the solo movement. Recall the observations about the tendency for muscles to cramp if asked to work in the contracted end of their range of movement, and how common this is with backwards-bending exercises.

Today's exercise avoids these problems because, unlike most backward bends, you can relax in the position completely. Look at the first photograph. To begin, we get into the exercise as usual. Once you are supported on your arms, ask your partner to sit on the back of your thighs (take care that this does not press the knees into the floor), and to place their hands on your shoulders, loose fingers cupping the muscles. Take in a deep breath.

On a breath out, ask your partner to lean back very slowly and carefully, until you feel the desired stretch. The mechanics of the position and the weight of your partner holding your hips onto the floor will help the very lowest part of the spine bend backwards. Make sure that you move into the final position very carefully; this can be an intense stretch. Most men will be able to get the trunk close to vertical using this strict form.

If you are extremely careful, a **C–R stretch** can be done by using the abdominal muscles to pull the shoulders forwards once in the stretch position. The final position that results is intense, so proceed carefully. Try to breathe deeply in the final position, and use one of the recovery poses to stretch the lumbar spine muscles forwards to finish.

The bottom frame shows an alternative way of doing the hanging version of exercise 2, shown on page 115. Get into the final position of exercise 2 and, with your partner in position, lift one arm off the floor. The partner takes this arm, leans back slightly to stabilise themselves, and you hang from their support and give them your other arm. Relax in this position for a moment, then on a breath out, let your whole body relax slowly. As you do, you will feel the front of the body being stretched. Once in this position, the effect can be increased by asking your partner to take your arms back further. This is one of the few backwards bending exercises that provides this lengthening, stretching sensation. Use a recovery pose to finish.

Exercise 47, Partner partial front splits, off support

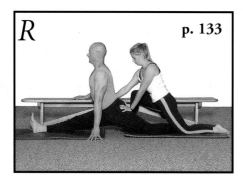

Review the instructions for this exercise, first met in lesson 7. Pay attention to alignment, and try to get as deep in the position as you can. Recall that there should be roughly equal stretch sensations in the back and front legs—if the hamstrings on the front leg are what you feel, make sure the trunk is vertical. You can lean back a fraction to intensify the effect in the back leg, if you wish.

Exercise 48, Floor forward bend over bent legs

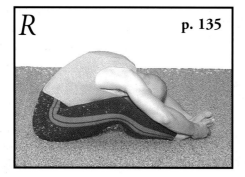

Also found in lesson 7, this minor movement will stretch the lower back wonderfully, especially if you add the alternate arm component, where you pull on the opposite foot with each arm in turn. Recall that, sometimes, exercises that stretch the hip flexors strongly (such as exercise 47) can cause the lower back to tighten.

Exercise 63, Legs apart, off support

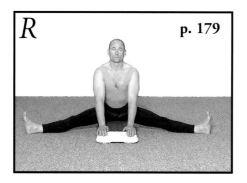

Review the instructions for this exercise, found in lesson 10. To do exercises 47 and 63 in the same session is intense, but no sequence of exercises will have the same effect on the legs. The end positions of each of these poses demonstrate the physiological limits of the hip's movements in these planes. Make sure that you use both foot positions (flat and vertical) and, as you improve, you may increase the contraction force used.

Exercise 64, Seated or standing bent leg rotation

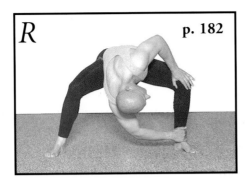

R   p. 182

Review the directions for this exercise, found in lesson 10. If you normally do the seated version, try the standing one, and vice versa. You may also vary the focus of the maximum stretch sensation by moving closer to each leg—have a play with this. Don't forget to use the **C–R stretches** to improve the final position.

Exercise 57, Lying legs behind

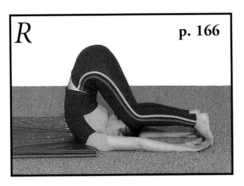

R   p. 166

Review the directions for this exercise in lessons 9 and 14, where walking the legs around was introduced. Let the body relax completely after this tough class.

Chapter three presents a number of additional end poses, and some new warm-ups, too. Do not be in too much of a hurry to achieve these positions. Challenge yourself—carefully.

END POSES

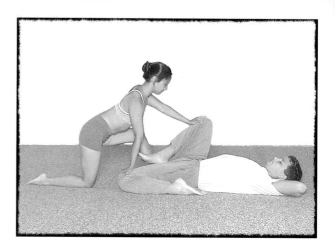

These are presented in no particular order. Some will be relatively simple; others are advanced exercises that may take you years to achieve. Introducing each pose are the exercises that we have found to be effective warm-up movements—but you may have others that are even more effective for you. If you have worked your way through the previous 15 lessons and can do most of the exercises in good form, you will be able to at least attempt all of these.

86. *The ultimate quadriceps stretch*

Warm-up for this exercise by doing your favourite hamstring stretches and follow with your preferred *quadriceps* stretches. Do at least two different exercises for both muscle groups.

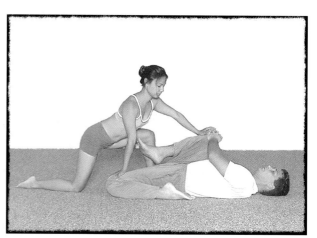

You will see that the start position for this sequence is the final position of exercise 26. Draw the support leg's knee as close as you can to the body, with the leg bent. Even though the hamstrings will not be stretched (because the knee is flexed) doing this will increase the stretch in the folded leg considerably, as the lower back is flattened. Julie and Mark are demonstrating the most intense position of this version in the bottom photograph. Three **C–R stretches** can be done from any of these positions: the first is to try to straighten the folded leg; the second is to try to lift the knee of the folded leg; and the third is to press the raised thigh back to your partner. Restretch after each contraction.

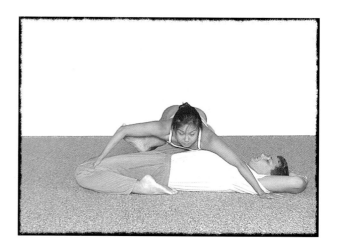

Once this position has been achieved, the stretch can be intensified by opening the knee angle of the leg next to the body. As the lower leg is moved (sequence on facing page) the stretch in the *quadriceps* of the folded leg is increased.

The third photograph opposite shows the beginning position of the full stretch. When the raised leg is straight, the stretch is intense. Various **C–R stretches** can be done.

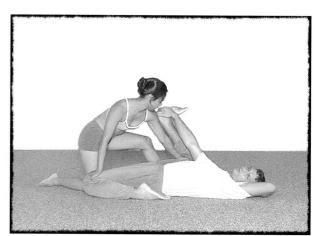

For the folded leg, the contractions are as described above. For the straight leg, you may try to pull the heel back to the bottom, and you can press the straight leg back to your partner. Restretch after both. The further the leg is moved back towards you, the more intense the stretch in the folded leg.

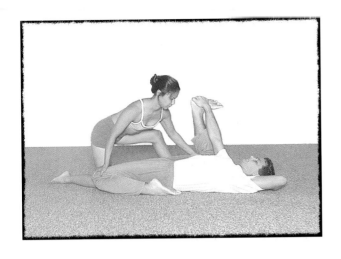

Greg and Carol are demonstrating the same exercise, but with variations in support positions. I find that the sensations of the stretch are easier to control if I am pulling on the raised leg myself. Others find the sensations easier to tolerate if the partner is in control of the movement. Try both and see which works best for you.

In addition to being a strong quadriceps stretch, these combined movements are intense hamstring stretches because the combined tension of quadriceps and the hip flexors hold the hips onto the floor, and because the lower back will be perfectly straight.

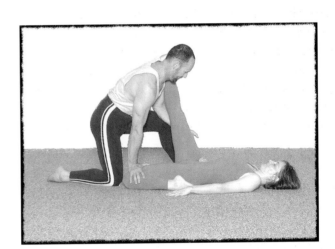

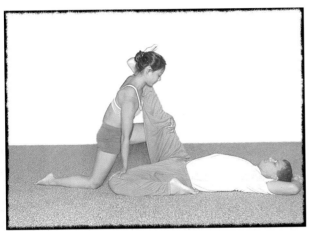

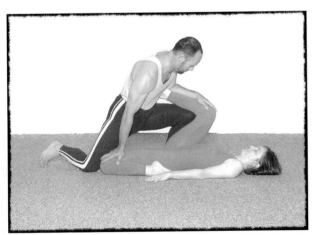

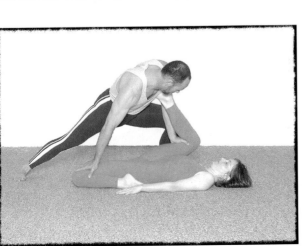

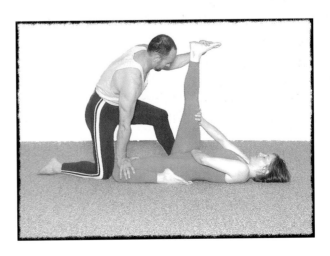

87. *Partner floor hamstring and lower back*

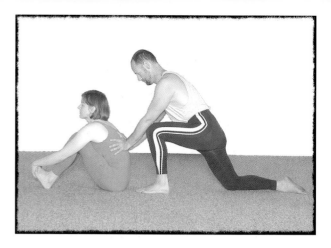

The end position of this exercise resembles exercise 96, forward bend over straight legs. However, because we get into this position via *bent* legs, the sensations are very different. For most people, bending forwards over both straight legs is difficult. Earlier, I suggested the reason was that the protective mechanisms of the body, the *proprioceptors*, are most directly stimulated in this position, and hence can limit the movement significantly.

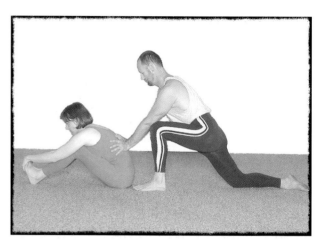

In contrast, everyone will be able to do this movement and, when we use it in class, usually in an *Intermediate* course, a dramatic improvement in the capacity to bend over both legs is the result. Carol and Greg are demonstrating the exercise: Carol holds her feet and pulls her body as close to her thighs as she can. Once the ribs are in contact with the legs, you will find that the body relaxes somewhat. Greg is supporting her middle and lower back, to help it maintain the shape it made getting into the first position.

Keeping her body firmly on her legs, Carol then tries to gently straighten her legs using *quadriceps*. Socks can be worn to help your feet slide, or you can place a mat under your heels. If the sensation of straightening both legs is too intense, try doing one at a time. The standard contractions to improve hamstring flexibility can be used: one **C–R stretch** involves pulling one or both heels to the floor; the other to press the back against your partner's support. Always restretch on a breath out—doubly significant here, as your spine will lift away from your thighs slightly as you breathe in.

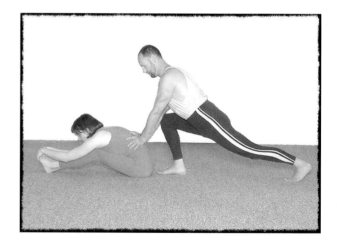

In the bottom frame, Greg is showing the preferred support position once you can get your upper body past 45 degrees from vertical; a partner's body weight is far better than force applied using their arms, as the force is far more stable and you can relax under it.

Don't think that the object of the exercise is to straighten the legs, although that will happen one day. A better objective is to explore the many feelings accompanying the process of getting to that position and the many stretch sensations that will be felt, from the calf muscles all the way up the back to the neck. Try to hold your end position for at least 10 breaths—20 would be better!

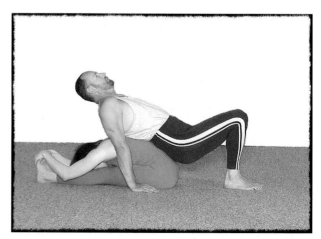

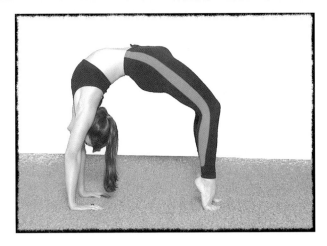

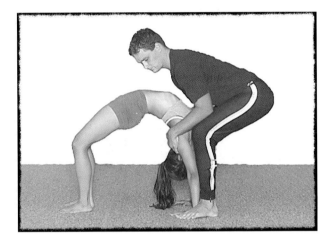

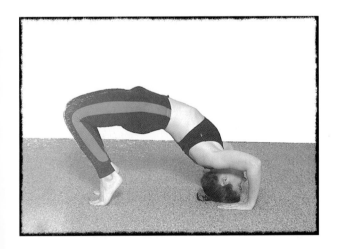

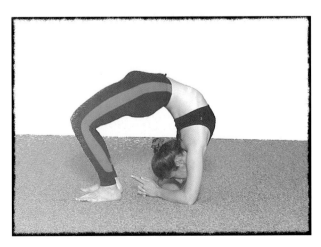

88. *The ultimate back bend*

This is a standard in dance, gymnastics, yoga, and both the traditional exercise forms I studied in Japan. If you can do this well, shoulder flexion movements, hip flexor stretches, upper, middle and lower-back backward-bending movements will be unnecessary. If you cannot, these are precisely the exercises you need to focus upon for your warm-ups. Exercise 88 stretches all the muscles on the front surface of the body. As I observed above when we first encountered backwards-bending exercises, for most people the emphasis will be in the lower back, and this is undesirable. For your first attempts, a partner is desirable, because your shape can be monitored and correction applied as necessary. The minimum warm-up should be exercise 83, partner floor back bend, off support. Review the instructions on how to use your arms to get into position to lift the hips up.

Look at Jennifer's demonstration of the movement in the top photograph: the whole of her spine is a smooth curve. Nonetheless, when Mark gently draws Julie's shoulders towards him as shown in the second frame, more of the stretch effect is experienced in the middle, or thoracic, spine, and the lumbar spine is not as curved as before. For men in particular, this assistance will transform the effects of exercise 88, as most men are particularly stiff in this area. As you are drawn back you will feel the chest being opened lengthways and sideways: this position is maximum expansion for the rib cage and a powerful stretch for the entire abdominal area. Huge sheets of *fascia* are stretched in the process—there are over 30 layers of fascia in the trunk alone.

Due to the position of the front ribs in the final position, breathing will be difficult. For the greatest benefits from the movement, accordingly, breathe as deeply and rhythmically as possible. You will be able to feel the intercostals, the muscles between the ribs, being stretched as you breathe.

Jennifer is demonstrating the ultimate back bend, her spine a smooth even curve. She starts the movement from the same support position as exercise 88, having lifted herself up onto her head, but then places her forearms on the ground. She is trying for maximum elevation by pushing up with her hips and, by applying a slight leg-straightening effort, is moving the stretch from the lower back into the middle and upper back. Use any of the recovery poses that bend the spine forwards to finish.

89. *The ultimate bent-leg hip adductor*

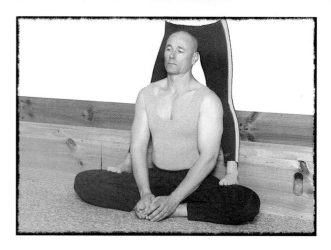

Warm-up for this movement by using a partner's weight to stretch the legs to the floor, as we did in exercise 61, partner wall seated knees apart. Olivia is standing on my thighs, about midway between hip and knee. For a stronger stretch, ask your partner to place their feet closer to your knees.

Look at the second frame. Mark is lying back on his elbows and Julie is helping him to open the legs. This is a gentle position that anyone will be able to do. If you feel too exposed in the stretch, by all means roll up two mats and place one under each knee: this will make you feel perfectly secure, and as you relax the mats will change shape slightly, letting the knees go to the floor.

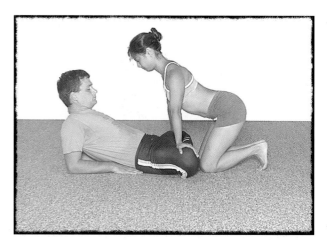

The final frame shows the strongest version, with the hips perfectly abducted and the legs hard on the floor. Rolled mats or similar supports may be used under both knees to facilitate early attempts. Additionally, if your partner stands closer to your hips, less stretch effect will be felt.

In either position, the **C–R stretches** will be the same: try to lift your knees up against your partner's weight, beginning with a gentle contraction and, in time, trying to lift the partner's whole weight. We are certain that the ultimate legs-apart positions require great strength in the adductors before the brain can signal to the muscles to let go. Try it for yourself.

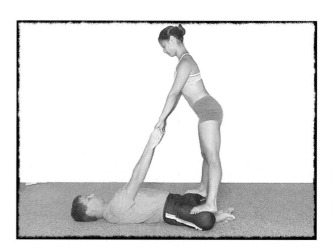

Cues

use mats under knees for first attempt

partner stands on thighs

let legs go to floor

C–R: squeeze knees together

restretch: let legs sink to floor

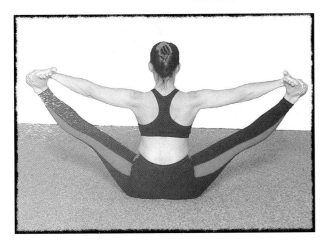

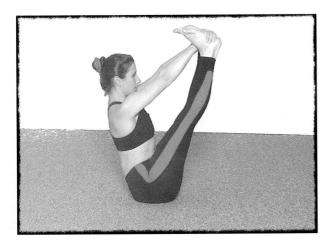

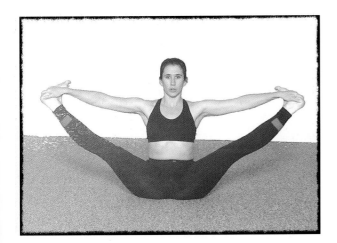

90. Balancing straight legs apart

One of the reasons I like the balancing poses so much as stretching movements is that, because you are focusing so strongly on staying balanced, you can more easily ignore the flexibility demands of any movement. Many students have reported that they either experienced breakthroughs immediately following such exercises, or that an unusual muscle soreness was experienced in the days following. By this I don't mean to imply that these sorts of exercises will leave you stiff and sore but, once you have become flexible, you will find that you can hit a plateau in your improvement, and a stronger stimulation will be required to move you onwards.

Begin by sitting on the floor with the legs bent and apart in front of you, holding the feet from the arch side. Lean backwards until you are balancing on the *ischial tuberosities*, or the bottom bones. Arch the lower back until the spine is a long, straight shape. Take in a breath.

On a breath out, slowly straighten the legs. I prefer to straighten one at a time; try both ways and see which you prefer. If you are very flexible, you may care to straighten both legs out in front of you while holding them together. If you cannot straighten the legs completely, you may loop a strap around each foot. Jennifer is demonstrating my preferred approach, which is to straighten the legs at the most comfortable angle. Balance there, making sure that the lower back is held straight, or better, slightly arched backwards.

Again on a breath out, and focusing closely on balancing, slowly take the legs out to the side as far as you can. Jennifer is demonstrating the ultimate final position, where legs and body are in the same line, and the trunk is held perfectly straight. Notice that, as you separate the legs, the angle of the body to the floor changes as your centre of gravity changes. You will need to feel how to come forwards slightly on the bottom bones to maintain balance: this is the point where most people topple forwards! This exercise is great fun to do.

Finish by doing any of the exercises that stretch the middle and upper back forwards: holding the spine straight against the combined forces of the adductors and both hamstrings is hard work.

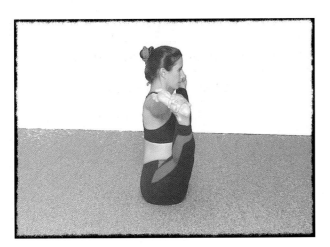

91. The ultimate legs-apart stretch

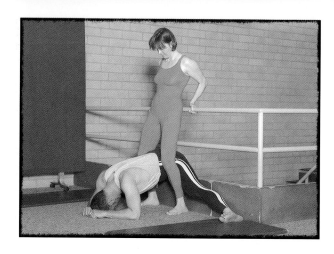

There are a number of benchmarks in stretching and, of them all, front splits and side splits (sometimes called straddle, or Chinese splits) probably rank the most highly in impressiveness. I am bound to say, though, now that I can do these myself (and having taken 20 years to achieve them!), I feel that these movements are not as important as I once thought. Of course, if you are a gymnast or martial artist, you must be able to do both of these fundamental movements, if only to demonstrate good technique. But if your main interest in flexibility is good health or the exploration of the mind–body connection, the relevance is much harder to argue and, as I mentioned in the unnumbered lesson, myriad minor positions—often in between the positions that most people regard as 'stretches'—may be of greater importance to you.

In this exercise, I shall group all the major warm-up and partial positions that I have found most useful in achieving side splits. For me, discovering that one might get into the side-splits position from above by opening the legs wider and wider from the standing position, rather than trying to open the legs further from the *seated* position, was the breakthrough that accelerated my progress. I cannot say that this approach will work for you—you will need to try all the assistance and partial approaches to find the key.

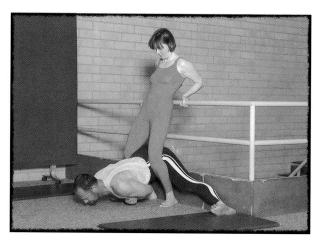

The first assistance position is being demonstrated by Greg and Carol. In the first frame, Carol has locked Greg into position against the wall by standing in such a way as to let her jam the back of his thighs against the support. The resulting friction allows him to stay in this position with far less discomfort, because the adductor muscles do not need to support nearly as much of his weight. Stay in this opening position for a minute or two.

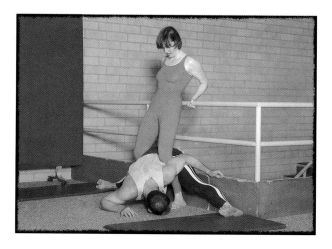

The **C–R stretch** is to contract the inner thighs while you support yourself on your arms, as though you are trying to squeeze the legs together through the floor. Begin with a gentle contraction and slowly increase it to your limit over 10 to 15 seconds. Relax and, on a breath out, ask your partner to let you go a little closer to the floor. The second frame shows Greg contracting sufficiently strongly such that he no longer needs to hold the upper body off the floor: such contractions should be built up to slowly, but they will yield excellent results. The third frame shows the sort of

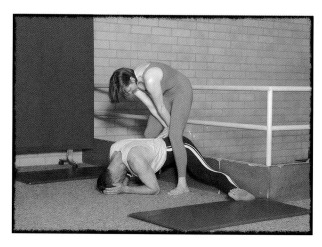

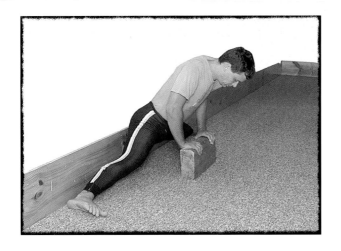

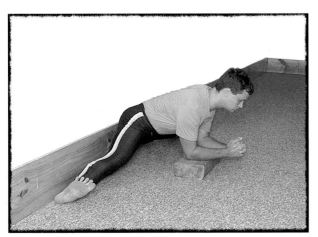

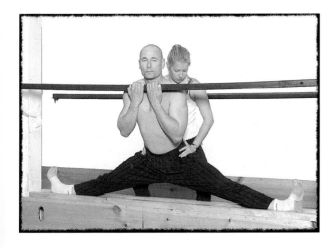

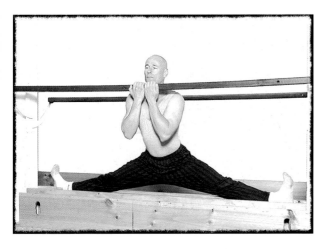

supplementary movements that may be added, and the last shows the assistance position to use in the **C–R** once you are strong enough to lift yourself out of the position by contraction force alone.

Mark is showing a position between side splits achieved by pure abduction (as Greg is demonstrating on the facing page) and the versions I am demonstrating overleaf (achieved by hyperextension and getting into the position via the plane of movement that emphasises stretching the hamstrings rather than the adductors). Mark's position is similar to the standing version Greg showed in exercise 63, legs-apart off support. Accordingly, adductors and the inner hamstrings are stretched in this position.

Mark is using a block to alter the angle between his body and the floor. Even small changes of trunk angle will change the stretch effects considerably. The contractions for the **C–R** are to try to bring the legs together. Use the strength of the arms to lower yourself closer to the floor. Try to stay in your best final position for a minute or so.

Using our purpose-built boxes, Olivia is helping me to bring the hips directly over the line of my legs in the third frame: this is the most difficult stretch angle by far, especially for men. Two **C–R stretches** are possible in this position: to help move the hips directly over the legs, contract the adductors (the inner thigh muscles) as though you were trying to bring the legs together *in front* of you. On a breath out, ask your partner to gently push your hips *forwards*. Once in your forward-most position, for the second **C–R** try to squeeze the legs *together*, as though you were trying to press them harder, directly down onto the surface of the box. For the restretch, let yourself go closer to the surface on a breath out, while your partner holds the hips in line with the feet, directly above them.

The final frame shows the solo version. If you concentrate, you will be able to keep the hips over the feet. To recover, you may use any of the *piriformis* stretches (these seem to make the hip joints feel good after a strong sideways stretch) or any of the exercises that stretch the spine forwards.

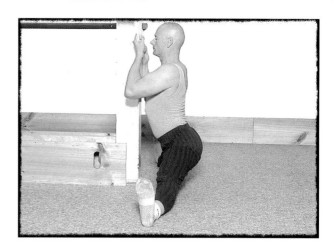

The top frame shows how any vertical support can be used for these sorts of warm-up movements. You can see here how the side-split position forces some hyperextension into the lumbar spine but, if you relax while lowering yourself, this will happen without effort. If the lower back is left feeling a little tight after this practice, stretch it forwards with exercise 48, floor forward bend over bent legs.

Once you have achieved some depth in the position, you may find that your progress stalls. I have found that using a support that will deform slightly under my weight can be helpful in getting over these 'sticking points'. In the second frame I am showing the legs-apart position off a low support, a height just above my maximum stretch position with the legs at 180 degrees. This lets you relax properly in the position, which you cannot do if the stretch is too intense. To add the adductors and inner hamstrings to the stretch, incline the body forwards, until the straight trunk is resting completely on the support if you can (frame three). The sensation of feeling your stomach and chest pressing on the support is excellent and you will be able to relax in the position.

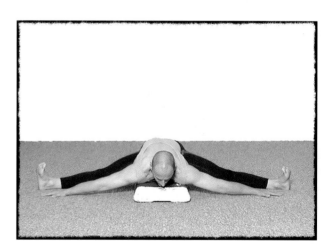

If you have good side splits, Olivia is demonstrating one way of ensuring that you are in the perfect position (last frame): with her body firmly on the floor, she has pushed herself back onto the support (a wall is good, too) until the backs of her legs are pressed hard against it. If you are close to this position but not quite on the floor, roll a mat and position it under the body lengthways.

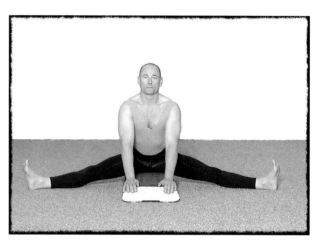

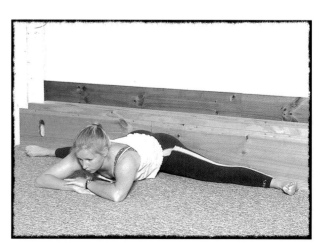

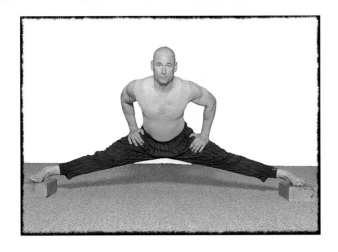

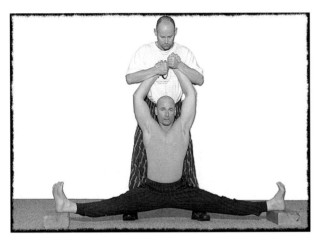

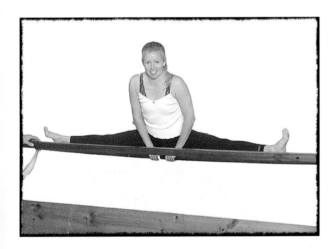

In the top two photographs, I am demonstrating my preferred approach to side splits. I am using two blocks to show the sort of strength required to hold these positions—there is no support from the floor in the final position. In the first frame, I have let my legs go apart, inclined my body forwards, and let the lower back hyperextend just enough for balance. All the muscles of the legs will be working hard in this position. If your knees do not like being stressed this way, try to relieve the pressure either by tensing the *quadriceps* (this is done by pulling the kneecaps upwards by tightening the thighs) or by using one of the other exercises. The previously shown movements that stress the knee joint from behind (the movements where you lower yourself into the position from directly above) will not have this effect, usually. Holding yourself as shown in the first frame, I find to be the best warm-up movement for the final position, and the weight of your body is a perfect resistance for a **C–R stretch**. The second frame shows the full side splits, in suspension off blocks. Greg is providing support for me—it's a bit hard to balance on the backs of your legs—he is not holding me up. You will notice that the calf muscles are below the level of the surface of the blocks, and the hips are directly in line with the feet. I do not recommend attempting this position unless you can hold yourself securely as shown in the first frame for at least half a minute or so.

Contractions in this position will ensure that you are able to do the movement on the floor. Use the muscles at the back of the legs to vigorously try to lift yourself straight up from the stretch position and, on a breath out, very slowly lower yourself to your limit. Working like this will remove the fear often associated with this movement, especially for men.

The third frame shows Olivia in full side-splits while sitting on a bar—a handy position for gymnasts. I have included this to show how easy the position will become for you one day (I'm still waiting for this day to come!). The final frame shows Jennifer in a totally relaxed side splits prone position—for her this is a warm-up. By all means make an effort to achieve similar positions yourself, but bear in mind my remarks at the beginning of this exercise, and be careful not to injure yourself in pursuit of a position that has little utility in daily life. My suggestion is to have no heed as to how long it might take you to get into these positions. Concentrate on the process rather than the outcome.

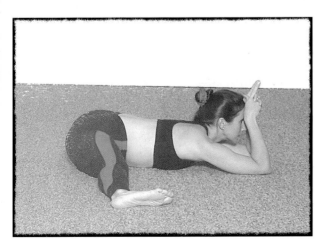

92. Sitting and standing peacocks

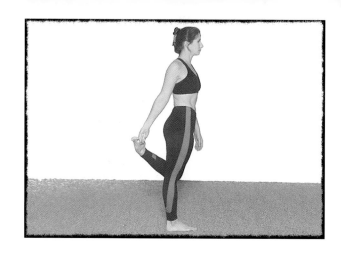

Jennifer is demonstrating a pair of beautiful poses from hatha yoga. The standing version requires great flexibility in spinal extension and shoulder flexion—but these poses are not good ways of achieving the required flexibility. I have included them here to show Jennifer's flexibility and balance, and to create the opportunity to suggest that, if you have come this far and want to go further than we have here, you may consider learning yoga from a good teacher.

The start position is achieved by holding a foot by the opposite shoulder's hand, and pulling the leg up behind you. As you do so, notice how you will need to incline the trunk forwards to keep balance; this will give you a good hamstring stretch in the support leg, too. Once the foot is close enough to the body, hold it with the other hand, too. The final position is shown in the last photograph in the right-hand column. Notice that Jennifer's hips are level—this is hard to do, as the held leg pulls the hip up with it. The seated version shown below is essentially the same, but without the balancing aspect.

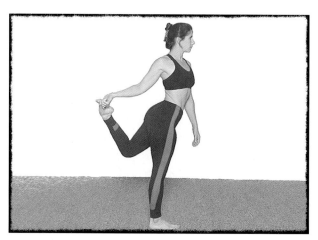

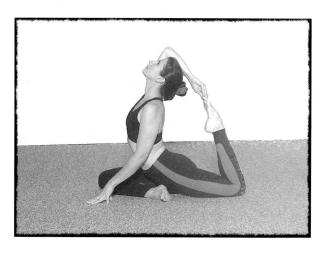

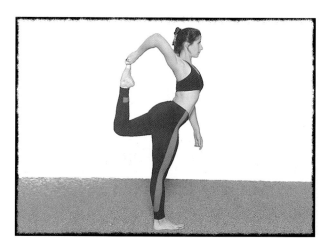

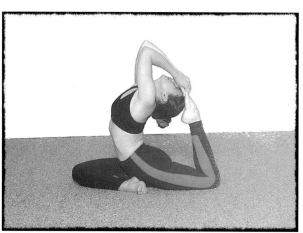

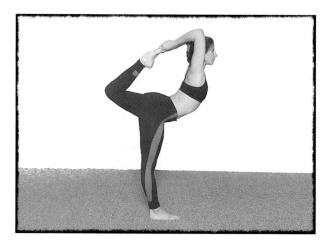

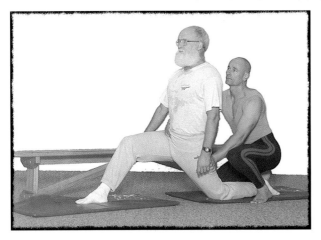

93. The ultimate front splits

I have asked Eldon, one of our senior students, to demonstrate the full front splits because he is a recreational athlete (a runner) and because he is middle-aged, chronologically speaking. People like Eldon are remaking the image we have of the term 'middle-aged'. At the time this sequence was taken, he had been attending *Posture & Flexibility* classes for about five years, and he was quite stiff when he began—he could not touch his toes.

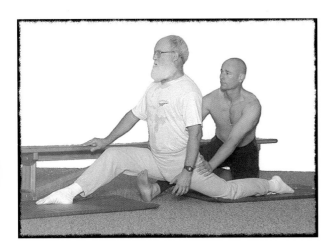

He is using the approach to get into this position that I described in exercise 47, partner partial front splits, off support, page 133. All contractions are the same, so turn back to this exercise to refresh your memory. I am holding his hips in perfect form, at 90 degrees to the line of his legs. In the final position, the front of his back leg is hard on the floor, and the back of the front leg is too, except where it is lifted away by the thickness of the mats. We use mats, or socks on a shiny floor from time to time, to help ensure that the transitions to the final position are very smooth and jerk free—it is easy to injure yourself as you get close to your limits.

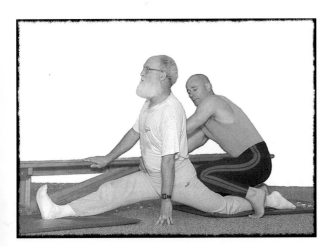

In the third frame I am showing the recommended support position for when you are working with someone who is physically much larger or stronger than you, or when the position needs to be held for a long time. Even small people will be able to use their weight to hold the partner in good form if this technique is used. The essence is to use your *weight*, not your strength, so hang off your partner as far as you can, pivoting yourself from the folded leg's knee, placed under the hip of your partner's back leg.

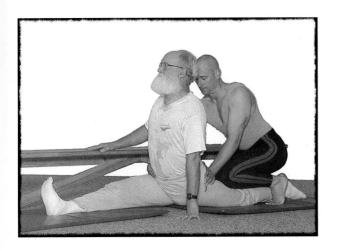

Cues

hips perfectly square
bent front leg to start
small supports under front leg if desired
straighten front leg using **C–Rs**
restretch: sink down onto floor

94. *The ultimate abdominal workout*

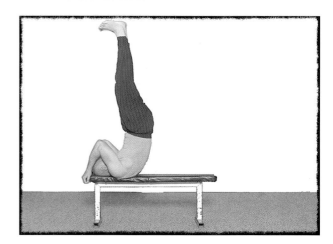

This sequence demonstrates the most difficult abdominal strengthening exercise that can be done without gymnastic equipment. All you need is a bench or a table. I caution against trying this movement if you are not already quite strong in this area of the body because, if your abdominal muscles are insufficiently strong, you will find your lower back hyperextending rapidly in the second-last or final position and you will not be able to control it. It is possible, however, to do a modified version of the movement, by folding the legs fully at the knees; this will mean that you are holding less weight, for leverage reasons.

Start by lifting yourself up into a loose shoulder-stand position, holding the edge of your support platform as shown. Try to elevate the body as far as possible (top frame). Once secure, lower the body and legs until you can feel their weight, and lift the hips (or lower the legs a little further) until the legs and body form a straight line (second frame). The exercise is much harder to do if the body is held straight, because the abdominal muscles do an increasing amount of the work as trunk and legs come into alignment.

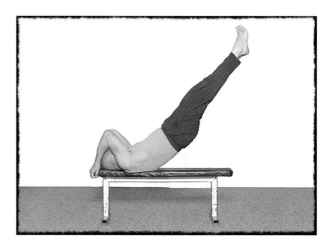

Once the body is straight, lower the whole body by pivoting around the shoulder joint, as shown in the third frame. To this point, the exercise will feel relatively easy. Pause in this position for a few seconds. Take in a breath and, while holding it in, lower yourself slowly as far as you can without resting your hips on the support. Once the body and legs are *under* a 45 degree angle (between shoulder and foot), the exercise rapidly becomes difficult—each position a degree lower seems twice as hard as the position above. Hold your best final position for at least five breaths in and out.

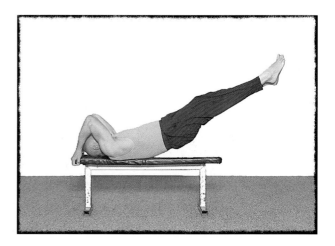

Once you have achieved the final position shown, there are two further movements that increase the strengthening effect. The first is to cautiously lower the legs *below* the level of the hips (be careful to do this very slowly to avoid straining the lower back); the other is to lift the whole straight body back up to the start position.

This sequence resembles the lever from men's gymnastics. If you are tall, or your legs are relatively long in relation to your trunk, this is the only abdominal exercise you will ever need to do. As we say in class, though, 'Rome wasn't built in a day!'. Don't be in too much of a hurry to accomplish this difficult exercise.

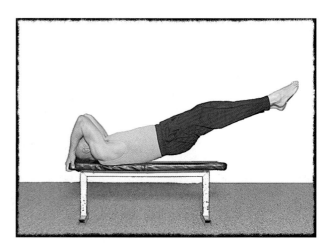

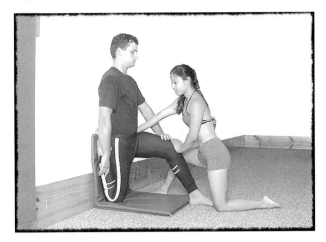

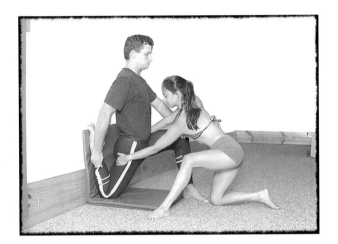

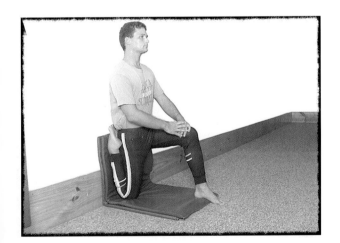

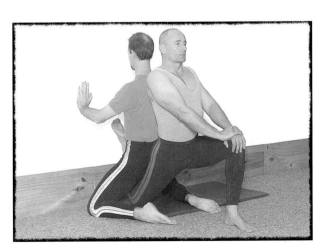

95. Ultimate quadriceps and hip flexor

This is a deceptive pose, for it looks easy compared with many others. As you try it, however, you will realise why it is here in chapter three rather than in chapter one. The combination of flexed thigh and movement of the body forward from this starting point will give you a stretch in *quadriceps* that is unparalleled. Additionally, whereas most *quadriceps* stretches have their main effect in the lower part of the thigh, and most combination *quadriceps* and hip flexor stretches have their effects high in the thigh, the exercises shown here affect the whole of the thigh with the focus in the middle, and hence is the perfect complement to the others.

Mark, assisted by Julie, is showing the start position. He has pushed the calf muscle of the folded leg out of the way before getting into position. Julie is holding the hip of the other leg against the wall. In the second frame, she is applying the necessary counter-rotation by pulling the hip of the folded leg away from the wall while pressing the hip of the support leg back. Mark is applying the abdominal brace. **C–R stretches** that may be done include Mark's trying to straighten the folded leg by pressing the foot into the wall and trying to pull the knee of the folded leg forwards. The third frame shows the start position of the solo exercise, intensified by applying both the abdominal brace and the tucking-the-tail-under movement.

The bottom frame shows a much stronger version, demonstrated by Kevin and myself. I have moved forward from the start position into approximately the same position as shown by Mark in frame two. Kevin has moved behind me and positioned his hips onto the back of my leg, just below the hip joint. By letting his weight bear down on my leg and pressing back to me gently, the best *quadriceps* and hip flexor stretch will be felt.

Contractions are the same as described above. The value of this version lies in the completely stable pressure your partner is able to apply, and the magnitude of the force itself. The sheer intensity of the final stretch sensation will have to be experienced to be appreciated. You can see from the photograph how far behind the line of the body the leg has been taken—and this is with the leg folded at the knee as well, which makes it very strong indeed.

96. Forward bend over straight legs

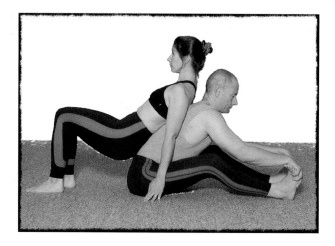

I have saved this pose until the end, because it is how we began. Recall that in the *Introduction* that I used this exercise as the example stretching movement, because it illustrated all the problems of conventional stretching. All that is a long way behind us, now. We are ready to attempt this excellent, whole-body movement.

Depending on your pattern of flexibility, this can be an intense hamstring stretch, a pleasant lower-back stretch, or simply a lovely movement to do. You may care to warm-up for this with a variety of hamstring stretches and, again depending on your pattern—which is well known to you now—a *piriformis* stretch, a calf muscle stretch, or one for the lower back.

The best single warm-up movement is exercise 87, partner floor hamstring and lower back. Do this now, emphasising the leg-straightening aspects.

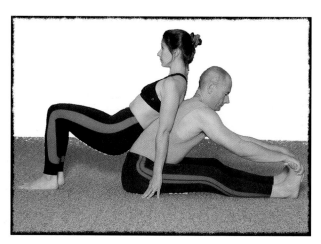

Various support positions are shown. There is no one correct way of doing this exercise, because it can be used to achieve different effects. I am showing the movement with Jennifer, going into the final position via exercise 87: starting with bent legs, I straighten one at a time to get used to the sensation. Three **C–R stretches** can be used: pulling one or both heels to the floor while holding the leg in position; pressing one or both straight legs into the floor; and pressing your upper back against your partner while lifting your chest (you will need to hold your feet for this). When restretching, try to pull yourself *along* the legs rather than trying to pull your face to your legs—this last movement stretches the back. Of course, if that is the effect you are after, do just that. My final position, simply relaxing over both straight legs, is a wonderful stretch for the whole of the back, and back of the legs. Deliberately, I have demonstrated this with my arms placed on the floor alongside my legs to show that once the ribs are in firm contact with the legs, your partner's weight is supported effortlessly.

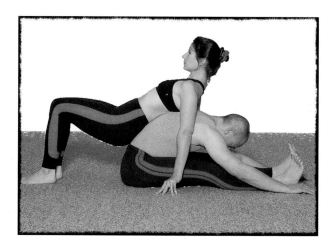

Cues

both legs bent

body hard on thighs

partner lies with full weight

all **C–Rs** may be used

restretch: let yourself relax onto legs

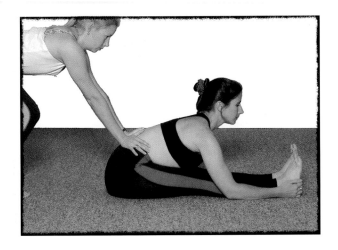

Jennifer is showing the exercise in a more conventional way, where the emphasis is on moving the hamstrings to their maximum stretch length. Various support positions may be used; a partner may simply apply a gentle straightening force to the lower back using their hands, or the most effective one, second frame, where Olivia is lying on Jennifer's back. All contractions are the same as described above. This is a wonderful stretch to finish any exercise session—let yourself relax completely.

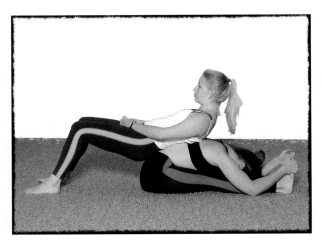

The third frame shows this exercise done perfectly, solo.

At this point, the formal teaching ends—and hence is a new beginning for you. You have the tools to design a program that's just right for you; all that is needed is to continue this process of self-exploration. I mentioned in the *Introduction* that, in time, our classes become self-teaching. This should be the goal of every teacher: to create the environment where the teacher is no longer necessary.

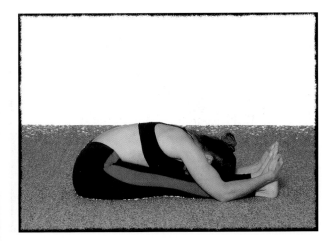

CHAPTER FOUR

RECOMMENDED EXERCISES FOR SPORTS

Different sports place different demands on the body and have different requirements for specific patterns of flexibility. This has lead to the wide prescription of specific exercises based on particular activities. I feel strongly, however, that the best overall results to be gained by stretching in terms of performance enhancement, injury reduction and self-awareness will occur by starting at lesson 1 and working through the material as presented because, as I have argued throughout, stretching is about far more than simply becoming flexible.

It may be helpful to arrange exercises by activity, though, if only to simplify the teaching of the exercises to groups of athletes of all ages, and to ensure that athletes are doing a bare minimum requirement of flexibility work. I have grouped sports and activities on the basis of more-or-less shared functions. The AFL football code, for example, with its requirement of high jumps, aerial activity, and spinal extension with shoulder flexion, resembles the requirements of the court sports more closely than it resembles Rugby League. These divisions are ones of convenience only and I encourage students to add any exercises to the groups shown here as they feel they need.

Bodybuilders and others who stress particular parts of the body in their workouts are advised to select exercises that stretch the muscles being worked, and to do these in between sets and as a cool-down. For example, if doing a chest workout, select those exercises that stretch *triceps,* the pectorals and the front shoulder muscles. The index provides exercises both by function and muscle name.

Racquet sports

Tennis, badminton and squash. Other activities requiring agility and overhead arm movements may use this group of exercises. Add any additional movements that work your tight or problem areas.

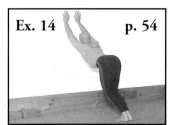

Ex. 14   p. 54

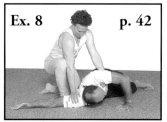

Ex. 8   p. 42

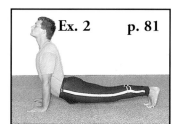

Ex. 2   p. 81

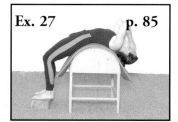

Ex. 27   p. 85

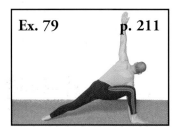

Ex. 79   p. 211

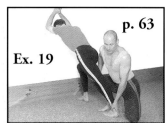

Ex. 19   p. 63

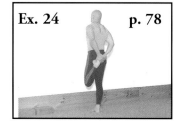

Ex. 24   p. 78

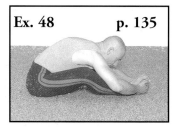

Ex. 48   p. 135

Football codes

Rugby League, Rugby Union, soccer and running activities in general. Cyclists may use this grouping, but emphasise the hip and *quadriceps* movements. Middle- and upper-back exercises can be added to relieve tension in these areas, too.

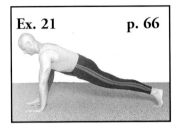

Ex. 21   p. 66

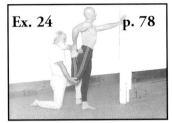

Ex. 24   p. 78

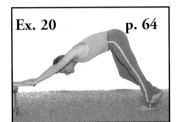

Ex. 20   p. 64

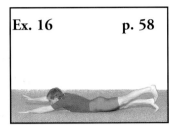

Ex. 16   p. 58

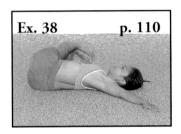

Ex. 38   p. 110

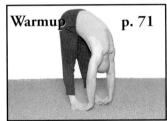

Warmup   p. 71

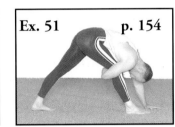

Ex. 51   p. 154

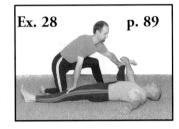

Ex. 28   p. 89

Court sports

Basketball, volleyball, netball and AFL. This group includes activities requiring jumping, extension and agility.

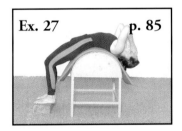

Ex. 27   p. 85

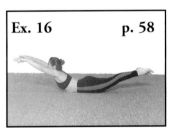

Ex. 16   p. 58

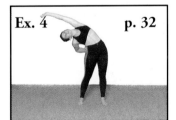

Ex. 4   p. 32

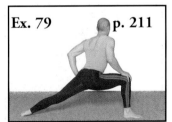

Ex. 79   p. 211

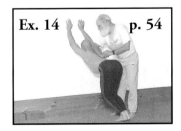

Ex. 14   p. 54

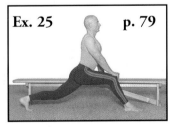

Ex. 25   p. 79

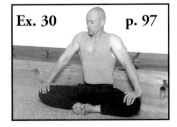

Ex. 30   p. 97

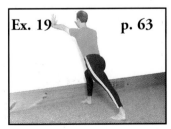

Ex. 19   p. 63

Martial arts and gymnastics

You need exceptional hip flexibility, side bending and rotation for good kicking technique. Include shoulder and arm exercises as necessary. Making *biceps brachii* and *biceps femoris* more flexible will improve punching and kicking speed.

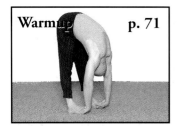
Warmup — p. 71

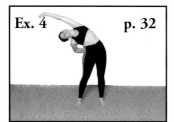
Ex. 4 — p. 32

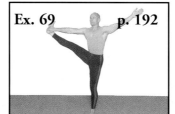
Ex. 69 — p. 192

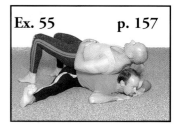
Ex. 55 — p. 157

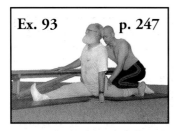
Ex. 93 — p. 247

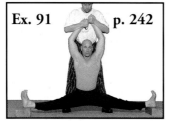
Ex. 91 — p. 242

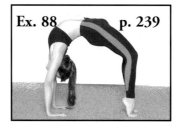
Ex. 88 — p. 239

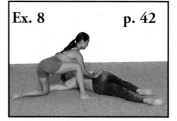
Ex. 8 — p. 42

Cricket

Baseball and softball players may use this group of exercises, too. Bowlers, pitchers and batsmen have different whole-body requirements—so make an appropriate selection. Bowlers and pitchers should concentrate on spinal extension, shoulder-flexion and hip-flexor suppleness; batsmen on spinal rotation and on loosening any of their tight areas.

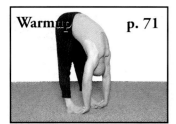
Warmup — p. 71

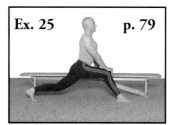
Ex. 25 — p. 79

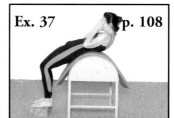
Ex. 37 — p. 108

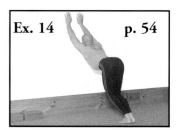
Ex. 14 — p. 54

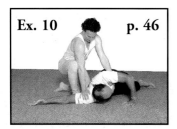
Ex. 10 — p. 46

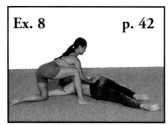
Ex. 8 — p. 42

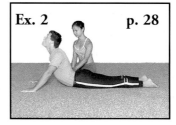
Ex. 2 — p. 28

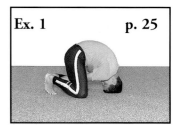
Ex. 1 — p. 25

Golf

The emphasis is on the development of whole-body rotational flexibility, essential to a good swing. In an activity like golf, where all the rotational power of the body is used in only one direction, asymmetry of both strength and flexibility are common, and can lead to back problems. Concentrate on balancing this pattern in all your stretching practice.

Ex. 3 p. 30 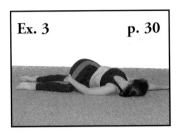	Ex. 38 p. 110 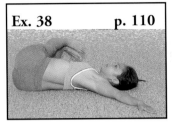	Ex. 2 p. 28 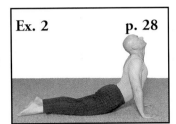	Ex. 14 p. 54 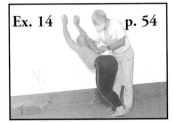
Ex. 37 p. 108 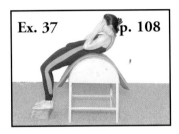	Ex. 25 p. 79 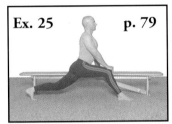	Warmup p. 71 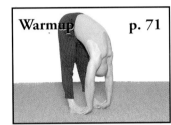	Ex. 43 p. 119 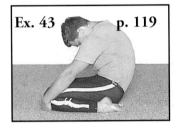

Swimming

Shoulder, hip-flexor and ankle flexibility are emphasised here. Different stroke specialists will need to add appropriate exercises, though—for example, the butterfly requires excellent lumbar and thoracic extension, so add these exercises.

Warmup p. 71 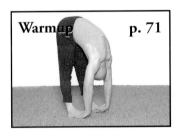	Ex. 2 p. 28 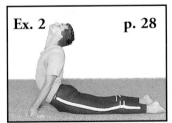	Ex. 37 p. 108 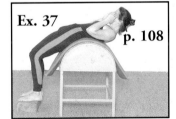	Ex. 23 p. 77 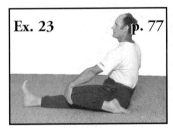
Ex. 18 p. 62 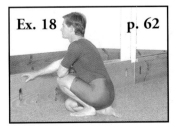	Ex. 19 p. 63 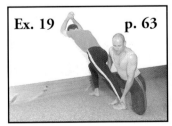	Ex. 35 p. 103 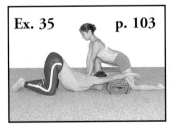	Ex. 3 p. 30 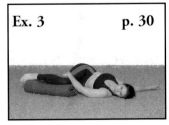

Acknowledgments

Many people helped me in the preparation of this book, directly and indirectly. I shall begin by thanking all the *Posture & Flexibility* teachers currently working at the Australian National University, and a few who travelled from afar to be present during the protracted shooting process. Two teachers, Jennifer Cristaudo (the senior instructor) and Dr Joe Hope, I would like to single out for special mention before the others for the time and effort spent in categorising the huge range of exercises, and for Jennifer's help in modelling for many of the photographs. Because we knew the material so well, the process was fast, and fun too. I have *never* accepted the wisdom of the old adage of not mixing business and pleasure—if you can't, you're in the wrong business!

My brother, Dr Greg Laughlin, helped by taking many of the photographs of me as well as demonstrating some of the more difficult exercises, dispelling once and for all the myth that you can't be big and strong and flexible at the same time. Dr Kevin Moore, Gary Williamson, Pierre Le Count and Alan Richardson (now famous as the teacher of the Over 40s class, many of the members of which inspire the younger students to work harder) all gave their time to model for the photographs, too. Dr Carol Wenzel travelled from Canada, complete with a photo album of the poses *she* wanted to see in the book—and many of the ones that make you feel good are among these. Olivia Allnutt, in addition to demonstrating many of the exercises, also proofread the manuscript and made many helpful suggestions. Additionally, she is the originator of the Dynamic Forms classes within *Posture & Flexibility*.

Julie Netto, one of the most recent additions to the teaching team, has set up classes at Sydney University. I give a special thank you to her here for all the research she did for the International edition of *Overcome neck & back pain*, too. Dr Mark Donohue made a special trip back from Irian Jaya to give his interpretation of some of the major and minor poses, and teaches in Sydney with Julie. Steve Burton modelled for pictures as well, and he, Jackie van der Neut and Julie organise the external *Posture & Flexibility* teaching program, to which all of the senior teachers from Canberra contribute. Sharon Clark organises the *Overcome neck & back pain* individual and practitioner workshops, the *Posture & Flexibility* workshops, teaches classes in Newcastle at the university and other locations, and took the time to model for some photos, too. Dr Petra Boevinck is working in Scotland at present, and organised to have photographs of herself done there—these images turned up at the Sports Union mysteriously one day—thank you! Ben Farrell teaches *Posture & Flexibility* at Adelaide University. I want to acknowledge my continuing debt to the entire team: much of the innovation and thoroughness of the *Posture & Flexibility* system is attributable directly to you all.

In terms of production, Jeremy Mears' contributions are found on every page. And Jeremy's personality deserves mention, as a model: no matter how frustrated I became at different stages of making the book, Jeremy embodied the concept 'cool', being entirely unflappable. His understanding of the Macintosh technology is legendary, too. His web-site address will be found on the back title page.

I wish to thank sincerely Jon Attenborough, David Rodrick, and editors Julie Stanton and Brigitta Doyle, from Simon & Schuster, Australia. We have evolved with each other over these past few years and enjoy a relationship of a kind that only the passage of time can yield. I wish to express my gratitude to Jason Gray, who was the external editor of the manuscript. I thank Grant Cole, Executive Officer of the Australian National University Sports Union, where most of the ACT classes are held, for being someone with whom one can genuinely negotiate, and who actively supports the *Posture & Flexibility* enterprise.

I reserve my final expression of appreciation for Dr Ross Gilham, who both edited and proofread the manuscript. He made copious suggestions regarding syntax, grammar and comma placement (many times!) and the book has benefitted greatly from his input. He took the time to explain the reasons for his suggestions and, as a result, not only was the book improved but I learned much, too. I feel fortunate that a man of his unique experience—both in the medical and linguistic fields—was able to review the entire manuscript, including illustrations and photographs, before we sent it to the printers: many errors were thereby avoided. Ross built the index, too. Remaining errors are my responsibility alone of course.

There is a growing number of teachers of *Posture & Flexibility*, both here and overseas. For an up-to-date listing with contact details, check our web page:

http://www.posture-and-flexibility.com.au

You can make contact with us through the web site, or write to my snail mail or e-mail address, found at the end of the book's *Introduction*. We will present workshops to any interested group, and an increasing number of sporting bodies are contacting us. Get in early!

Last, I wish to thank you, the reader, the essential final partner in the relationship, and to whom I have two things to say. To illustrate what I mean about being a partner in the relationship, I shall mention that at the end of our *Posture & Flexibility* classes, the teacher and the class face each other, kneel, and bow. This is a habit I brought back from Japan. My teacher, Okamoto Hisama, explained it like this:

> 'We bow to each other to show respect, and to make explicit the mutual
> necessity of the relationship. Without students, there can be no teachers—
> and without teachers there can be no students. So, I thank you.'

Finally, as I recounted at the end of *Overcome neck & back pain*, don't be like the businessman who rushed up to me at Melbourne airport when the book was first released, and said, 'Didn't I see you on TV the other day talking about back problems? I've got your book; it's a fantastic book!' Quite naturally, as a brand-new author I was very gratified by this, so I asked what exercises he had found the most helpful. He said, 'Oh, I don't do any of the exercises, but it's a beautiful book!' The moral? Holding the book in your hand is an essential first step, but if you want the benefits, you have to do the work. Good luck.

TECHNICAL NOTES

Stretching & Flexibility is still one of the few books written, photographed, illustrated, laid up, and printed all-digitally—that is, none of the images involved the standard silver-halide film process, except the few shots of Petra. All the text was written on a Macintosh PowerBook in *ClarisWorks*, e-mailed to Jeremy (the graphics guru who sensibly lives an hour away from me in the country), who poured it into *Quark Express* 4.04 for the final layout. Illustrations were done in Adobe *Illustrator* and *Photoshop*. Photographs were taken using a Nikon CoolPix 900s, the images first being recorded on a 24-megabyte flash memory card in the camera, downloaded onto the laptop's hard drive and transferred to Iomega Zip Disk at the same time, all on location. The Zip Disk was sent to Jeremy and, because it was copied at the same time, we both had identical copies of the images, each identified by a unique set of folder and photo numbers. This becomes important when trying to keep track of more than 1,300 images—over 700 of which are used in the book. We used *Graphic Converter* to make single-screen thumbnail summaries of each photo session (43 images will fit on a 24-megabyte flash memory card at the finest resolution). These thumbnail images are big enough to see sufficient detail to know what's in each shot. As each photograph had a unique folder number and shot number (the latter automatically appended in the camera), finding the right images was a relatively simple matter of paging through the 30 or so folders.

For an experienced photographer, the current generation of affordable digital cameras has good and bad points. On the good side is the capacity to instantly review images, by TV screen if you wish, as you take them. This allows the photographer to assess the images to be certain that the required content is there and that exposure and framing are acceptable (and the model's eyes really *were* open when the flash went off). As you cannot control aperture directly through the camera unless you use a proprietory flash unit (none of which had the power we needed to light our large room), any desired exposure and saturation must be found by experimentation. In contrast to the silver-halide process, where aperture can be minutely controlled in half-stop increments, and where particular combinations of aperture and shutter speed can give the same exposure to the film yet with quite different aesthetic effects (providing, for example, control over depth of field) the digital cameras have no such analogue. To illustrate, we found that over-lighting and underexposing manually did absolutely nothing for depth of field, so that creative tool could not be used. The reason for this is that the lens on this camera has a 17-mm focal length. I used the fine setting (1.3 million pixels per image) on all shots, because we wanted the best possible final images. Annoyingly, you cannot select camera-to-subject distance manually either, which means that you must rely on the auto-focus mechanism. In low light this can be a little slow, or the camera may refuse to focus until you realign it onto part of the subject that triggers the mechanism into action. In the studio situation, measuring the distance to the subject (especially if most of the images will be recorded from the same position) gives perfect focus and perfect exposure every time, once you have found the best subject distance and flash intensity settings.

We wanted the photos to look as natural as possible—but as anyone who has done this kind of photography knows, what looks natural and uncontrived takes a lot of time and effort. I made a huge wood and paper background to shoot against (4.5 by 2.7 metres; it was still too small for some shots) and we used this for most of the images, to avoid the background clutter of an exercise studio. I used a blue background because blue is furthest away from flesh tones, with the intention that Jeremy would drop it out electronically to the manufactured white background that we wanted in the final pictures to give us maximum creativity in the final look of the photos.

I used a single studio Hensel flash unit to light the sets, bouncing the light out of an umbrella, and mostly aligned directly above the camera lens, to avoid shadows on the background walls (we shot against them if they were necessary to the exercises) and on the paper background. I decided that we needed to show the actual room and equipment we use in the classes for some of the exercises, and this created a number of lighting problems, which this on-axis approach (while having a flattening effect admittedly) mostly bypasses. I blocked off the flash light sensor and the red-eye light on the camera with gaffer tape, so the on-camera flash would fire at full power. An aluminium foil reflector taped on to the camera body bounced all of this light up to the studio strobe trigger unit. The umbrella, as sole light source, helped achieve a softer modelling of the teachers' faces (while not doing much for mine!). Additionally, by eliminating the flash light coming from the camera and shooting manually (not using the automatic exposure facility) I was able to control the final exposure more directly. Flash synchronisation trigger-voltage incompatibility meant that I had to use the on-camera flash to trigger the big unit, and this was an additional reason for using the on-camera hand-made reflector.

In a book with this many photographs, the time for developing original film and having proofs made, then transferring the negatives to Compact Disc (which was the method Jeremy and I used for *Overcome neck & back pain*), and the sheer expense of conventional photography meant that we could not use it, even if we had wanted to. In using digital images, the main cost (in addition to the equipment) is how much time the graphic artist needs to spend to make the images acceptable, both aesthetically (does the image show sufficient detail to allow someone to imitate the form of the movement and is it pleasing to the eye?) and technically (how will it look when converted to dot screen and printed using conventional printing presses?). This meant that we needed to run a few tests and shoot at specific distances to get as close as possible to even and repeated exposure on all images (recall that we were not using automatic exposure).

The teachers and I decided to show the exercises wearing the sort of clothes we teach and practise in—and this is an interesting mixture. As we were using our usual room (apart from the background) we felt that the clothes represented gave more of a feeling of being in the classes than a studio background with everyone wearing leotards would have. You will have to let us know whether this was a good choice!

To anyone contemplating doing something similar, I recommend insisting on asking the publisher to run tests of your images *before* you commit the entire book to CDRom (or whichever medium you are using). This is because printing presses vary considerably and, for example, the presses being used by the publisher may not be able to hold the resolution of the images you supply. Too fine a dot will not print; accordingly, the printed images will be too light. On some illustrations for the USA edition of *Overcome neck & back pain*, for example, this meant we had to lower the screen ruling of the mezzotint to the point where the dots could be held by the presses to produce images of acceptable density.

RECOMMENDED READING LIST

All of the references mentioned here have helped me to understand what happens to us as we stretch. Some readers may be surprised by the age of the books mentioned in this list, as there is a widespread tendency to place greater reliance on more recent publications, on the assumption that the scientific enterprise moves forwards continually. In my experience, however, the earliest possible sources are often the best, even if subsequent work reveals errors of various kinds. Innovators create fields of enquiry; subsequent researchers provide refinement of detail. Both kinds of enquiry are necessary to fuller understanding. The big ideas usually appear in earlier works.

Albrecht, K., 1979. **Stress and the Manager: making it work for you.** Simon & Schuster, New York, Touchstone edition, 1986. Foreword by Hans Selye. One of the earliest texts in the field of occupational stress; relevant and practical. Contains a good relaxation script.

Alter, M. J., 1988. **Science of Stretching.** Human Kinetics Books, Champaign, Illinois. A wealth of scientific detail underlying the practical dimensions of stretching.

Benson, H., 1976. **The Relaxation Response.** Collins, London. This very small book is a minor gem, condensing a great deal of technical research into meditation and similar practices.

Chiba, S., Ishibashi, Y., and Kasai, T., 1994. Perforation of dorsal branches of the sacral nerve plexus through the piriformis muscle and its relation to changes of segmental arrangements of the vertebral column and others. *Kaibogaku Zasshi (Acta Anatomica Nippon).*

Damasio, A. R., 1994. **Descartes' Error: emotion, reason and the human brain.** Macmillan, London, Papermac edition, 1996. The most influential book I read in 1997, and which provides a deep understanding of the relation between the 'mind' and the 'body'. It is my sincere hope that *Stretching & Flexibility* can provide some of the tools to alter the perception of, and the function of, this dualism.

Jerome, J., 1987. **Staying Supple: the bountiful pleasures of stretching.** Bantam Books, New York. The 'Unnumbered lesson' derives much from this slim but rich publication. I had extolled the pleasure of stretching long before I found this book, but Jerome made me think again about how the points between the cardinal points on our stretching compass need to be explored. His insistence on the necessity of *listening* to what the body is trying to tell you cannot be overemphasised in achieving the goal of flexibility. Are you listening?

Johnson, M., 1987. **The Body in the Mind: the bodily basis of meaning, imagination, and reason.** University of Chicago Press, Chicago. This brilliant book examines the ways in which our body and its movement through time and space is constitutive of thought, from basic awareness to abstract concepts, via image schemata and metaphor. Although Johnson's focus is different, his insights are compatible with Damasio's. Perhaps the negative prejudice accorded the body (in comparison with the mind) explains why Johnson's ideas are not more central to mainstream philosophy.

Juhan, D., 1987. **Job's Body: A Handbook for Bodywork.** Station Hill Press, New York. Foreword by Ken Dychtwald. I read this wonderful book many years before Damasio's; when I read the latter I was reminded of the many insights Juhan had achieved without the new biochemical and neurological evidence presented in *Descartes' Error.* The understanding provided by direct experience, and acts of imagination constrained by this experience, can be far-reaching indeed. Juhan's book should be read by all who describe themselves as body workers.

Kapandji, I. A., 1974. **The Physiology of the Joints.** Volumes I–III. Churchill Livingstone, Edinburgh. This is the first and finest exposition of the anatomy and physiology of the bones and muscles of the body, presented from an engineering and Newtonian physics perspective. The sheer comprehensiveness of these texts is humbling and they are beautifully and innovatively illustrated. Kapandji's capacity to draw the fundamental physical principles involved in joint movement in a simple, though anything but simplistic, way is an inspiration. This is a must-have set of books for anyone interested in exercise or rehabilitation.

Keleman, S., 1985. **Emotional Anatomy: the structure of experience**. Center Press, Berkeley. Keleman argues persuasively that one's own body shape is a dynamic interaction between one's genetic inheritance and one's personal emotional history. His work is a considerable elaboration of Reich's insights (see below) into character armoring. Of particular interest is his analysis of the *internal* implications of this history, and its effect on organ function, the musculoskeletal dimension, and the emotional choices that are made as a result, all of which constrain options for future adaptation. Remarks made above in relation to Damasio's work are relevant here, too.

Kendall, H. O., Kendall, F .P., and Wadsworth, G. P., 1971. **Muscles, Testing and Function**. Williams and Wilkins, Baltimore, 2nd edition. Again, the original and, in many ways, the best. A newer revised edition is available.

Knott, M., and Voss, D. E., 1968. **Proprioceptive Neuromuscular Facilitation**. Harper & Row, New York. The first of its kind; two subsequent editions have been released.

Kurz, T., 1994. **Stretching Scientifically: a guide to flexibility training**. Stadion, Island Pond, Vermont, USA, revised 3rd edition. Kurz's book has some useful ideas on developing dynamic flexibility; athletes in sports requiring this kind of flexibility would do well to read it. He is critical of partner stretching, though: too dangerous and inefficient, on his account. His theory chapter is brief and excellent.

Laughlin, K., 1998. **Overcome Neck & Back Pain**, first published 1995, by BodyPress, Canberra; second edition Simon & Schuster, Sydney; revised third edition, Simon & Schuster, New York. All relevant details of how we approach the treatment of neck and back problems will be found here, as will the references on which the approach draws. For example, the Chiba *et al.* research that revealed the high percentage of the general population whose *piriformis* muscle is pierced by the sciatic nerve will be found here. This reference is included, above.

Reich, W., 1989. **The Function of the Orgasm.** Souvenir Press, London. First published in English, 1942, as *The Discovery of the Orgone, Volume I: the function of the orgasm*, Orgone Institute Press. Through his insistence that 'muscular attitudes and character attitudes have the same function in the psychic mechanism ... they cannot be separated ... [and] are identical in their function', Reich gave modern voice to what are now called schools of body work.

Selye, H., 1976. **The Stress of Life**. McGraw-Hill Book Co., New York. Revised edition 1976, paperback edition 1978. This book, first published in 1956, spawned a major field of research and remains relevant today. Selye's insights are one of the longest-lasting major revisions in modern medicine and the full weight of his research is yet to be felt.

Travell, J. G., and Simons, D. G., Volume 1, 1983; Volume 2, 1992. **Myofascial Pain and Dysfunction: the trigger point manual**. Williams & Wilkins, Baltimore. Another monument of scholarship, Travell and Simons's two volumes are, in my experience, owned by many but understood by few. Like Kapandji, these books repay constant revisiting, and one cannot help feeling awed by the sheer hard work involved in their preparation. The illustrations of muscles and bones by Barbara Cummings are the best I have ever seen.

GENERAL INDEX

Notes:

1. Page locators in *italics* indicate pages located in a named exercise

2. Page locators with an *asterisk indicate diagrams

3. Page locators in **bold** indicate pages of major entries

4. Word entries in *italics* indicate (Latin) named anatomical structures

5. A separate index of named exercises follows this general index

abdominal muscles 108, *197*
   see also *rectus abdominis* ('abs')
abductors (general)
   see also individual named muscles
     shoulder *170*
     thigh *32, 92–3, 98, 177, 179–80, 182, 187, 195, 240, 243–4*
acetabular rim 93
Achilles tendon *23, *61, 63*
adductor brevis 92
adductor longus *66, 92
adductor magnus *60, 92
adductor pollicis 199
adductors of thigh (general) *66–7, 70, 88*, 92–3, *97, 98, 100, 126, 152, 157, 179, 187, 195, 226, 240, 241, 243*
   see also individual named muscles
   see also hip movements & muscles
aerobics 15
AFL football & footballers 252, 253
ageing 54, 55, *247*
agonist muscle groups 57
anatomy
   connective tissue 18–19
   fascia 18
   importance of (in technique) 16
   muscles 18–19
   skin 18
ankle
   flexion *62, 64*, 195, *196, 197, 209*
   general 216, 255
   inversion & eversion *147, 196*
   sprain *196*

antagonist muscle groups 57
aponeurosis 23
arches (of foot) *189, 220*
athletes 10, 15, 57, 75
autogenic inhibition 18

back pain 34
badminton & badminton players 252
balancing exercises *241*
baseball & baseball players 254
basketball & basketballers 253
benzodiazepines 17
biceps brachii ('biceps') *21, *42, 46–7, 48, 54–5, 122, 164, 183, 254*
biceps femoris *23, *60, *61, 60–1, 92, 156, 213, 254*
biofeedback 17
bodybuilders 252
Bol, René 10
brachial plexus 40, 45, 48
brachialis 47
brachioradialis *22, 47
breathing **16–17**
   contract–relax and 11
   posture & flexibility and **16–17**, 20
   tension and 16–17
   tidal 17
   Valsalva manouevre 11

C–R see contract–relax
calf muscles (general) **57, 58–74**, 139, *176, 195, 209, 213, 220, 225, 226, 238*
   see also individual named muscles
cervical spine *25, *108, 166*
Chinese splits *242*
collagen 18–19
connective tissue 18–19
contract–relax (C–R) (general) **11–13**
   see also posture & flexibility
   see also C–R stretches in individual exercise descriptions
     advantages of 12–13, 18
     agonist/antagonist imbalance and 57
     breathing and 11
     contraction and 11, 13, 150

flexibility and 13
history of 7–9
isometric contraction and 13
isotonic contraction and 13
posture & flexibility (C–R as element of) 10, 11–13
principles (ten) of **20–1**
relaxation and 11, 15
repetitions of 12
restretch and 11, 150
safety/cautions and 4–5, 10, 12, 14, 15, 20, 21, 25, *83*
steps of 11–12
strength and 13
stretching and 11, 12, 150
contractions, isometric 9, 13, *72*
contractions, isotonic 9, 13
contraction of muscles *see* contract–relax
cool-down exercises *224*
cricket & cricketers 254
cycling & cyclists 253

daily five (plus two) **25–41**, *57*
dancing & dancers 7, 75, 93, *97*, 124, 151, *153*, 174, *230*, *239*
deltoid ('delts'), *anterior* and *posterior* *22–3, *37–8, *42–3, 46, 50, 54–5
dynamic forms classes 15

elastin 18
emotion 16–17, 19–20, *39*, *121*, *230*
erector spinae *72*, 95
eversion (of ankle) *147*, *196*

facet joints (of back) *28*
fascia
    general 8, 18, *105*, *157*, *239*
    latissimus dorsi *23*
    shoulder stretches and 42
fascia lata *60*
femur *60*, *68*, *69*, *75*, *92*, 93, *113*
fibula *61*
fingers 195, *198–9*
flexibility *see* posture & flexibility
'flight or fight' syndrome 25

foot *188–9, 198, 220–1*
football
    AFL 252, 253
    rugby league 252, 253
    rugby union 253
forearms 195
form 150
fungal infections (feet) *188*

gastrocnemius 13, *22–3, *60–1, *63*
glenohumeral joint *170*
glenoid fossa *170*
gluteus maximus ('glutes') 13, *23, *34, *60, *61, 66–7, 131*
gluteus medius *23, *66, 88, 201*
gluteus minimus *60, 88, 201*
golf & golfers 108, 255
gracilis *60, *66, 92, *102*
groove, intertubercular *46*
ground substance 18–19
gymnastics & gymnasts 75, 93, 97, 124, *153, 170, 174, 230, 239, 242, 248*, 254

hamstrings (general) **57, 58–74**, 89–90, 124, **125–38**, 139, **154–8**, *166*, 174, *180, 187, 190, 195, 197, 202, 210, 212, 213, 214, 224, 226, 234, 236–7, 238, 241, 243–4, 250–1*
see also specific muscles
    description of h 57, 60, 75
    duration of contraction of h 11
    frequency of stretching of h 10
    hip movements and h 57, 60, 75, 92–3, *154*
    knee movements and h 57, 60, 75
    partial poses and h 13
    partner assisted and h 14
    'pulled' hamstring 57
    tension and h *39*
    thrust (negative) and h *34*
hands *see* wrist *and* fingers
hip movements & muscles (general)
    see also individual named muscles
    abduction *32*, 92–3, *98, 177, 179–80, 182, 187, 195, 240, 243*

adductors (general) *66–7, 70, 88, 92–3, 97, 98, 100, 126, 152, 157, 179, 187, 195, 226, 240, 241, 243–4*
awareness of hip flexors 11
back pain and 34
calf muscles and 57, *61, 62, 63, 64*
daily five and 25, *34–5*
external rotators 34, 68, 195, *206–7*
flexion *64–5, 66–7, 68–9, 72–3, 75, 75–6, 79–80,* 108, *113, 115, 117, 128, 129, 154, 185, 190, 197, 202, 205, 210, 214, 225, 230, 234, 237, 239, 249, 254, 255*
hamstrings and 57, *60, 75*
partial movements and 13
piriformis syndrome 68
seated forward bend and 5
hurdling & hurdlers 174, *210*
hypnosis (self) 17

iliacus 11, *60, *66, 66–7, *75*
ilio-psoas 75, 75–6, 79–80, 113
iliofemoral ligaments *93, *113, 113*
*ilium *68, *69, *113*
*infraspinatus *23, *43, 50, 170*
intercostales (intercostals) *54–5, 239*
intertubercular groove *46*
intervertebral disc *75
inversion (of ankle) *147, 189, 196*
ischial tuberosity 34, 57, *113, 124, 241
isometric contractions 9, 13, *72*
isotonic contractions 9, 13

Jikyo Jutsu 8

knee (general) 8, 13, *46, 57, 60, 63, 75, 83, 89, 97*
knee ligament, medial *83, 210*
kneecap (*patella*) *60, 63, *66, 70*
Knott & Voss (physical therapists) 9, 20

latissimus dorsi (lats) *23, 32, 40, *42, *43, 52–3, 95, 123, 157, 165*
levator scapulae 25, *37, *38, *56, *122, 121–2, 137–8*
ligaments (named)

iliofemoral *93, *113, 113*
medial (knee) 83, *210*
pubofemoral 93, *97, *113, 113*
lower-back problems 28, *190, 221*
lumbar spine *see* spine, lumbar

martial arts 15, *126–7,* 151, *152, 153,* 174, *185, 195, 242,* 254
masseter 38
meditation 17
metatarsals *189*
muscles (general)
see also individual named muscles
agonist/antagonist muscle groups 57
anatomy & physiology **17–20**
diagrams of *22–3, *37, *38, *39, *42, *43, *56, *60, *61, *62, *66, *68, *69, *75*
insertion of *60*
origin of *60*
'pulling' of 19, 57
tone (tonus) 17, 19–20

neck muscles (general) *37–9, 40–1, 56, 166–7, 216, 219–20*
see also individual named muscles
see also spine, cervical
daily five and 25
diagrams of *37, *38, *39, *56*
duration of contraction of 11
emotion and *39, 121*
flexibility 195
neck, shoulder & relaxation classes 15
overcome neck and back pain workshops *95*
netball & netballers 253

obliquus externus (obliques) *22, *32, 95, 110, 157*
opponens pollicis 199
oriental medicine 8, 195
over-40s classes 15
overuse injuries *40, 199*

paravertebrals *see* spinal muscles
partial poses **13–14**
see also posture & flexibility
calf muscles and *60*

effectiveness of 13–14

functional units and 13–14

hamstrings and 13, *60*

partner-assisted exercises (general) **14–15**

 see also posture & flexibility

 advantages of 14

 choice of partner 14–15

 hamstrings and 14

 quadriceps and 14

 safety of 14, 15

patella (kneecap) *60, 63, *66, *70*

pectineus *66, 92

pectoralis (pecs), *major* and *minor* *22, *38, *42, *54–5*, *56, *182–3, 252*

pelvis *34, 78*, 92, *108, *113, *129, 179, 200*

physiology (of stretching) **17–20**

physiotherapy 15

pilates 15

piriformis 13, 16, *34*, *60, *68, *69, *68–9, 135*, 139, 150, 195, *203, 205, 207, 227, 228, 232, 243, 250*

piriformis syndrome *68*

postcontractive reflex depression 18

posture & flexibility (technique) **10–21**

 aerobics and 15

 anatomy and 16, **17–20**

 athletics and 15

 breathing and **16–17**, 20

 constraints on 10, 15

 contract–relax and 10, **11–13**

 dynamic forms classes 15

 effectiveness of 10, 15

 elements of 10, 11–15

 evolution of training **15–16**

 hatha yoga and 10

 history of 10

 martial arts and 15

 neck, shoulder & relaxation classes 15

 objective of 15, 16

 over-40s classes 15

 partial poses and 10, **13–14**

 partner-assisted and 10, **14–15**

 physiology of **17–20**

 physiotherapy and 15

 pilates and 15

principles (ten) of **20–1**

proprioception and 12, 19–20

relaxation and 11, 15

safety/cautions and 4–5, 10, 12, 14, 15, 20, 21, 25, *83*

tension and 16–17, 19–20

tradition of 15–16

yoga and 15

pronation (of ankle) *62, 63, 189*

proprioception 12, 19–20, *134, 191, 238*

proprioceptive neuromuscular facilitation (PNF) 9, 11, 20

prostate gland *153*

psoas 11, *60, *66, 66–7, *75

pubofemoral ligaments 93, 97, *113, *113*

psychological aspects *see* emotion; tension

quadratus lumborum 32, *75, 95, 110, 157, 201*

quadriceps (quads) *66–7, 75–6, 77, 78, 81, 83–4, 90, 102, 115, 116, 117, 126, 129–30, 132, 143, 177, 184, 187, 190–1, 205, 210, 229, 230, 236–7, 238, 245, 249, 253*

 see also individual named component muscles

 contraction (duration of) 11

 diagram *22

 hip flexor 75

 partner-assisted and 14

 stretching (frequency of) 10

 tension and 39

racquet sports 252

rectus abdominis ('abs') *22, 57

rectus femoris *60, *66, 66–7, 79–80, 113*

relaxation *see* contract–relax; posture & flexibility

reproductive organs *153*

rhomboideus major & minor 25, 82, 119, *122

rock climbers *170*

rotation of spine *see* spine, rotation

rotator cuff 46, *170, 172*

rugby league 252

running & runners *246, 253*

sacrum *68, *69

safety/cautions 4–5, 10, 12, 14, 15, 20, 21, 25, *83*

sartorius *60, *66, 79, 113*

scalenus group *121*

scalenus posterior *37, 38

sedentary occupations 54

segmental nerves 68, 69

self-hypnosis 17

sciatic nerve & sciatica pain
    calf muscles and *61, 209*
    diagrams *68, *69, *75
    piriformis syndrome *68*

semimembranosus *23, *60, *61, *60–1, 156*

semitendinosus *23, *60, *61, *60–1, 92, 156*

serratus anterior *22, *42

shin splints *77*

Shoshin Centre 10

shoulder *25*, **42**, **42–56**, *70, 162–3, 168–72, 239, 252, 255*
    see also individual named muscles
    abduction *170*
    diagrams *42, *43
    external rotators *50, 170–1*
    fascia and *42*
    flexion *239, 254*
    glenohumeral joint *170*
    glenoid fossa *170*
    internal rotators *170*
    intertubercular groove and *46*
    pectorals and *42*
    rotator cuff and *46*

skin 18

soccer 253

softball 254

soleus *23, *60, *61, *61, 62*

spinal muscles (paravertebrals) *21, 25, 32, 54, 72, 78, 119*

spine
    cervical *25, *108, *166*
    lumbar *75, 78, *108, *133, 166, 177, 201, 230, 232, 233, 239, 243, 244, 255*
    rotation of *20, 21, 30–1, 42, 58–9, 90, 105–6, 110–11, 136–7, 144, 145, 157, 162–4, 181, 193, 200, 212, 224, 228, 232, 253, 255*
    thoracic *103–4, *108, *113, 166, 230, 239, 255*

splenius *37, *38

splits *242*

squash & squash players *108, 252*

sternoclavicular joint *122, *122*

sternomastoid *37, *38, *39, *56, *56*

sternum *183*

stress *see* tension

stretching
    see also contract–relax; posture & flexibility
    ballistic 12
    breathing and **16–17**
    cautions/safety *4–5, 10, 12, 14, 15, 20, 21, 25, 83*
    rationale for *1–2*
    tension and 17
    static 12

straddle *242*

subscapularis 170

supraspinatus 170

swimming & swimmers 255

tennis & tennis players 108, 252

tension
    body and emotion **19–20**, *39, 230*
    breathing and **16–17**
    'flight or fight' syndrome 25
    muscle groups and *39, 121*

tensor fasciae latae *22, *32*, *60, *61, *66, *88*

teres major *23, *43

teres minor *43, *50, 170*

thixotropy 18

thoracic spine *103–4, *108, *113, 166, 230, 239*

thrust (negative/positive) 34

thumb *see* fingers

tibia 61

tibialis anterior *22, *77*

toes *148, 188–9, 196, 220–1*

tonus *see* muscles–tone

trapezius *22, *23, *25, *37, *38, *39, *43, *56, *122, *121–2, 138*

triceps brachii *23, *42, *43, *52, 100, 252*

tuberosity(ies)
    intertubercular groove (*humerus*) *46*
    ischial (pelvis) *34, 57, *113, 124, 241*

Valsalva manouevre 11

vastus intermedius *60

vastus lateralis *60, *61, *66

vastus medialis *60, *66
vertebral body *75, *75*, *113*, *166*
volleyball 253
Voss, Knott & (physical therapists) 9, 20

wrist 195, *198–9*, 216
writer's cramp *199*

yoga 10, 15, 25, *97*, 151, *153*, *166*, 174, *211*,
230, *239*, *246*

INDEX OF NAMED EXERCISES

Notes:

1. Numbers in (**bold**) are the numbers given to the exercises as listed in Contents

2. Some exercises are unnumbered in Contents

(**37**) abdominal curls over support 108–9, 254, 255

(**9**) arm across body 44–5, 107, 169

(**13**) arm behind head 52–3, 173

(**90**) balancing straight legs apart 241

(**2**) backward bend from floor 28–9, 81, 117, 178, 227, 252, 254, 255

(**21**) buttock & hip flexor 66–7, 128, 185–6, 189, 210, 253

(**6**) chin to chest 37, 122, 168, 218, 229, 255

daily five (plus two) 25–41

(**1**) floor clasped feet middle and upper back 25–6, 82, 161, 215, 254

(**16**) floor face down arm & leg lifts, & abdo. curls 58–60, 95, 163, 253

(**42**) floor feet held back bend 118, 191, 229

(**67**) floor feet sequence warm-up 188–9, 196, 221

(**18**) floor folded leg calf (soleus) 62, 196, 255

(**48**) floor forward bend over bent legs 135, 183, 193, 222, 234, 244, 252

(**78**) floor forward bend over straight leg, hurdler's variation 210

(**23**) floor instep 77, 196, 220, 255

(**15**) floor neck rotation 56, 169, 220

(**29**) floor side bend over straight leg; other folded 95

(**20**) floor single leg calf 64, 253

(**71**) floor wrist and hand sequence 198–9, 220

(**43**) folded legs clasped knees upper back 119–20, 169, 191, 204, 255

(**96**) forward bend over straight legs 250–1

free squat ankles clasped bottom position 202

free squat bottom position, ankles clasped, straighten legs sequence 224

free squats warm-up, knees apart, revisited 184–5

free squats warm-up, knees pressed apart by elbows 151

free squats warm-up, partner or solo 75–6

free squats warm-up, with held positions 125, 174, 208

(**72**) kneeling elbow on floor rotation 200

(**63**) legs apart, off support 179–80, 234

(**22**) lying hip 68–9

(**57**) lying legs behind 166–7, 183, 215, 218, 235

(**3**) lying rotation 30–1, 181, 255

(**38**) lying rotations 110, 164, 253, 255

martial arts warm-up, one foot flat; solo, bars or partner 152, 174, 185, 195

martial arts warm-up with partner 126–7, 185

middle and upper back (floor clasped feet) 25–6, 29, 222

middle and upper back (from chair) 27, 29

(**7**) neck side bend 40, 55, 107, 122, 169, 218

(**49**) partner all fours rotation 136–7, 173, 193, 215

(**12**) partner arm up behind shoulder blade 50–1, 106, 173

(**11**) partner arms up behind back 48–9, 107, 172

(**27**) partner backward bend over support 85–7, 112, 160, 178, 202, 223, 252, 253

(**58**) partner bar shoulder flexion with hip traction 168–70, 229

(**77**) partner bar standing calf 209

(**83**) partner floor back bend, off support 230–1, 239

(**85**) partner floor backward bend 233

(**76**) partner floor external hip rotator 205

(**87**) partner floor hamstring & lower back 238

(**46**) partner floor hip & hamstring 129–31

(**35**) partner floor middle & upper back bend 103–4, 255

(**70**) partner floor single leg, both legs calf 197, 225

(**17**) partner floor single leg forward bend 60–1, 72–3, 132

(**73**) partner floor wall seated side bend 201–2

(**10**) partner front arm 46–7, 164, 254

(**39**) partner hip flexor 113–15, 214

(**65**) partner kneeling arms up & behind 182–3

(**28**) partner lying hamstring, knee flexed 89–90, 187, 253

(**8**) partner lying rotation 42–3, 70, 90, 160, 224, 252, 254

(**66**) partner lying 'Y' 187, 214

(**47**) partner partial front splits, off support 133–4, 214, 234, 247

(**55**) partner seated legs apart 157–61, 176, 181, 222, 254

(**40**) partner seated/lying single leg *quadriceps* 115, 209

(**44**) partner shoulder depress 121–2, 218

(**50**) partner shoulder depress with flexion & lateral flexion 137–8, 164, 204, 219

(**36**) partner/solo floor lying bottom leg folded rotation 105–6, 118, 161

(**31**) partner/solo kneeling knees apart 98–9

(**60**) partner/solo shoulder external rotation 171–2

(**59**) partner/solo shoulder internal rotation 170–1

(**52**) partner/solo standing single leg forward bend 155

(**31**) partner/solo wall lying bent legs apart 100

(**41**) partner standing suspended hip flexor, with support 116–17

(**81**) partner wall reverse legs apart forward bend 226

(**61**) partner wall seated knees apart 175–6, 240

(**62**) partner wall seated legs apart, facing wall 177

(**53**) partner wall standing hamstring 156

(**54**) partner wall squat knees apart 156

(**75**) seated clasped bent leg upper back 204

(**5**) seated hip 34–7, 227

(**55**) seated legs apart, solo version 222

    see also partner seated legs apart

(**74**) seated legs folded knees apart forward bend 203

(**26**) seated/lying single leg *quadriceps* 83–4, 132,   209

(**64**) seated or standing bent leg rotation 182, 184–5, 235

(**56**) sideways bend across support 165, 223

(**92**) sitting and standing peacocks 246

solo external hip rotator; with support 206–7

standing alternate leg forward bend warm-up

71, 163, 208, 253, 254, 255

(**51**) standing clasped single bent leg hamstring 154, 253

(**79**) standing forward bend over bent and straight leg 211–12, 252, 253

(**68**) standing horizontal one leg support 190–1

standing legs apart warm-up, bent & straight legs 93–5, 152

(**24**) standing *quadriceps* 78, 252, 253

standing rag-doll warm-up 162–3, 217

(**4**) standing side bend 32–3, 88, 112, 181, 253, 254

(**25**) standing suspended hip flexor 79–80, 127, 185–6, 205, 210, 214, 225, 253, 254, 255

(**69**) standing 'Y' one leg support 192–3, 254

(**94**) ultimate abdominal workout 248

(**88**) ultimate back bend 239, 254

(**89**) ultimate bent-leg hip adductor 240

(**93**) ultimate front splits 247, 254

(**91**) ultimate legs-apart stretch 242–5, 254

(**95**) ultimate *quadriceps* and hip flexor 249

(**86**) ultimate *quadriceps* stretch 236–7

(**45**) upper back on all fours 123

(**80**) wall and floor kneeling/straight leg outer hamstring 213

(**82**) wall lunge rotation 228, 232

(**33**) wall lying straight legs apart 101

(**14**) wall middle and upper back backward bend 54–5, 161, 252, 253, 254, 255

(**30**) wall seated knees apart 97–8, 153, 253

(**34**) wall seated straight legs apart 102, 221

(**84**) wall squatting rotation 232

(**19**) wall standing calf (*gastrocnemius*) 63, 195, 197, 208, 220, 252, 253, 255

(**9**) wall standing legs apart warm-up 176